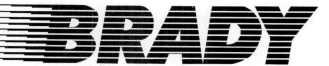

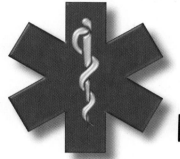

PREHOSPITAL
EMERGENCY
PHARMACOLOGY

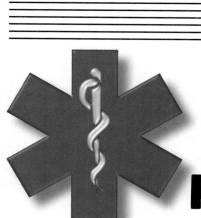

BRADY

PREHOSPITAL EMERGENCY PHARMACOLOGY

FIFTH EDITION

BRYAN E. BLEDSOE, D.O., F.A.C.E.P., F.A.A.E.M., F.A.E.P., EMT-P

Emergency Department Staff Physician
Baylor Medical Center—Ellis County
Waxahachie, Texas
            and
Clinicial Associate Professor of Emergency Medicine
University of North Texas Health Sciences Center
Fort Worth, Texas

DWAYNE E. CLAYDEN, EMT-P, M.E.M.

EMS Chief
Airdrie Emergency Services
Airdrie, Alberta, Canada
Team Leader—Paramedic Outreach Program
Southern Alberta Institute of Technology
Calgary, Alberta, Canada

FRANK J. PAPA, D.O., Ph.D., F.A.C.E.P.

Professor of Emergency Medicine and Medical Education
Department of Medical Education
University of North Texas Health Sciences Center
Fort Worth, Texas

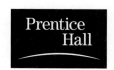

Prentice
Hall

Upper Saddle River, New Jersey 07458

Library of Congress Cataloging-in-Publication Data

Bledsoe, Bryan E.
  Prehospital emergency pharmacology / Bryan E. Bledsoe, Dwayne E. Clayden,
Frank J. Papa.—5th ed.
    p. cm.
  Includes bibliographical references and index.
  ISBN 0-13-025950-0
    1. Medical emergencies. 2. Chemotherapy. 3. Drugs. I. Clayden, Dwayne E.
II. Papa, Frank J., III. Title.

RC86.7 .B597 2001
616.02'5—dc21   00-064258

Publisher: Julie Alexander
Executive Editor: Greg Vis
Acquisitions Editor: Katrin Beacom
Director of Manufacturing and Production: Bruce Johnson
Managing Editor: Patrick Walsh
Production Editor: Amy Gehl, Carlisle Communications
Production Liaison: Cathy O'Connell
Manufacturing Manager: Ilene Sanford
Director of Marketing: Leslie Cavaliere
Marketing Manager: Tiffany Price
Editorial Assistant: Kierra Bloom
Creative Director: Marianne Frasco
Cover Design: Lafortezza Design Group
Cover Photos: Eddie Sperling
Interior Design and Composition: Carlisle Communications
Printing and Binding: Courier Westford

Prentice-Hall International (UK) Limited, *London*
Prentice-Hall of Australia Pty. Limited, *Sydney*
Prentice-Hall Canada Inc., *Toronto*
Prentice-Hall Hispanoamericana, S.A., *Mexico*
Prentice-Hall of India Private Limited, *New Delhi*
Prentice-Hall of Japan, Inc., *Tokyo*
Prentice-Hall Singapore Pte. Ltd.
Editora Prentice-Hall do Brasil, Ltda., *Rio de Janeiro*

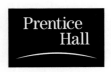

ISBN 0-13-025950-0

Dedication

Emergency medical services (EMS) is a profession that takes us away from our families. Often birthdays and holidays are missed due to shift work. Writing texts for EMS further erodes the family time. I am fortunate to have a family that not only supports but also encourages my efforts in EMS and specifically in the revision of this text. Without the love and support of my wife, Nancy, the successes I have enjoyed in this great profession would not have been possible.

Our children, Meagan, Lauren, Matthew, and Kaitlyn, have always encouraged my writing and are concerned about the progress of a book.

I appreciate the support of very good EMS friends. I especially want to thank Baxter Larmon, Bryan Bledsoe, Thom Hillson, Mike Pirie, and Brenda Beasley for their support and friendship.

Dwayne E. Clayden, EMT-P, M.E.M.

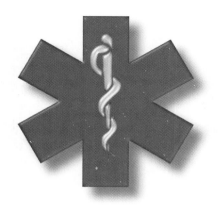

CONTENTS

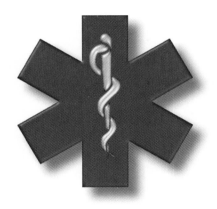

PREFACE

Modern emergency medical service (EMS) is based on sound principles, practice, and research. The paramedic of today must be knowledgeable in all aspects of prehospital emergency medicine. Nowhere is this more important than in the knowledge and administering of medications. *Prehospital Emergency Pharmacology* is a complete guide to the most common medications used in prehospital emergency care. This comprehensive text is designed with two purposes in mind: First, it is a complete pharmacology teaching text. Second, it is a handy reference to the most common drugs and fluids used in prehospital care.

The fifth edition of *Prehospital Emergency Pharmacology* adds to the extensive revisions of the fourth edition. It has been updated to reflect current trends in prehospital care. Each chapter has been revised. We hope that *Prehospital Emergency Pharmacology* will prove a valuable aid to both the practicing paramedic and the paramedic student.

It is the intent of the authors and publishers that this textbook be used as part of a formal paramedic education program taught by a qualified instructor and supervised by a licensed physician. The knowledge and skills outlined in this textbook are best learned in the classroom, skills laboratory, and then the clinical field setting. It is important to point out that this or any other text cannot teach skills. Care skills are only learned under the watchful eye of a paramedic instructor and perfected during clinical and field internships.

The care procedures presented here represent accepted practices in the United States and Canada. They are not offered as a standard of care. Paramedic-level care is to be performed only under the authority and guidance of a licensed physician. It is the reader's responsibility to know and follow local care protocols and standing orders as provided by medical advisers directing the system to which he or she belongs. Also, it is the reader's responsibility to stay informed of emergency care procedures and changes.

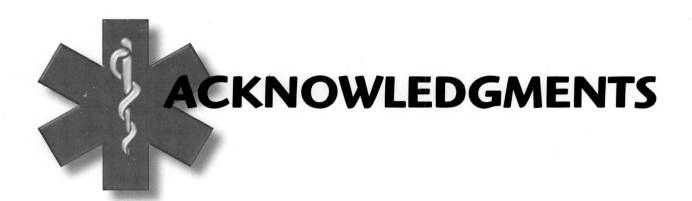

ACKNOWLEDGMENTS

We wish to acknowledge the talents and efforts of the following people who contributed to *Prehospital Emergency Pharmacology.*

Chapter Authors

Two new authors contributed to the revision of this text. First, we would like to thank Alan Mikolaj for his outstanding chapter on drug calculations. His work on this completely rewritten chapter provides easy-to-use instructions for both the paramedic student and the seasoned veteran.

Second, we would like to thank Andy Anton, M.D., F.R.C.P.C., for his work on the toxicology chapter. He has written a chapter that provides the essential information for a paramedic dealing with complicated overdose and poisoning situations.

Revised Text Reviewers

We appreciate the dedication of the text reviewers to this profession and especially appreciate their efforts in reviewing the revision of this text. The quality of the reviews has been outstanding. The reviewers' comments and suggestions were invaluable as we revised this text. The assistance provided by these EMS experts is deeply appreciated.

Beth L. Adams, M.A., R.N., NREMT-P
ALS Coordinator, EMS Program
The George Washington University
Fairfax, VA

Jan Auerbach, R.N., MSN, EMT-P
Associate Professor
University of Texas Southwestern Medical Center
Dallas, TX

Anne E. Clouatre, EMT-P, MHS
Centura Health-Porter/Littleton Adventist Pre-Hospital Service
Denver, CO

JoAnn Cobble Ed.D., NREMT-P, R.N.
Chair, Department of EMS
University of Arkansas for Medical Sciences
Little Rock, Arkansas

R. Scott Crawford, NREMT-P, EMSI
Lead Instructor, Advance EMS Programs
Nebraska Methodist College
Omaha, NE

James F. Gross, B.S., MICP
Hemer, CA

John Eric Powell, M.S., NREMT-P
Paramedic Instructor
Roane State Community College
Knoxville, Tennessee

Regina Twisdale
Director, School of Paramedic Sciences
Camden County College
Blackwood, New Jersey

Richard A. Craven, M.D., F.A.C.E.P.
Clinical Director
East Coast Clinical Research
Virginia Beach, Virginia

Mike Pirie, EMT-P
Medical Education Coordinator
Airdrie Emergency Services
Airdrie, Alberta, Canada

Development and Production

We would like to acknowledge the efforts and support of many talented individuals who assisted with the fifth edition.

First, we would like to thank Julie Alexander, publisher at Brady, for her assistance in this project. We would also like to thank the following editors at Brady who worked with us on this text: Judy Streger, Laura Edwards, and especially Katrin Beacom, who brought this project to completion.

We would also like to thank Amy Gehl of Carlisle Publishers Services for her persistence and hard work in seeing this manuscript through production.

ABOUT THE AUTHORS

Bryan E. Bledsoe, D.O., F.A.C.E.P., F.A.A.E.M., F.A.E.P., EMT-P

Dr. Bryan Bledsoe is an emergency physician with special interest in prehospital care. He received his bachelor of science degree from the University of Texas at Arlington and received his medical degree from the University of North Texas Health Sciences Center/Texas College of Osteopathic Medicine. He completed his internship at Texas Tech University and residency training at Scott and White Memorial Hospital/Texas A&M College of Medicine. Dr. Bledsoe is board certified in emergency medicine and family practice. He is presently a Ph.D. candidate at Charles Sturt University at Wagga Wagga, New South Wales, Australia.

Prior to attending medical school, Dr. Bledsoe worked as an emergency medical technician (EMT), paramedic, and paramedic instructor. He completed EMT training in 1974 and paramedic training in 1976 and worked for 6 years as a field paramedic in Fort Worth, Texas. In 1979, he joined the faculty of the University of North Texas Health Sciences Center and served as coordinator of EMT and paramedic education programs at the university. Dr. Bledsoe is active in emergency medicine and serves as medical director for several emergency medical service (EMS) agencies and educational programs.

Dr. Bledsoe has authored several EMS books published by Brady including *Paramedic Emergency Care, Intermediate Emergency Care, Atlas of Paramedic Skills, Prehospital Emergency Pharmacology,* and *Pocket Reference for EMTs and Paramedics.* He is married to Emma Bledsoe. They have two children, Bryan and Andrea, and live in Midlothian, Texas, a suburb of Dallas. He enjoys saltwater fishing and listening to Jimmy Buffett.

Dwayne E. Clayden, EMT-P, M.E.M.

Dwayne Clayden is currently the Emergency Medical Services Chief for the City of Airdrie Emergency Services in Airdrie, Alberta, Canada, and the Provincial Team Leader of the Paramedic Outreach Program for the Southern Alberta Institute of Technology (SAIT), Calgary, Alberta, Canada.

In 1998, the Alberta Prehospital Professions Association presented Mr. Clayden with the Award of Excellence for his contributions to emergency medical services (EMS) in Alberta. In 2000, Mr. Clayden received the

Exemplary Service Medal, authorized by the governor general of Canada, for his contributions to EMS in Canada. He is currently studying for his bachelor of science degree in paramedicine at Charles Sturt University at Wagga Wagga, New South Wales, Australia.

Mr. Clayden began his career as a police officer in Calgary. In 1980 he joined the Calgary Fire Department, Ambulance Division, as an emergency medical technician (EMT). Following his paramedic education he became a member of the Staff Development Division of the City of Calgary Emergency Medical Services. In 1987 he began his teaching career at SAIT, first in the EMT program and then in 1988 in the paramedic program. After more than 20 years in EMS, Mr. Clayden cannot think of a more rewarding or challenging career.

Mr. Clayden is a founding member of the Prehospital Care Research Forum and active in educating paramedics on how to do prehospital research.

Mr. Clayden has coauthored two books with Bryan Bledsoe for Brady, *Prehospital Emergency Pharmacology* and *Pocket Reference for EMTs and Paramedics.* He is currently working on two other titles for Brady. He is also the author of more than 75 EMS articles appearing in *JEMS* and *ON SCENE Canada.* He lives in Airdrie, Alberta, Canada, with his wife, Nancy, and their children, Meagan, Lauren, Matthew, and Kaitlyn.

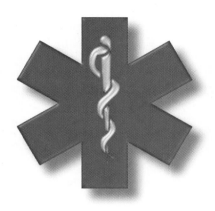

NOTICES

NOTICE ON DRUGS AND DRUG DOSAGES

Every effort has been made to ensure that the drug dosages presented in the textbook are in accordance with nationally accepted standards. When applicable, the dosages and routes are taken from the American Heart Association's Advanced Cardiac Life Support Guidelines. The American Medical Association's publication *Drug Evaluations,* the *Physicians' Desk Reference,* and Appleton & Lange's *Health Professions Drug Guide 2000* are followed with regard to drug dosages not covered by the American Heart Association's guidelines. It is the responsibility of the reader to be familiar with the drugs used in his or her system, as well as the dosages specified by the medical director. The drugs presented in this text should only be administered by direct order, whether verbally or through accepted standing orders, by a licensed physician.

NOTICE ON GENDER USAGE

The English language has historically given preference to the male gender. Among many words, the pronouns "he" and "his" are commonly used to describe both genders. Society evolves faster than language and the male pronouns still predominate in our speech. The authors have made great effort to treat the two genders equally, recognizing that a significant percentage of paramedics and patients are female. However, in some instances, male pronouns may be used to describe both male and female paramedics and patients solely for the purpose of brevity. This is not intended to offend any readers.

PRECAUTIONS ON BLOODBORNE PATHOGENS AND INFECTIOUS DISEASES

Prehospital emergency personnel, like all health care workers, are at risk for exposure to bloodborne pathogens and infectious diseases. In emergency situations it is often difficult to take or enforce proper infection control measures. However, paramedics must recognize their high-risk status. Readers should study the following information on infection control before turning to the main portion of this book.

Infection control is designed to protect emergency personnel, their families, and their patients from unnecessary exposure to communicable diseases.

Laws, regulations, and standards regarding infection control include the following:

- *Centers for Disease Control (CDC) Guidelines.* The CDC has published extensive guidelines regarding infection control. Proper equipment and techniques that should be used by emergency response personnel to prevent or minimize risk of exposure are defined.

- *The Ryan White Act.* The Ryan White Act of 1990 allows emergency personnel to find out if they were exposed to an infectious disease while rendering patient care. Employers are required to name a "designated officer" to coordinate communications with the treating hospital.

- *Americans with Disabilities Act.* This act prohibits discrimination against individuals with disabilities, including those with contagious diseases. It guarantees equal employment opportunities and job protection if the infected individual can perform essential job functions and does not pose a threat to the safety and health of patients and coworkers.

- *Occupational Safety and Health Administration (OSHA) Regulations.* OSHA enacted a regulation entitled Occupational Exposure to

Bloodborne Pathogens that classifies emergency response personnel as being at the greatest risk of occupational exposure to communicable diseases. This regulation requires employers to provide hepatitis B (HBV) vaccinations free of charge, maintain a written exposure control plan, and provide personal protective equipment (PPE). These requirements primarily apply to private employers. Applicability to local and state governmental employees varies by locality. Many states have developed their own OSHA plans.

- *National Fire Protection Association (NFPA) Guidelines.* This is a national organization that has established specific guidelines and requirements regarding infection control for emergency response agencies, particularly fire departments and emergency medical service agencies.

BODY SUBSTANCE ISOLATION PRECAUTIONS AND PERSONAL PROTECTIVE EQUIPMENT

Emergency response personnel should practice *body substance isolation (BSI)*, a strategy that considers *all* body substances potentially infectious. To avoid contact with body substances, all emergency personnel should utilize *personal protective equipment (PPE)*. Appropriate PPE should be available on every emergency vehicle. The minimum recommended PPE includes the following:

- *Gloves.* Disposable gloves should be donned by all emergency response personnel *before* initiating any emergency care. When an emergency incident involves more than one patient, paramedics should attempt to change gloves between patients. When gloves have been contaminated, they should be removed as soon as possible. To remove gloves, the gloved fingers of one hand are first hooked under the cuff of the other glove. Then that glove is pulled off without letting the gloved fingers come in contact with bare skin. Then the fingers of the ungloved hand are slid under the remaining glove's cuff. That glove is pushed off without contact between the glove's exterior and the bare hand. Hands should always be washed after gloves are removed, even when the gloves appear intact.

- *Masks and Protective Eyewear.* Masks and protective eyewear should be present on all emergency vehicles and used in accordance with the level of exposure encountered. Proper eyewear and masks prevent a patient's blood and body fluids from spraying into paramedics' eyes, nose, and mouth. Masks and protective eyewear should be worn together whenever blood spatter is likely to occur, such as during arterial bleeding, childbirth, endotracheal intubation, invasive procedures, oral suctioning, and cleanup of equipment that requires heavy scrubbing or brushing. Both the paramedic and the patient should wear masks whenever the potential for airborne transmission of disease exists.

- *High-Efficiency Particulate Air (HEPA) Respirators.* Due to the resurgence of tuberculosis (TB), prehospital personnel should protect themselves from TB infection through use of a HEPA respirator, a design approved by the National Institute of Occupational Safety and Health (NIOSH). It should fit snugly and be capable of filtering out the tuberculosis bacillus. The HEPA respirator should be worn when caring for patients with confirmed or suspected TB. This is especially true when performing "high hazard" procedures such as administration of nebulized medications, endotracheal intubation, or suctioning on such a patient.

- *Gowns.* Gowns protect clothing from blood splashes. If large splashes of blood are expected, such as with childbirth, impervious gowns should be worn.
- *Resuscitation Equipment.* Disposable resuscitation equipment should be the primary means of artificial ventilation in emergency care. Such items should be used once, then disposed of.

Remember, the proper use of personal protective equipment ensures effective infection control and minimizes risk. *All* protective equipment recommended for any particular situation should be used to ensure maximum protection.

All body substances should be considered potentially infectious, and body substance isolation should *always* be practiced.

HANDLING CONTAMINATED MATERIAL

Many of the materials associated with the emergency response become contaminated with possibly infectious body fluids and substances. These include soiled linen, patient clothing and dressings, and used care equipment, including intravenous needles. It is important that prehospital personnel collect these materials at the scene and dispose of them appropriately to ensure their safety as well as that of their patients, their family members, bystanders, and fellow caregivers. Contaminated materials should be disposed of according to the following recommendations:

- Handle contaminated materials only while wearing the appropriate personal protective equipment.
- Place all blood- or body-fluid-contaminated clothing, linen, dressings, and patient care equipment and supplies in properly marked biological hazard bags and ensure they are disposed of properly.
- Ensure that all used needles, scalpels, and other contaminated objects that have the potential to puncture the skin are properly secured in a puncture-resistant and clearly marked sharps container.
- Do not recap a needle after use, stick it into a seat cushion or other object, or leave it lying on the ground. These practices increase the risk of an accidental needle stick.
- Always scan the scene before leaving to ensure all equipment has been retrieved and all potentially infectious material has been bagged and removed.
- If prehospital personnel are exposed to an infectious disease, have contact with body substances with a route for system entry (such as an open wound on a hand when a glove tears while moving a soiled patient), or receive a needle stick with a used needle, the receiving hospital should be alerted and the service's infection control officer contacted immediately.

Following these recommendations will help protect paramedics and the people they care for from the dangers of disease transmission.

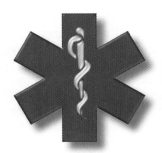

chapter 1

GENERAL INFORMATION

OBJECTIVES

After completing this chapter, the reader should be able to

1. List four drug sources and give examples of each source.
2. Define the terms *pharmacology, pharmacologists,* and *pharmcognosy.*
3. Identify drugs by their chemical name, generic name, trade name, and official name.
4. List four sources of drug information and demonstrate how to find a medication in one of these references.
5. List several examples of both liquid and solid drugs.

INTRODUCTION

Drugs are chemical agents used in the diagnosis, treatment, or prevention of disease. The study of drugs and their actions on the body is called *pharmacology.* Scientists who study the effects of drugs on the body are called *pharmacologists.* It is through experimental pharmacology that medicine has made many of its most profound advances.

Historical Considerations

The use of herbs and minerals to treat various medical disorders is as old as the practice of medicine itself. Written records of drug use date back to early Egyptian times. Ancient Egyptians, Arabs, and Greeks probably passed formulations down through generations by word of mouth for centuries until they were recorded in pharmacopoeias. Hippocrates, generally considered the father of modern medicine, wrote extensively on the use of drugs, although he rarely used them in the care of his patients. After the Renaissance, healers began to take a somewhat more scientific approach to disease and found that certain drugs were useful in treating some disorders but not others. Drug therapy was based largely on observation, and physicians were frequently unsure which body systems the drugs affected. Pharmacology was now a distinct and growing discipline, separate from medicine.

One common additive to early medications was the purple foxglove plant. A common flowering plant, the purple foxglove was first described in A.D. 1250 by Welsh physicians. It was long thought to be a diuretic because of its role in the treatment of dropsy, an old term used to describe the generalized body edema associated with congestive heart failure. In 1785 William Withering described the use of the purple foxglove plant in the treatment of dropsy and other disorders. Although he did not associate the improvement seen in the treatment of dropsy with the foxglove's effect on the heart, he did note its effectiveness. He wrote, "It has a power over the motion of the heart to a degree yet unobserved in any other medicine." It was not until 1800 that the effect of foxglove specifically on the heart was actually described and its suspected action as a diuretic was finally discarded.

Digitalis is the active agent in foxglove. Digitalis tends to increase myocardial contractile force. It is this increase in cardiac performance, with subsequently improved renal perfusion and filtration, that causes a reduction in the body swelling and not its diuretic effect as earlier thought. Even today digitalis remains one of the most commonly prescribed medications in the treatment of congestive heart failure and other cardiovascular disorders.

During the seventeenth and eighteenth centuries, tinctures of opium, coca, and digitalis were available. The related concept of vaccination from biologic extracts began in 1796 with Edward Jenner's smallpox inoculations. By the nineteenth century, atropine, chloroform, codeine, ether, and morphine were in use. The discoveries of animal insulin and penicillin in the early twentieth century dramatically changed the treatment of endocrine/metabolic and infectious diseases. Now, at the start of the twenty-first century, recombinant DNA technology has produced human insulin and tissue plasminogen activator (tPA). These drugs have markedly changed the treatment of diabetes and cardiovascular disease.

Medicine changed dramatically in the early part of the twentieth century with the discovery of antibiotics. Prior to the introduction of the sulfa-class antibiotics in 1935, physicians had virtually no effective therapy for infections. Penicillin became widely available in the early 1940s, thus providing physicians a versatile yet inexpensive antibiotic. Additional antibiotics were subsequently developed. The introduction of antibiotic therapy resulted in a significant decrease in mortality and a resultant increase in life expectancy in the United States and other developed countries.

Pharmacognosy

Traditionally, *pharmacognosy* refers to the study of natural drug sources, such as plants, animals, or minerals and their products. Today, however, chemicals developed and used in the laboratory allow researchers to increase the number of drug sources. For example, oral contraceptives, which are synthetic analogues of human sex hormones, are manufactured chemically. Chemically developed drugs are free of the impurities found in natural substances.

Researchers and drug developers also can now manipulate the molecular structure of substances, such as antibiotics, so that a slight change in chemical structure makes the drug effective against different organisms.

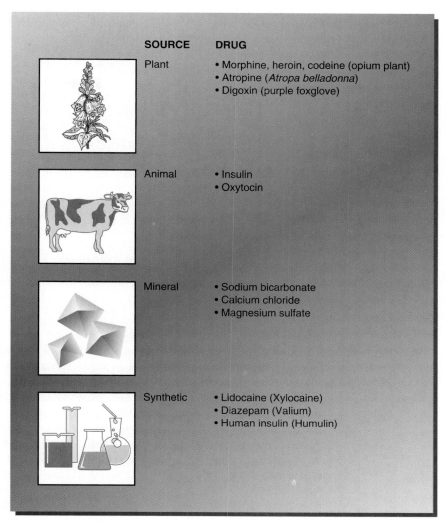

SOURCE	DRUG
Plant	• Morphine, heroin, codeine (opium plant) • Atropine (*Atropa belladonna*) • Digoxin (purple foxglove)
Animal	• Insulin • Oxytocin
Mineral	• Sodium bicarbonate • Calcium chloride • Magnesium sulfate
Synthetic	• Lidocaine (Xylocaine) • Diazepam (Valium) • Human insulin (Humulin)

FIGURE 1–1 Drug sources.

The hormone insulin, used to treat diabetes mellitus, was customarily obtained from the pancreas of slaughtered animals, mainly cattle and pigs. Although animal insulin is not chemically identical to human insulin, it is physiologically active in humans. Porcine insulin (insulin derived from pigs) most nearly resembles human insulin. The chemical alteration of three amino acids in porcine insulin makes it identical to human endogenous insulin. The chemically altered porcine insulin is marketed and usually referred to as "human insulin." Drug developers also can manufacture human insulin from bacteria.

The four main sources of drugs are plants, animals, minerals, and laboratory (synthetic) (see Figure 1–1).

Plant Sources of Drugs

Plants may be the oldest source of medications.

The earliest concoctions using plants as drug sources consisted of the entire plant, including leaves, roots, bulb, stem, seeds, buds, and blossoms. Some of the extra material was harmful to human tissues. As the understanding of plants as a drug source became more sophisticated, researchers sought to isolate the active components (the components that caused the drug's effect) and avoid the harmful material.

The active components consist of several types and vary in character and effect. The most important are alkaloids (one of the largest groups of active components), which act as alkali. The organic alkaloids react with acids to form a salt. This salt, a neutralized or partially neutralized form, is more readily soluble in body fluids. The names of alkaloids and their salts usually end in *-ine;* examples include atropine, caffeine, and nicotine. Atropine sulfate is used in the treatment of slow heart rates and in certain types of toxicological emergencies. Atropine is derived from the deadly nightshade plant (*Atropa belladonna*). This plant is native to central and southern Europe but cultivated widely in North America.

Another emergency medication derived from *plant sources* is morphine sulfate. Morphine is used to treat moderate to severe pain. It is made from parts of the opium plant, which is native to Turkey and other parts of the Middle East. In addition to morphine, heroin, codeine, and many other analgesic preparations are derived from the opium plant. However, because of their psychotropic effects, narcotic analgesics are subject to abuse. They also can result in physical and psychological dependence.

Animal Sources of Drugs

The body fluids or glands of animals can act as sources of drugs. The drugs obtained from animal sources include hormones, such as insulin (as previously discussed); oils and fats (usually mixed), such as cod-liver oil; and enzymes, produced by living cells, which act as catalysts. Enzymes include pancreatin and pepsin. Vaccines (suspensions of killed, modified, or attenuated microorganisms) also are obtained from animal sources. Examples of hormone drugs derived from *animal sources* include insulin and oxytocin. Both of these agents are extracted from the desiccated endocrine glands of mammals. Insulin is used in the treatment of diabetes mellitus, whereas oxytocin is used to induce labor and treat certain types of vaginal bleeding. Cod-liver oil is an example of an oil derived from animals.

Mineral Sources of Drugs

Metallic and nonmetallic minerals provide various inorganic material not available from plants or animals. The mineral sources are used as they occur in nature or are combined with other ingredients to yield acids, bases, or salts. Two emergency medications come from *mineral (inorganic) sources.* They are sodium bicarbonate ($NaHCO_3$) and magnesium sulfate ($MgSO_4$). Sodium bicarbonate is occasionally used to treat severe metabolic acidosis and is an adjunct in certain toxicological emergencies. Magnesium sulfate is used in the treatment of eclampsia, a life-threatening seizure disorder associated with pregnancy, and in some cardiac emergencies.

Laboratory-Produced Drug Sources

Researchers today produce an ever-increasing number of drugs in the laboratory. The new drugs may be natural (from animal or plant sources), synthetic, or a combination of the two. Examples of drugs produced in the laboratory include thyroid hormone (natural), cimetidine (synthetic), and anistreplase (combination of natural and synthetic). Recombinant deoxyribonucleic acid (DNA) research has led to another chemical source of organic compounds: The reordering of genetic information enables scientists to develop bacteria that produce insulin for humans. This technology is used to

TABLE 1-1

Sources of Drug Information

Pharmacopeia: Official

The United States Pharmacopeia (USP) and National Formulary (NF)
The British Pharmacopoeia (BP)
The British National Formulary (BF)
Compendium of Pharmaceuticals and Specialties (CPS) Canada

Compendia: Nonofficial

Martindale: The Extra Pharmacopoeia
(Drug information/hospital formulary) American Hospital Formulary Service,
published by authority of the American Society of Hospital Pharmacists
Facts and comparisons
USP dispensing information
Pharmaceutical companies
Physicians' Desk Reference (PDR)
Package inserts: brochures required by law; content is approved by Food and
Drug Administration

Journal

The Medical Letter on Drugs and Therapeutics

manufacture insulin, hepatitis B vaccine, and several other products. Insulin
is manufactured by taking the genetic code for human insulin and placing it
into the cells of selected bacteria. These bacteria can then be grown in large
quantities, thus producing a large amount of insulin at relatively low cost.

Many drugs on the market today are synthetically derived. Common examples of emergency drugs that are synthetically manufactured include lidocaine (Xylocaine), bretylium tosylate (Bretylol), and diazepam (Valium). Lidocaine and bretylium tosylate are used to treat cardiac dysrhythmias. Valium
is used to treat seizures, anxiety, and other neuropsychiatric disorders.

Sources of Drug Information

Obtaining information on drugs can be difficult. Using multiple sources of
information about drugs is usually a good idea. Every book about drugs, including this one, has a disclaimer regarding doses and current uses, referring the reader to local medical direction for the final word. Using multiple
sources and comparing the author's statements about a drug may lead you
to the best available information. EMS providers generally like small, short
guides that they can carry in a shirt pocket. These usually include important details about drugs that the prehospital providers administer along
with a long list of commonly prescribed drugs and their classes. These EMS
guides will be useful if you clearly understand the drugs used in your system and have a working knowledge of commonly prescribed drug classes.

There are many sources of drug information available to the prehospital provider (see Table 1–1).

DRUG RESEARCH AND BRINGING A DRUG TO MARKET

The pharmaceutical industry is highly motivated to bring profitable new
drugs to market. Proving the safety and reliability of these new drugs, however, requires extensive research. While better understanding of biology is

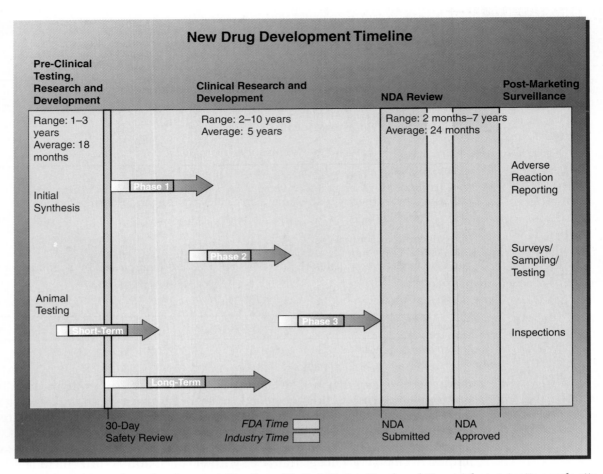

New Drug Development Timeline

| Pre-Clinical Testing, Research and Development | | Clinical Research and Development | NDA Review | Post-Marketing Surveillance |

Range: 1–3 years
Average: 18 months

Range: 2–10 years
Average: 5 years

Range: 2 months–7 years
Average: 24 months

Initial Synthesis

Phase 1

Adverse Reaction Reporting

Phase 2

Surveys/ Sampling/ Testing

Animal Testing

Short-Term

Phase 3

Inspections

Long-Term

30-Day Safety Review

FDA Time
Industry Time

NDA Submitted

NDA Approved

CHART 1–1 New drug development timeline. (United States Food and Drug Administration web site, http://www.ida.gov/fdac/special/newdrug/testing.html.)

shortening the time needed to bring a new drug to market, the process still takes many years. To assure the safety of new medications, the U.S. Federal Drug Administration (FDA) has developed a process for evaluating their safety and efficacy. The process, illustrated in Chart 1–1, adds even more time to the development cycle. Initial drug testing begins with the study of both male and female mammals. After testing a drug's toxicity, researchers evaluate its pharmacokinetics—it is absorbed, distributed, metabolized (biotransformed) and excreted—in animals. These animal studies also help determine the drug's therapeutic index (the ratio of its lethal dose to its effective dose). If the results of the animal testing are satisfactory, the FDA designates the drug as an investigational new drug (IND) and researchers can then test it in humans. Human studies take place in four phases.

Common Pharmacological Terminology and Abbreviations

It is common to use abbreviations in pharmacology. Abbreviations serve to expedite paperwork and promote efficiency. The abbreviations used in pharmacology are fairly standard. It is important to be familiar with these abbreviations and with some of the common terminology applicable to the field of emergency pharmacology (see Table 1–2).

TABLE 1–2

Common Abbreviations

Abbreviation	Meaning	Abbreviation	Meaning
$\bar{a}$	*ante* (before)	IC	intracardiac
a.c.	*ante cibos* (before meals)	IM	intramuscular
ACh	acetylcholine	IO	intraosseous
ACLS	advanced cardiac life support	IV	intravenous
admin.	administer	IVP	intravenous push
a	alpha	IVPB	intravenous piggyback
ALS	advanced life support	K^+	potassium
AMA	against medical advice	kg	kilogram
AMI	acute myocardial infarction	KO	keep open
Amp.	ampule	KVO	keep vein open
APAP	acetaminophen	L	liter
ASA	aspirin	lb	pound
b	beta	$<$	less than
bid	*bis in die* (twice a day)	LR	lactated Ringer's solution
c	*cum* (with)	$MgSO_4$	magnesium sulfate
Ca^{++}	calcium ion	♂	male
$CaCl_2$	calcium chloride	MAX	maximum
caps	capsules	MDI	metered-dose inhaler
cc	cubic centimeter	μ	micro
CC	chief complaint	μgtt	microdrop
CHF	congestive heart failure	μg	microgram
Cl^-	chloride ion	μcg	microgram
cm	centimeter	μm	micrometer
cm^3	cubic centimeter	mEq	milliequivalent
c/o	complains of	mg	milligram
CO	carbon monoxide	min	minute
CO_2	carbon dioxide	mL	milliliter
COPD	chronic obstructive pulmonary disease	mm	millimeter
		MS	morphine sulfate
CSM	carotid sinus massage	MSO_4	morphine sulfate
CVA	cerebrovascular accident	N_2O	nitrous oxide
°	degree	Na^+	sodium ion
°C	degrees Celsius	$NaHCO_3$	sodium bicarbonate
°F	degrees Fahrenheit	nitro	nitroglycerin
D/C	discontinue	NKA	no known allergies
↓	decrease	NKDA	no known drug allergies
D_5W	5 percent dextrose in water	NTG	nitroglycerin
$D_{10}W$	10 percent dextrose in water	∅	null or none
$D_{50}W$	50 percent dextrose in water	O_2	oxygen
dig	digitalis	OD	overdose
Dx	diagnosis	OD	*oculus dexter* (right eye)
ECG	electrocardiogram	OS	*oculus sinister* (left eye)
EKG	electrocardiogram (from German)	OU	*oculus utro* (both eyes)
elix	elixir	oz	ounce
EOA	esophageal obturator airway	p	post (after)
=	equal to	pc	*post cibos* (after eating)
et	and	PAC	premature atrial contraction
ET	endotracheal	PAT	paroxysmal atrial tachycardia
ETC	endotracheal combitube	PEA	pulseless electrical activity
ETOH	alcohol (ethyl)	pedi	pediatric
♀	female	PJC	premature junctional contraction
g	gram	po	*per os* (by mouth)
gr	grain	pr	*per rectus* (by rectum)
$>$	greater than	prn	*pro re nata* (when necessary)
gtt	*gutta* (drop)	PSVT	paroxysmal supraventricular tachycardia
gtts	*guttae* (drops)		
HHN	handheld nebulizer	q	*quisque* (every)
hs	*hora somni* (at bedtime)	qd	*quisque die* (every day)
↑	increase	qh	*quisque hora* (every hour)

(continued)

TABLE 1–2 *(continued)*

Common Abbreviations

Abbreviation	Meaning	Abbreviation	Meaning
qid	*quarter in die* (four times a day)	SpO$_2$	oxygen saturation (oximetry)
qod	*tertio quoque die* (every other day)	SQ or SC	subcutaneous
qt	quart	stat	*statim* (now or immediately)
®	registered trademark	SVN	small-volume nebulizer
RL	Ringer's lactate solution	tid	*ter in die* (three times a day)
Rx	treatment	t-PA	tissue plasminogen activator
s̄	*sine* (without)	TKO	to keep open
SC	subcutaneous	u	unit
SK	streptokinase	ut dict	*ut dictum* (as directed)
sol	solution	y/o	year old

FDA CLASSIFICATION OF NEWLY APPROVED DRUGS

The FDA has developed a method for immediately classifying new drugs. This method of drug classification utilizes a number and a letter for each new drug in the IND phase or upon New Drug Application (NDA) review by the FDA. The manufacturer has a right to contest this classification and have it changed before the final classification is established.

Numerical Classification (Chemical)

1. A new molecular drug
2. A new salt of a marketed drug
3. A new formulation or dosage form not previously marketed
4. A new combination not previously marketed
5. A drug that is already on the market, a generic duplication
6. A product already marketed by the same company (This designation is used for new indications for a marketed drug)
7. A drug product on the market without New Drug Application approval (drug was marketed prior to 1938)

Letter Classification (Treatment or Therapeutic Potential)

A. Drug offers an important therapeutic gain (P-priority)
B. Drug that is similar to drugs already on the market (S-similar)

Other Classifications

A. Drugs indicated for AIDS and HIV-related disease
B. Drugs developed to treat life-threatening or severely debilitating illness
I. An orphan drug

NEW DRUG DEVELOPMENT

In the past, drugs were found by trial and error. Now they are developed primarily by systematic research. Scientists still search for new organic and inorganic sources; however, they now focus most of their attention on the laboratory to discover needed drugs.

The U.S. Food and Drug Administration (FDA) carefully monitors new drug development, which can take many years to complete. Testing of new drugs begins with animals to evaluate a drug's pharmacological use, dosage ranges, and possible toxic effects. Only after reviewing extensive animal studies and data on the safety and effectiveness of the proposed drug will the FDA approve the application for an Investigational New Drug (IND).

Four phases of clinical evaluation involving human subjects follow approval of the IND. The clinical studies are intended to provide information on purity, bioavailability, potency, efficacy, safety, and toxicity. Depending on the results of testing, the studies can be stopped at any phase.

Phase I

The primary purposes of phase I testing is to determine the drug's pharmacokinetics, toxicity, and safe dose in humans.

In phase I, a clinical pharmacologist supervises studies involving a small number of healthy volunteers. All effects of the drug on the volunteers are recorded. The recorded clinical data determine the need for further testing.

Phase II

The primary purpose of phase II testing is to find the therapeutic drug level and watch carefully for toxic and side effects.

A small number of individuals who have the disease for which the drug is purported to be diagnostic or therapeutic are then given the drug. Supervisors carefully document toxic effects and adverse reactions to determine the drug's proper dosage. Researchers then review and compare data from the animal studies and human studies, closely monitoring effects on animal and human fertility and reproduction.

Phase III

The main purpose of phase III testing is to refine the usual therapeutic dose and to collect relevant data on side effects.

In phase III, large numbers of patients in medical research centers receive the drug. This larger sampling provides information about infrequent or rare adverse effects. Information collected during this phase helps determine risks associated with the new drug. Researchers also must perform various tests that take into account those patients who are so emotionally involved that they experience relief of symptoms based on suggestion. The administration of a placebo, a medically inert substance, to some patients provides control for such psychological responses. In one frequently used procedure, one-half of the patients receive the drug and one-half receive the placebo. To remove all bias, neither the patient nor the physician knows who has received the drug and who has received the placebo until completion of the study; this type of study is known as a double-blind study. In another type of study (crossover study) patients receive the drug for part of the time and a placebo for the rest of the time.

After the three phases, the FDA evaluates the results. If the FDA announces a favorable evaluation, the company developing the drug then completes a New Drug Application (NDA). FDA approval of the company's NDA means that the new drug has been accepted and can be marketed exclusively by its sponsoring company.

Phase IV

Phase IV testing involves post-marketing analysis during conditional approval. Once the drug is being used in the general population, the FDA requires the drug's maker to monitor its performance.

Phase IV is voluntary. After the NDA is approved, the drug company begins surveillance or post-market surveillance. It receives reports about the therapeutic results of the drug from physicians. The company must communicate adequately with the FDA and with the public during the drug's use. Some medications, such as benoxaprofen (Oraflex), have been found to be toxic and have been removed from the market after their initial release. At times, manufacturers have contended that a drug's benefits for a certain segment of the population outweigh its risks. Such was the manufacturer's response when the antidepressant tranylcypromine was withdrawn from the market. Eventually, but with certain restrictions, the FDA reinstated tranylcypromine in the market for use by patients with severe depression.

Expedited Drug Approval

Although most INDs undergo all four phases of clinical evaluation, a few can receive expedited approval. For example, because of the public health threat posed by acquired immunodeficiency syndrome (AIDS), the FDA and drug companies have agreed to shorten the IND approval process, allowing physicians to give qualified AIDS patients so-called Treatment INDs not yet approved by the FDA. Sponsors of drugs that reach phase II or III clinical trials can apply for FDA approval of Treatment IND status. When the IND is approved, the sponsor supplies the drug to physicians whose patients meet appropriate criteria.

Orphan Drugs

Some drugs useful to treat various diseases never reach the market. Drug companies do not adopt and develop these medications, appropriately referred to as orphan drugs. The reasons vary. Some orphan drugs useful for rare diseases have a limited market; others produce high-risk adverse reactions that make insurance costs prohibitive. Many useful drugs remain orphans because manufacturers cannot hope to recover the huge amounts of money spent in developing a new drug.

In 1983, Congress signed the Orphan Drug Act, which offers substantial tax credits to companies that develop orphan drugs. Small companies may receive federal financial grants to help them research and develop orphan drugs. As a result, thousands of patients may now use drugs that until recently were unavailable. Despite legislation, many orphan drugs remain without developers.

UNLABELED USES OF DRUGS

When approving a new drug, the FDA accepts it only for the indications for which phase II and phase III clinical studies have shown it to be safe and effective. These indications are approved (labeled); all others are not approved (unlabeled).

For example, the FDA may approve a new drug to treat hypertension if phase II and phase III studies showed that it was safe and effective for use in patients with hypertension. If the drug also works as an antianginal agent, the FDA cannot approve it for this indication unless formal studies in patients with angina pectoris are completed successfully. Such a drug is unapproved for treatment of angina pectoris, yet it may be used for this unlabeled indication, based on empirical evidence.

After prescribing a new drug approved to treat hypertension, a physician may discover that it also decreases the patient's angina. Then the physician may share this finding with colleagues in medical journals or at meetings, and they, too, may prescribe it for unlabeled uses.

The FDA recognizes that a drug's labeling does not always contain the most current information about its usage. Therefore, after the FDA approves a drug for one indication, a physician legally may prescribe it, a pharmacist may dispense it, and a nurse or paramedic may administer it for any labeled—or unlabeled—indication.

Although clinicians are not prohibited from prescribing, dispensing, or administering a drug for an unlabeled use, the FDA forbids the manufacturer from promoting a drug for any unlabeled indications. That is why drug package inserts and the *Physicians' Desk Reference* (a collection of drug manufacturers' product labeling) contain no information about unlabeled uses, and pharmaceutical sales representatives cannot discuss such uses.

Nevertheless, many drugs commonly are prescribed for unlabeled uses.

MEDICAL OVERSIGHT

Prehospital care has evolved as an extension of health care provided within the hospital setting. As such, all aspects of prehospital care have traditionally fallen under the supervision of medical doctors. This role is referred to as medical oversight and is currently enforced by legislation throughout Canada and the United States. Although the specifics of this legislation vary from state to state, it is based on a common theme involving all prehospital care providers acting under the direction and control of a physician. The prehospital care provider is acting as a delegate for the physician and is, in essence, working under the medical license of the physician providing medical control.

The Medical Director

The individual physician who assumes the medical oversight role described in the previous section is designated the medical director. The medical director is typically a licensed physician active in emergency medicine with an understanding of, and experience in, prehospital care. The specific duties of the medical director include development and implementation of medical control guidelines, education, quality assurance, equipment and medication review, and assessment of competency. The role of the medical director has also evolved in recent years to include some scene response and field triage at mass casualty incidents. The medical director is responsible for the actions of care providers working under his or her medical control and, as such, is the ultimate authority with respect to all medical control and competency issues. Because prehospital care providers work under the license of the medical director, the medical director can be found medicolegally liable in cases of litigation involving prehospital care. In some systems, the medical director receives input from a medical control or medical advisory board, which generally has physician representation from the various institutions served by the emergency medical services (EMS) system. The roles and authority of these types of committees are system specific. Although the level of involvement of the medical director within an EMS system varies, ideally that individual should have ongoing exposure to activities in the field as a means of staying abreast of medical and operational issues. Care providers should view the medical director as a resource who can provide constructive feedback and answer questions as they arise. At the same time, the medical director must serve as a patient advocate, ensuring that patient care is the foremost priority.

Medical Control

Medical control constitutes one of the components of medical oversight and can be further subdivided into direct (on-line) and indirect (off-line) medical control.

Direct Medical Control

Direct medical control refers to orders given directly to prehospital care providers by a physician, generally via radio or telephone. Typically the prehospital care provider speaks to a physician in the emergency department to which the patient is being transported. Also known as a "base" physician, this individual is generally well acquainted with local medical control guidelines and the overall capabilities of the local EMS system and personnel.

Indirect Medical Control

Indirect medical control essentially includes all aspects of medical oversight that do not involve direct medical control, including system design, protocol development, education, and quality improvement. To be effective, medical control must have the authority to discipline or limit the activities of those who deviate from an established standard of care. As an advancing field, prehospital care demands a commitment to lifelong learning, and it is the responsibility of both the care provider and the medical director to ensure that this process is ongoing. The education component of prehospital care is becoming increasingly important as the complexity of care, including medications and equipment, increases. The importance of training and education can be demonstrated by the ever-increasing number of medications and interventions provided in the field that have lethal potential if used inappropriately.

Medical Control Protocols and Guidelines

All treatments and interventions in the prehospital field are provided under the direct or indirect orders of a physician. Many of these orders are provided in the form of medical protocols that provide an algorithm for treating patients in the field. Many systems provide standing orders or standing protocols that allow the care provider to treat patients without speaking to a physician. These protocols are designed to facilitate management of specific presenting signs and symptoms rather than a specific diagnosis. Certain treatments and presenting problems may require base physician contact prior to implementation. Recently some EMS systems have implemented treat-and-release protocols that allow staff to release patients who respond to treatment and meet certain preestablished criteria. This is an example of the ever-increasing responsibility that prehospital care providers face, and it emphasizes the importance of education, judgment, and critical-thinking skills.

Legal Regulations, Standards, and Legislation

As a society develops and uses drugs, it needs to establish controls regulating the manufacture, distribution, and use of those drugs. In many cases a society's attitude and values, rather than formal controls, determine the acceptable limits of drug use. Formal drug controls range from individual institutional policies to governmental legislation.

International Controls

The United Nations, through its World Health Organization, attempts to influence international health by providing technical assistance and encouraging research for drug use. One committee has been established to cope with the problems associated with habit-forming drugs. Drug enforcement agencies in various nations cooperate, but no administrative or judicial structures enforce controls. As a result, control of international drug trade depends largely on the voluntary cooperation of nations.

Controls in the United States

Before a drug can be marketed, it must undergo extensive testing. This testing generally involves two phases, animal studies and clinical patient studies. Only after these extensive tests, and with governmental approval, can drugs be placed on the market. Even after clinical usage, the effectiveness of the drugs must be closely monitored. The U.S. Food and Drug Administration (FDA) is the federal agency responsible for approval of drugs before they are made available to the general public.

Legislative control in the United States began in 1906, when Congress enacted the Pure Food and Drug Act. In addition to establishing the FDA, this act prohibited the sale of medicinal preparations that had little or no use and restricted the sale of drugs with a potential for abuse. The Pure Food and Drug Act named the *United States Pharmacopeia (USP)* and the *National Formulary (NF)* as official drug standards. Any drug bearing the official title USP or NF must conform to rigid standards regarding purity, preparation, and dosage.

The Pure Food and Drug Act was not as all-encompassing as its planners had envisioned it to be. For several years stronger drug laws were debated in both Congress and state legislatures. In the 1930s more than 100 people died from ingesting sulfanilamide, an antibacterial drug. Researchers discovered that the sulfanilamide had been prepared with a previously uninvestigated toxic substance called diethylene glycol. Finally in 1938, Congress enacted the Federal Food, Drug, and Cosmetic Act. Among the most important features of this act was the truth-in-labeling clause. The act required the following:

1. A statement accurately describing the package's contents
2. The usual names of the drugs, for official drugs (preparations listed in the pharmacopeia and adopted by the government as meeting pharmaceutical standards) and nonofficial drugs (drugs not listed in the pharmacopeia)
3. Indication of the presence, quantity, and proportion of certain drugs (such as alcohol, atropine, and bromides)

4. Warning of habit-forming drugs in the product and of their effects
5. The names of the manufacturer, packager, and distributor
6. Directions for use and warnings against unsafe use, including recommendations for dosage levels and frequency

Narcotics

A problem almost as old as medicine itself is abuse and addiction to certain drugs. Narcotics are among the drugs most frequently abused. Recognizing the need to control the sale of narcotics, the federal government enacted the Harrison Narcotic Act in 1914. This act served to control the importation, manufacture, and sale of the opium plant and its derivatives. It also controlled the derivatives of the coca plant. The primary drug derived from the coca plant is cocaine. As a result of this act, these drugs, as well as other drugs added to the list later, could be obtained only with special prescriptions. Only physicians who qualified and attained a special narcotic license could prescribe this class of drugs.

In 1970 major revisions were made in the use and control of narcotics and other drugs. This law, the Comprehensive Drug Abuse Prevention and Control Act of 1970 (commonly called the Controlled Substance Act of 1970), classifies the drugs used in medicine into five different schedules. A summary of the five schedules is found in Table 1–3.

The Controlled Substances Act

The Controlled Substances Act mandates that prescriptions for Schedule II drugs cannot be refilled. Moreover, it requires that prescriptions for Schedule II drugs be filled within 72 hours. Prescriptions for drugs in this class cannot be called into the pharmacy over the telephone (except in special situations). Prescriptions for drugs in Schedules III and IV may be refilled up to five times within 6 months. Prescriptions for Schedule V drugs may be refilled at the discretion of the physician.

Responsibility for enforcing the Controlled Substances Act rests with the Drug Enforcement Administration (DEA). Only physicians approved by the DEA may write prescriptions for scheduled drugs. The physician must indicate his or her DEA number on the prescription. Many states have enacted laws further regulating controlled substances.

Canadian Drug Legislation

Drug control in Canada falls under the direct supervision of the Department of National Health and Welfare. The Food and Drug Act, passed in 1941, empowers the governor-in-council to prescribe drug standards and limit variation in any food or drug. The 1953 Canadian Food and Drugs Act (amended yearly) provides regulations for drug manufacture and sale. A comparison of the drug schedules in the United States and Canada is found in Table 1–3.

Canadian Narcotic Control Act and Regulations

In 1965, the Canadian Narcotic Control Act restricted the sale, possession, and use of narcotics. It further restricted narcotics to authorized personnel. This act defines who may prescribe a narcotic drug, such as physicians, dentists, research personnel, and their agents, and places conditions on the

TABLE 1–3

Schedule of Controlled Drugs

United States		Canada	
Category	Examples	Category	Examples
Schedule I No recognized medical use High abuse potential Research use only	**Opiates** Heroin **Hallucinogens** LSD Mescaline **Depressants** Methaqualone	**Schedule H** Restricted drugs No recognized medicinal properties	**Hallucinogens** Peyote LSD Mescaline
Schedule II Written prescriptions required No telephone renewals In an emergency, a prescription may be renewed by telephone	**Opiates** Codeine Morphine Meperidine **Stimulants** Amphetamines Phenmetrazine **Depressants** Secobarbital	**Narcotics schedule** Stringently restricted drugs The letter N must appear on all labels and professional advertisements	**Coca leaf derivatives** Cocaine **Opiates and opiate derivatives** Morphine Codeine Methadone Hydromorphone Meperidine **Other drugs** Phencyclidine Cannabis
Schedule III Prescriptions required to be rewritten after 6 months or five refills Prescriptions may be ordered by telephone	**Opiates** Codeine of less than 1.8 g/dl Opium of less than 25 mg/5 ml **Stimulants** Benzphetamine Mazindol **Depressants** Butabarbital Glutethimide Talbutal **Anabolic steroids** Ethylestrenol Fluoxymesterone Methyltestosterone Nandrolone decanoate	**Schedule G** Controlled drugs Prescriptions are controlled because of the abuse potential of these drugs	**Narcotic analgesics** Nalbuphine Butorphanol **Stimulants** Amphetamines **Barbiturates** Phenobarbital Amobarbital Secobarbital
Schedule IV Prescriptions required to be rewritten after 6 months or five refills	**Opiates** Pentazocine Propoxyphene **Stimulants** Fenfluramine Phentermine **Depressants** Benzodiazepines Chloral hydrate	**Schedule F** Prescription drugs Although not controlled drugs, agents in this category include some with a relatively low abuse potential The symbol Pr must appear on their labels	**Anxiolytics** Benzodiazepines
Schedule V Dispenses as any (nonnarcotic) prescription Some may be dispensed without prescription unless additional state regulations apply	Primarily small amounts of opiates, such as opium, dihydrocodeine, and diphenoxylate, when used as antitussives or antidiarrheals in combination products	**Nonprescription drug schedule (group 3)** Drugs available only in the pharmacy and used only on a physician's recommendation Limited public access	**Analgesics** Low-dose codeine preparations **Other drugs** Insulin Nitroglycerin Muscle relaxants

recipient of a narcotic prescription, requiring disclosure of all previous narcotics received within the past 30 days. In addition, the act describes procedures for record keeping and dispensing by pharmacists. Hospital regulations are also outlined.

Methadone is covered individually in this act, which sets requirements for authorized practitioners who prescribe and dispense this drug.

Drug Standards

The federal government establishes and enforces drug standards to ensure the uniform quality of drugs. Because some generic drugs affect patients differently than their brand name counterparts, standardization of drugs is necessary. Despite FDA standards, drugs sold or distributed by various manufacturers may have biological or therapeutic differences. An assay determines the amount of purity of a given chemical in a preparation in the laboratory (in vitro). While two generically equivalent preparations may contain the same amount of a given chemical (drug), they may have different therapeutic effects. This relative therapeutic effectiveness is determined by a bioassay, which attempts to ascertain their bioequivalence. The United States Pharmacopeia (USP) is the official standard for the United States. These standards pertain to the following drug properties:

Purity refers to the uncontaminated state of a drug containing only one active component. In reality, a drug consisting of only one active compound rarely exists because manufacturers usually must add other ingredients to facilitate drug formation and to determine absorption rate. As a result, standards of purity do not demand 100 percent pure active ingredients but specify the type and acceptable amount of extraneous material.

Bioavailability describes the degree to which a drug becomes absorbed and reaches general circulation. Factors affecting bioavailability include the particle size, crystalline structure, solubility, and polarity of the compound. The blood or tissue concentration of a drug at a specified time after administration usually determines bioavailability.

Potency of a drug refers to its strength or its power to produce the desired effect. Potency standards are set by testing laboratory animals to determine the definite measurable effect of an administered drug.

Efficacy refers to the effectiveness of a drug used in treatment. Objective clinical trials attempt to determine efficacy, but absolute measurement remains difficult.

Safety and toxicity are determined by the incidence and severity of reported adverse reactions to the use of a drug. Some harmful effects may not appear for a considerable time. Safety and toxicity standards are being refined constantly as past experiences illuminate deficiencies in the standards.

Drug Names

Drugs are identified by four different names: chemical, generic, trade, and official. A drug's chemical name precisely describes its atomic and molecular structure. Because drugs are usually chemically complex in nature, so too are the chemical names. When a manufacturer decides to market a new drug, the United States Adopted Names (USAN) Council selects a generic name. The *generic name,* usually an abbreviated version of the chemical name, is frequently used. Manufacturers of pharmaceuticals rarely refer to drugs by their generic names. Instead, they select a name for a drug that is based on its chemical name or on the type of problem it is used to treat. This is referred to as the *trade name.* Trade names are always capitalized, whereas generic names are not. Trade names are protected by copyright. The symbol ® after the trade name means it is registered by and restricted to the drug manufacturer. The fourth method of naming a drug is the *official name.* The official name is followed by the initials USP or NF, which are official publications that list drugs conforming to standards set forth by the publication. The official name is usually the same as the generic name. Following is an example of the four names of a specific drug:

Chemical name: Ethyl 1-methyl-4-phenylisonipecotate hydrochloride
Generic name: Meperidine hydrochloride
Trade name: Demerol Hydrochloride
Official name: Meperidine hydrochloride, USP

Proprietary (Trade) Names

In recent years, controversy has developed regarding generic and non-generic drugs. When writing a prescription, a physician can order the drug by either the trade name or the generic name. Until recently, the pharmacist had to fill the prescription as written. Now, in many states, the pharmacist may substitute a less-expensive generic drug for the prescription. As a rule, generic drugs are not inferior in quality. They are usually cheaper because lesser-known companies with minimal advertising and production costs manufacture them.

Most pharmaceutical houses market their drugs primarily under trade names rather than under generic names. Today there may be a number of trade names under which a single drug may be sold. The practice of using these brand names is often confusing to the medical provider and sometimes even to the physician, to say nothing of the inconvenience to the pharmacist, who must stock four or five different brands of the same drug. Currently, there is a trend to return to the use of official or generic names on prescriptions. When a physician orders a specific trade name, however, the pharmacist must dispense it. No other brand, even if the product is exactly the same as the one ordered, may be substituted without the physician's knowledge and consent.

Drugs that share similar characteristics are grouped together as a pharmacological class (family), such as beta-blockers. A second grouping is the therapeutic classification, which groups drugs by therapeutic use, such as antihypertensives. Thiazides and beta-blockers are both antihypertensives, but they share few characteristics.

COMPONENTS OF A DRUG PROFILE

A drug's profile describes its various properties. As a paramedic or paramedic student, you will become familiar with drug profiles as you study specific medications. A typical drug profile will contain the following information:

Names.   These most frequently include the generic and trade names, although the occasional reference will include chemical names.

Classification.   This is the broad group to which the drug belongs. Knowing classifications is essential to understanding the properties of drugs.

Mechanism of Action.   The way in which a drug caused its effects; its pharmacodynamics.

Indications.   Conditions that made administration of the drug appropriate (as approved by the Food and Drug Administration).

Pharmacokinetics.   How the drug is absorbed, distributed, and eliminated; typically includes onset and duration of action.

Side effects/adverse reactions.   The drug's untoward or undesired effects.

Routes of administration.   How the drug is given.

Contraindications.   Conditions that make it inappropriate to give the drug. Unlike when the drug is simply not indicated, a contraindication means that a predictable harmful event will occur if the drug is given in this situation.

Dosage.   The amount of the drug that should be given.

How supplied.   This typically includes the common concentrations of the available preparations; many drugs come in different concentrations.

Special considerations.   How the drug may affect pediatric, geriatric or pregnant patients.

Drug profiles may also include other components, such as its interactions with other drugs or with foods, when appropriate.

Drug Forms

Drugs come in many forms and are packaged in numerous styles. Each form and each style has advantages and disadvantages. For example, drugs taken by mouth tend to have a slow and unpredictable rate of absorption and thus a slower rate of onset of effect. Drugs given intravenously, although rapidly acting, are much more difficult to administer. Drugs may be packaged in unit-dose form, in which one dose of a drug comes in a labeled container or wrapper. They may also be packaged in bulk form, in which multiple doses of a drug are packaged in a container, bottle, or wrapper.

Drugs are manufactured in many different forms including liquids, solids, suppositories, inhalants, sprays, creams, lotions, patches, and lozenges. To administer drugs safely, you must be knowledgeable about the different effects of the many drug forms. For example, nitroglycerin administered sublingually (allowing it to dissolve under the tongue) can relieve anginal pain in less than 1 minute. The same drug administered as an ointment applied to the chest wall may not relieve acute pain at all; however, it may be used prophylactically for anginal pain. Common drug preparations are described in the following sections.

Liquid Drugs

Liquid drugs usually consist of a powder dissolved in a liquid. The drug is referred to as the *solute.* The liquid into which it is dissolved is called the *solvent.* In liquid drug preparations, the primary difference between one preparation and another is the solvent.

Solutions.   Solutions are preparations that contain the drug dissolved in a solvent, usually water (for example, 5 percent dextrose in water).

Tinctures. Tinctures are drug preparations whereby the drug was extracted chemically with alcohol. They usually contain some dilute alcohol (for example, tincture of iodine).

Suspensions. Suspensions are drugs that do not remain dissolved. After sitting for even short periods, these drugs tend to separate. They must always be shaken well before use (for example, penicillin preparations).

Spirits. Spirit solutions contain volatile chemicals dissolved in alcohol (for example, spirit of ammonia).

Emulsions. Emulsions are preparations in which an oily substance is mixed with a solvent into which it does not dissolve. When mixed, it forms globules of fat floating in the solvent. An example of a common emulsion outside of medicine is oil and vinegar salad dressing.

Elixirs. Elixirs are preparations that contain the drug in an alcohol solvent. Flavoring, often cherry, is added to improve the taste (for example, Tylenol Elixer).

Syrups. Often drugs are suspended in sugar and water to improve the taste. These are referred to as syrups (for example, cough syrup).

Liquid drugs administered into the body through intramuscular, subcutaneous, or intravenous routes are called *parenteral drugs.* Most drugs used in emergency medicine are parenteral. Because they are introduced into the body, they must be sterile.

Liquid drugs given parenterally are available in four packaging styles: vials, ampules, self-contained systems or syringes, and nebules. Sterile parenteral containers designed to carry a single patient dose are called *ampules* (see Figure 1–2). An ampule is a glass container with a thin neck, which usually is scored so it can be snapped off. After the tops are broken, the drug is drawn into a syringe for administration.

In emergency medicine many drugs given parenterally are in self-contained systems or *prefilled syringes* (see Figures 1–3 and 1–4). These preparations save time by avoiding the problems inherent with ampules. Self-contained systems or prefilled syringes contain a single dose of a drug in a plastic bag or in a prefilled syringe with an attached needle. Prefilled

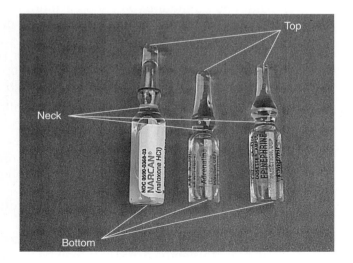

FIGURE 1-2 Ampules.

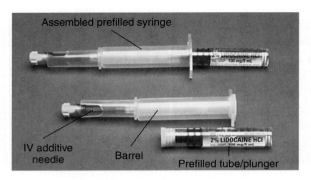

FIGURE 1-3 Prefilled syringes.

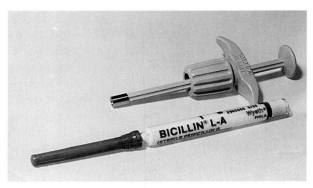

FIGURE 1-4 Tubex syringes.

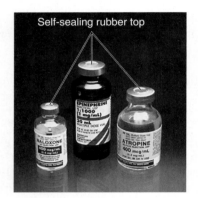

FIGURE 1-5 Multidose vials.

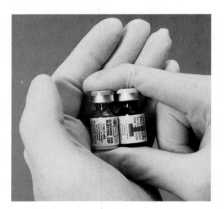

FIGURE 1-6 Single dose vials.

syringes are often used during cardiopulmonary resuscitation and other advanced life support activities.

Vials are another type of container for parenteral drugs (see Figures 1–5 and 1–6). Vials are bottles sealed with a rubber diaphragm and may contain a single or multiple doses. Multidose vials contain preservatives that enable them to be used for more than one dose, whereas single-dose vials do not contain such agents. Many drugs used in emergency medicine are supplied in vials.

Nebules are used for medications that are premixed. For example, salbutamol (Ventolin) and ipratropium bromide (Atrovent) are both administered to the patient by nebulizer. Each nebule is filled with the amount of medication generally administered to an adult patient.

Solid Drugs

Solid drugs are usually administered orally, although many can be administered rectally. They include the following:

Pills. Pills are drugs that are shaped into a form that makes them easy to swallow.

Powders. Powders are drugs in powdered form. They are not as popular as pills, but some are still in use (for example, B.C. powder).

Capsules. Capsules consist of gelatin containers into which a powder is placed. The gelatin dissolves, liberating the powder (for example, Dalmane capsules) into the gastrointestinal tract.

Tablets. Tablets are similar to pills. They are composed of a powder that has been compressed into an easily swallowed form and are often covered with a sugar coating to improve taste.

Suppositories

Administered rectally and vaginally, suppositories carry medications in a solid base that melts at body temperature. Suppositories produce local (analgesic, laxative, and anti-infective) and systemic (antiemetic, antipyretic, and analgesic) effects. Usually bullet shaped, most suppositories are about 1 inch (2.5 cm) long and require lubrication for insertion. Because they melt at body temperature, suppositories require refrigeration until administration. When placed into the body, either rectally or vaginally, they dissolve and are then absorbed into the surrounding tissue.

Inhalants

Inhalants are powered or liquid forms of a drug that are given using the respiratory route and are absorbed rapidly by the rich supply of capillaries in the lungs. Several frequently used methods of inhalation are nebulizers, metered-dose aerosol, or turbo inhalers or vaporizers.

IMPORTANT PHARMACOLOGICAL TERMINOLOGY

Important pharmacological terminology includes the following:

Antagonism. Antagonism signifies the opposition between two or more medications (for example, between Naloxone and morphine).

Bolus. A bolus is a single, oftentimes large dose of medication (for example, lidocaine bolus, which is often followed by a lidocaine infusion).

Contraindications. Contraindications are the medical or physiological conditions present in a patient that would make it harmful to administer a medication of otherwise known therapeutic value.

Cumulative action. A cumulative action occurs when a drug is administered in several doses, causing an increased effect. This increased effect is usually due to a quantitative buildup of the drug in the blood.

Depressant. A depressant is a medication that decreases or lessens a body function or activity.

Habituation. Habituation is physical or psychological dependence on a drug.

Hypersensitivity. Hypersensitivity is a reaction to a substance that is normally more profound than seen in a population not sensitive to the substance (for example, allergic reaction to penicillin).

Idiosyncrasy. An idiosyncrasy is an individual reaction to a drug that is unusually different from that seen in the rest of the population.

Indication. An indication refers to the medical condition or conditions in which the drug has proven to be of therapeutic value.

Potentiation. Potentiation is the enhancement of one drug's effects by another (for example, barbiturates and alcohol).

Refractory. Patients or conditions that do not respond to a drug are said to be refractory to the drug (for example, a patient with premature ventricular contractions who does not respond to lidocaine).

Side effects. Side effects are the unavoidable, undesired effects frequently seen even in therapeutic drug dosages.

Stimulant. A stimulant is a drug that enhances or increases a bodily function (for example, caffeine in coffee).

Synergism. Synergism is the combined action of two drugs. The action is much stronger than the effects of either drug administered separately.

Therapeutic action. A therapeutic action is the desired, intended action of a drug given in the appropriate medical condition.

Tolerance. When patients are receiving drugs on a long-term basis, they may require larger and larger dosages of the drug to achieve a therapeutic effect. This increased requirement is termed *tolerance.*

Untoward effect. An untoward effect is a side effect that proves harmful to the patient.

SUMMARY

Drugs are chemical agents used in the diagnosis, treatment, or prevention of disease. They are necessary for successful emergency care. It is important to be familiar with the commonly used emergency medications and with the terminology and abbreviations used in medicine so that communication with other medical personnel will be efficient and professional. Overall, it is essential to appreciate the inherent danger of any and all drugs and to use them properly. The rule to remember is, *When in doubt, do no harm.*

KEY WORDS

assay. A test that determines the amount and purity of a given chemical in a preparation in the laboratory.

bioequivalence. Relative therapeutic effectiveness of chemically equivalent drugs.

bioassay. Test to ascertain a drug's availability in a biological model.

controlled drug. Federal, state, and local laws control a drug that may lead to drug abuse or drug dependence and therefore its use.

drug. Any substance introduced into the body that changes a body function.

drug abuse. The self-directed use of drugs for nontherapeutic purposes, a practice that does not comply with a culture's sociocultural norms.

drug dependence. Condition in which a person cannot control drug intake; may be physiological, psychological, or both.

Drug Enforcement Administration (DEA). Federal agency with responsibility for enforcing the Controlled Substances Act.

empirical. Skill or knowledge based entirely on experience.

enteral. Administration of a drug via the gastrointestinal tract.

Food and Drug Administration (FDA). The federal agency responsible for approval of drugs before they are made available to the general public.

genetic engineering. Also called recombinant DNA technology; involves taking genetic material (DNA) from one organism and placing it into another.

medical director. A licensed physician who serves as the chief medical officer of an EMS or educational program system. Each paramedic functions under the license of the system medical director.

National Formulary. The Pure Food and Drug Act named the National Formulary (NF) and the United States Pharmacopeia (USP) as official drug standards. Any drug bearing the official title NF or USP must conform to a rigid set of standards regarding purity, preparation, and dosage.

off-line medical control. Also known as *indirect medical control;* the establishment of system policies and procedures, such as training, chart review, protocol development, audit, and quality improvement.

on-line medical control. Also known as *direct medical control;* communication between field personnel and a medical control physician, with the medical control physician providing immediate direction for on-scene care.

parenteral. Routes of administering drugs into the body without going through the digestive tract.

pharmacologist. Scientist who studies the effects of drugs on the body.

pharmacology. The study of drugs and their actions on the body.

recombinant DNA technology. Also called genetic engineering; involves taking genetic material (DNA) from one organism and placing it into another.

solute. A powder (drug) that is dissolved in a liquid (solvent).

solvent. The liquid into which a drug (solute) is dissolved.

standing orders. Written directives that may be carried out without, or prior to, contacting medical control.

synthetic. Substance made by combining two or more simpler compounds.

treatment protocols. Treatment guidelines for prehospital care. They may incorporate standing orders or may require contact with medical control prior to initiating advanced life support therapy.

United States Pharmacopeia. The Pure Food and Drug Act named the United States Pharmacopeia (USP) and the National Formulary (NF) as official drug standards. Any drug bearing the official title USP or NF must conform to a rigid set of standards regarding purity, preparation, and dosage.

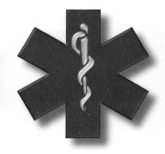

PHARMACOKINETICS AND PHARMACODYNAMICS

OBJECTIVES

After completing this chapter, the reader should be able to

1. Define pharmacokinetics and pharmacodynamics.
2. Define drug absorption.
3. Explain the factors involved in drug absorption.
4. Explain the factors that can affect drug distribution.
5. Explain biotransformation.
6. List and explain how a drug is eliminated from the body.
7. Explain the special considerations in drug therapy.

INTRODUCTION

To exert its desired biochemical and physiological effects on the body, a drug must reach its targeted tissues in a suitable form and in a sufficient concentration. The study of how drugs enter the body, reach their site of action, and are eventually eliminated is termed *pharmacokinetics*. Once drugs reach their targeted tissues, they begin a chain of biochemical events that ultimately lead to the physiological changes desired. These biochemical and physiological events are called the drug's *mechanism of action*.

After describing pharmacokinetics this chapter describes pharmacodynamics, or the mechanisms by which drugs produce biochemical or physiological changes in the body. It describes the interaction between drugs and receptors as well as drug action and drug effect. Pharmacotherapeutics addresses the different types of therapy and identifies factors that influence the choice of drug therapy and the patient's response to drugs during therapy.

This chapter addresses the fundamentals of pharmacokinetics, pharmacodynamics, and pharmacotherapeutics as they apply to prehospital emergency care.

PHARMACOLOGY

Pharmacology is the study of drugs and their interaction with the body. Drugs do not confer any new properties on cells or tissues; they only modify or exploit existing conditions. They may be given for their local action (in which case systemic absorption of the drug is discouraged) or for systemic action. Although generally given for a specific effect, drugs tend to have multiple actions at multiple sites, so they must be thought of in terms of their systemic effects rather than in terms of an isolated single effect. Pharmacology's two major divisions are pharmacokinetics and pharmacodynamics. Pharmacokinetics addresses how drugs are transported into and out of the body. Pharmacodynamics deals with their effects once they reach the target tissues.

PHARMACOKINETICS

Strictly defined, pharmacokinetics is the study of the basic processes that determine the duration and intensity of a drug's effect. These four processes are absorption, distribution, biotransformation and elimination.

To produce its desired effects, a drug must be present in the appropriate concentration at its various sites of action. Lidocaine, a drug commonly used in the treatment of life-threatening ventricular dysrhythmias, must reach its target—cardiac tissue—rapidly and in a sufficient concentration to suppress the dysrhythmia. Several factors influence the concentration of a drug at its site of action. These factors include *absorption* of the drug into the circulatory system; *distribution* of the drug throughout the body; *biotransformation* of the drug into its active form, if required; and, finally, *elimination* of the drug from the body. All of these factors do not play a role in every medication used in prehospital care, but a fundamental understanding of each of these factors is essential.

REVIEW OF PHYSIOLOGY OF TRANSPORT

Pharmacokinetics is dependent upon the body's various physiological mechanisms that move substances across the body's compartments. These mechanisms can be broken down into two broad categories based on their energy requirements then further classified. A mechanism is referred to as *active transport* if it requires the use of energy to move a substance. This energy is achieved by the breakdown of high-energy chemical bonds found in chemicals such as ATP (adenosine triphosphate). ATP is broken down into ADP (adenosine diphosphate) liberating a considerable amount of biochemical energy. A common example of an active transport mechanism is the sodium-potassium ($Na^+ - K^+$) pump. This is a protein pump that actively moves sodium ions into the cell and potassium ions out of the cell. Because this movement goes against the ion's concentration gradients, it must use energy. Large molecules, such as glucose and most of the amino acids, do not readily pass through the cell membrane because of their size. These molecules are moved across the cell membrane with the help of special "carrier" proteins found on the surface of the target cells. These large molecules are "carried" across the cell membrane in a special transport process called carrier-mediated diffusion or facilitated diffusion. Once the molecule to be transported binds with the carrier protein, the configuration of the cell membrane changes, allowing the large molecule to enter the target cell. Insulin, an important hormone secreted by the endocrine pancreas, can increase the rate of carrier-mediated glucose transport from 10 to 20-fold. This is the principle mechanism by which insulin controls glucose use in the body.

Most drugs travel through the body by means of passive transport, the movement of a substance without the use of energy. This requires the presence of concentration gradients in a solution. Diffusion and osmosis are forms of passive transport. Diffusion involves the movement of solute in the solution, while osmosis involves the movement of the solvent (usually water). In diffusion, the solute's molecules or ions move down their concentration gradients from an area of higher concentration to an area of lower concentration. Conversely, in osmosis the solvent's molecules move up the concentration gradient to an area of higher concentration. Another way of looking at this is to think of osmosis as simply the diffusion of solvent from an area of high solvent concentration to an area of low solvent concentration. A final type of passive transport is filtration. This is simply the movement of molecules across a membrane down a pressure gradient, from an area of high pressure to an area of low pressure. This pressure typically results from the hydrostatic force of blood pressure.

Drug Absorption

Drug absorption encompasses a drug's progress from its pharmaceutical dosage form to a biologically available substance that can then pass through or across tissues. The transformation from dosage form to a biologically available substance must occur before the active drug ingredient reaches the systemic circulation. After a tablet or capsule disintegrates in the stomach or small intestine, enough liquid must be available for the active drug ingredients to dissolve before systemic absorption can occur. The body requires a solution of the drug's active ingredients to dissolve before systemic absorption can occur because tissues cannot absorb dry powders or dry crystals. Because syrups and suspensions occur in dosage form as solutions, their progress from drug administration to drug absorption is more rapid, leading to a quicker onset of drug action.

Absorption is the process of movement of a drug from the site of application into the body and into the extracellular compartment. The duration and intensity of a drug's action are directly related to the rate of absorption of the drug. Many factors affect drug absorption, including

1. Solubility of the drug
2. Concentration of the drug
3. pH of the drug
4. Site of absorption
5. Absorbing surface area
6. Blood supply to the site of absorption
7. Bioavailability

The *solubility* is the tendency of a drug to dissolve. To facilitate drug absorption, the solubility of the administered drug must match the cellular constituents of the absorption site. Lipid-soluble (fat-soluble) drugs can penetrate lipoid (fat-containing) cells; water-soluble drugs cannot. For example, a water-soluble drug such as penicillin cannot penetrate the highly lipoid cells that act as barriers between the blood and brain. However a highly lipoid-soluble drug such as thiopental can penetrate the lipoid cells, cross into the brain, and induce an effect such as anesthesia. The human body is approximately 60 percent water. Thus, drugs given in water solutions are more rapidly absorbed than those given in oil-based solutions, suspensions, or solid forms.

The *concentration* of a drug also affects the rate of absorption. Drugs administered in high concentrations are absorbed much more rapidly than drugs administered in low concentrations.

Another factor that affects drug absorption is the *pH* of a drug. The pH refers to how acidic or how basic (alkaline) the drug is. Most drugs are either weak acids or weak bases. Acidic drugs tend to be more rapidly absorbed when placed into an acidic environment (such as the stomach). Alkaline drugs, on the other hand, are more rapidly absorbed when placed into an alkaline environment (such as the kidneys).

The *site of absorption* directly affects the rate of drug absorption. Once administered, drugs must pass through the various biological membranes until they reach the circulation. Drugs placed on the skin (transdermal route) must pass through several cell layers before reaching the circulatory system. On the other hand, drugs placed on mucous membranes (intranasal route) have many fewer cell layers through which to pass. Thus, drug absorption through mucous membranes is faster than drug absorption through the skin. It is sometimes useful to have slow absorption of a drug. A common emergency drug for which prolonged absorption is desired is nitroglycerin; nitroglycerin can be placed on the skin, where it is slowly absorbed over a prolonged period.

The *surface area* of the absorbing surface is an important determinant of the rate of drug absorption. Drugs are absorbed quite rapidly from large surface areas. Inhaled medications are quickly distributed across the vast pulmonary epithelium. Drugs administered by this route are rapidly absorbed into the circulation. In fact, some studies have shown that the rate of drug absorption through the inhaled route is nearly as rapid as administration by the intravenous route.

Finally, drug absorption is related to *blood supply* to the site of absorption. Some areas of the body have very rich blood supplies, whereas other areas do not. Medications placed in areas with rich blood supplies, such as the tissues under the tongue (sublingual), are absorbed rapidly. Medications placed in areas with poor blood supply, such as the fatty tissues (subcutaneous), are absorbed slowly. Muscle, as a rule, is more richly supplied with blood vessels than is subcutaneous tissue. Therefore, one would expect a drug to be absorbed more rapidly from muscle than from subcutaneous tissue (see Figure 2–1).

Knowledge of the various rates of drug absorption from each of the various routes is essential. (Routes of drug administration are discussed in detail in Chapter 3.) Epinephrine 1:1000, a drug commonly used in the management of acute allergic reactions, is generally given by the subcutaneous route. The reasons for choosing this site are many. First, epinephrine 1:1000 is a potent and concentrated drug. Rapid absorption of a large quantity of this drug into the circulation would certainly accentuate epinephrine's side

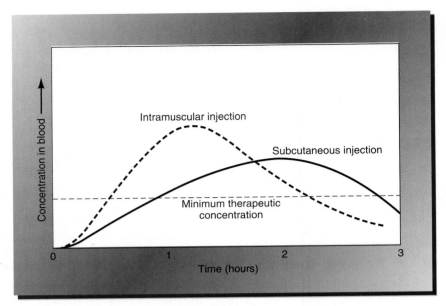

FIGURE 2–1 Comparision of drug levels following IM and SC injections.

effects such as tachycardia, trembling, and elevated blood pressure. Second, the therapeutic effects of epinephrine are fairly brief. The slower absorption obtained with subcutaneous injection allows prolonged release of the drug into the circulation, thus maintaining the desired effects for a longer period (see Table 2–1).

Systemic blood flow can also affect drug absorption. Factors that may *delay* absorption from parenteral sites include shock, acidosis, and peripheral vasoconstriction secondary to such things as hypothermia. Factors such as peripheral vasodilation, which can occur in hyperthermia and fever, may *increase* the rate of drug absorption.

Drug absorption may be minimized by injecting the medication directly into the circulatory system by the intravenous route. The desired effects are seen much sooner, and the eventual blood levels of the drug are

TABLE 2–1

Comparison of Rates of Drug Absorption
of Various Routes of Administration

Route	Rate of Absorption
Oral	Slow
Subcutaneous	Slow
Topical	Moderate
Intramuscular	Moderate
Intralingual	Rapid
Rectal	Rapid
Sublingual	Rapid
Endotracheal	Rapid
Inhalation	Rapid
Intraosseous	Immediate
Intravenous	Immediate
Intracardiac	Immediate

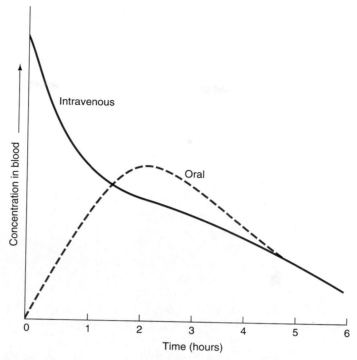

FIGURE 2–2 Comparison of drug levels following IV and oral drug administration.

much more predictable. Consequently, most critical-care medications are given intravenously (see Figure 2–2).

Bioavailability is the measure of the amount of a drug that is still active after it reaches its target tissue. This is the bottom line as far as absorption is concerned. The goal of administering a drug is to assure sufficient bioavailability of the drug at the target tissue in order to produce the desired effect, after considering all of the absorption factors.

Distribution

Once a drug has entered the blood stream, it must be distributed throughout the body. Most drugs will pass easily from the blood stream, through the interstitial spaces, into the target cells. Distribution is the process whereby a drug is transported from the site of absorption to the site of action.

Several factors can affect drug distribution:

1. Cardiovascular function
2. Regional blood flow
3. Drug storage reservoirs
4. Physiological barriers

As with drug absorption, drug distribution depends on *cardiovascular function.* Following administration and absorption, the drug is initially distributed to highly perfused body areas such as the brain, heart, kidneys, and liver. Delivery of the drug to the gastrointestinal system, skin, muscles, and fat is generally much slower. In certain conditions, such as shock and congestive heart failure, cardiac output will fall. When it does, drug distribution becomes much slower and much more unpredictable. When cardiac output is markedly diminished, some body areas are minimally perfused, and drug delivery to these areas is negligible.

Variances in *regional blood flow* can also affect drug distribution. For example, in cardiogenic shock, blood flow to the kidneys is often diminished. Medications that act specifically on the kidneys, such as diuretics, may not reach the kidneys in an adequate concentration to be effective.

In the body, a drug may be stored in various sites known as *drug reservoirs.* These reservoirs store drugs by binding the drugs to proteins present within the tissue in question. This action tends to delay the drug's onset of action and prolongs its duration of effect. There are two types of storage reservoirs: *plasma reservoirs* and *tissue reservoirs.*

During drug distribution through the vascular or lymphatic system, the drug comes in contact with proteins and remains free or binds to plasma carrier protein, storage tissue protein, or receptor protein. The portion of the drug that is bound to plasma proteins is called the *bound drug,* and the unbound portion is often referred to as the *free drug.* As soon as a drug binds to plasma carrier protein or storage tissue protein, it becomes inactive, rendering it unavailable for binding to a receptor protein and incapable of exerting therapeutic activity. However, a bound drug can free itself rapidly to maintain a balance between the amounts of free and bound drug. Only the free, or unbound, percentage of the drug remains active.

The percentage of drug that remains free and available for activity depends on the amount of plasma protein available for binding. The most common plasma protein involved in drug binding is *albumin.* However, other plasma proteins, such as hemoglobin and globulins, are utilized as well. This binding of drug to protein is usually reversible. The extent of binding depends on the physical properties of the drug itself. Some drugs are highly bound, whereas others have limited binding. The degree to which a drug is bound is referred to as the *binding capacity.* Binding of a drug to plasma proteins tends to limit its concentration in the tissues.

Drugs can also accumulate in the various tissues of the body. Common tissue reservoirs include fat, bone, and muscle tissue. Once in these compartments, the drug binds to proteins and similar substances. As with plasma protein binding, tissue binding is usually reversible. Some body compartments, such as the muscle tissue, can represent a sizable drug reservoir. Many drugs are lipid soluble (fat soluble). These drugs concentrate in the fatty tissues of the body, resulting in a prolonged drug effect.

Physiological barriers also affect drug distribution. Physiological barriers inhibit the movement of certain substances while permitting the passage of others. One of the most important physiological barriers is the *blood-brain barrier.* The blood-brain barrier refers to a network of capillary endothelial cells in the brain. These cells have no pores and are surrounded by a sheath of glial connective tissue that makes them impermeable to water-soluble drugs. The network excludes most ionized drug molecules, such as dopamine, from the brain. However, it allows nonionized, unbound drug molecules, such as barbiturates, to pass readily and enter the brain. The blood-brain barrier is an effective boundary between the central nervous system and the peripheral nervous system. Delivery of drugs and other substances to the brain is limited by the blood-brain barrier. It allows entry of certain drugs and is considered a protective mechanism of the brain.

The so-called **placental barrier** can likewise prevent drugs from reaching a fetus, although it is not the solid barrier that its name implies. The fetus is exposed to almost every drug that the mother takes. But because any drug must traverse the maternal blood supply and cross the capillary membranes into the placenta (fetal) circulation, delivering drugs to a fetus requires them to be lipid soluble, non-ionized and non-protein-bound. This may slow some drugs or reduce their placental transfer to benign levels.

Biotransformation

Like other chemicals that enter the body, drugs are metabolized, or broken down into different chemicals (metabolites). The special name given to the **metabolism** of drugs is **biotransformation.** Biotransformation has one of two effects on most drugs: 1) it can transform the drug into a more or less active metabolite, or 2) it can make the drug more water soluble (or less lipid soluble) to facilitate elimination. Some drugs, such as lidocaine, are totally metabolized before eliminating, others only partially, and still others not at all. The body will transform some molecules of most drugs and eliminate others without transformation. Protein-bound drugs are not available for biotransformation. Some so-called **prodrugs** (or parent drugs) are not active when administered, but biotransformation converts them into active metabolites.

Many biotransformation processes occur in the liver. The endoplasmic reticula of hepatocytes (liver cells) contain microsomal enzymes that perform much of the metabolizing. (Smaller quantities of the enzymes are also found in the kidney, lung, and GI tract.) Because the blood supply from the GI tract passes through the liver via the portal vein, all drugs absorbed in the GI tract pass through the liver before moving on through the systemic circulation. The first pass through the liver may partially or completely inactivate many drugs. This **first-pass effect** is why some drugs cannot be given orally but instead must be given intravenously to bypass the GI tract and prevent first-pass hepatic metabolism. It is also why drugs that can be given either orally or intravenously may require a much higher oral dose than IV dose. Because we can observe the extent of first-pass metabolism, we can predict how much to increase a dose of an oral medication to deliver an effective amount of the drug into the general circulation.

Through biotransformation, the body detoxifies and disposes of foreign substances. Because drugs are unnatural to the body, they are disposed of, as are other toxins. In most cases, the enzyme system increases the water solubility of a drug so that the renal system can excrete it. The lipid solubility of some drugs may be altered enzymatically so that the end products enter into and are excreted through the biliary system. Using the renal or the biliary pathway for disposal, the body usually transforms the drug into a readily eliminated, pharmacologically inactive product.

Biotransformation begins immediately following introduction of the drug into the body. Certain drugs are rapidly biotransformed, and others are not. For example, the emergency drug epinephrine is active as administered. However, it is very rapidly metabolized to inactive forms before elimination. Because of this rapid biotransformation, epinephrine must be readministered approximately every 3 to 5 minutes if still required.

Some drugs are inactive when administered. Once they have been absorbed, they must be converted to an active form, either in the blood or by the target tissue. The inactive precursor is referred to as a *prodrug*. Several

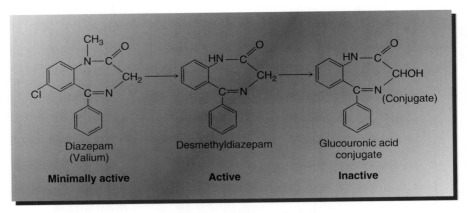

FIGURE 2–3 Metabolites of Diazepam.

drugs used in prehospital care must be converted into an active form before they can exert their desired effects. Diazepam (Valium), a drug used in the treatment of seizures, is relatively inactive as administered. Once in the body it is converted to its active metabolite, *desmethyldiazepam*, which then induces the desired effects (see Figure 2–3).

Elimination

Drugs are eventually eliminated from the body in either their original form or as metabolites. Drug excretion refers to movement of a drug or its metabolites from the tissues back into the circulation and from the circulation into the organs of excretion. Drugs may be excreted by the kidneys into the urine, by the liver into the bile, by the intestines into the feces, or by the lungs with the expired air. Additionally, drugs may be excreted through sweat, saliva, and breast milk. Excretion through sweat glands is rarely a significant mechanism for elimination. Excretion through mammary glands becomes a concern when nursing mothers take medications. Drugs may also be removed artificially by direct interventions, such as peritoneal dialysis or hemodialysis. The rate of elimination varies with the medication and the state of the body. During shock states, the kidneys are poorly perfused. Drugs that are primarily eliminated by the kidneys then remain present in the body for longer periods. The slower the rate of elimination, the longer the drug stays in the body.

Elimination can be affected by the following:

1. Drug half-life
2. Accumulation
3. Clearance
4. Onset, peak, and duration

Drug Half-Life

To predict the frequency of the drug dosage schedule, the physician must determine how long a drug will remain in the body. Usually the rate of drug loss from the body can be estimated by determining the drug's half-life. Drug half-life is the time required for the total amount of a drug in the body to diminish by one-half. If a patient receives a single dose of a drug with a half-life of 5 hours, the total amount of the drug in the patient's body would diminish by one-half after 5 hours. The drug amount would continue to decrease accordingly with each subsequent half-life. Most drugs are essentially eliminated after five half-lives because the amount remaining is too low to exert a beneficial or adverse effect. This concept is useful in many situations. For example, if a drug overdose occurs and the excretion rate of the drug is not compromised, about 97 percent of the original dose will be eliminated after five half-lives.

Accumulation

Drug half-life is also useful when assessing drug accumulation. A drug that is not readministered is eliminated almost completely after five half-lives, but a regularly administered drug reaches a constant total body amount, or steady state, after about five half-lives.

Having reached a steady state, the drug's concentration in the blood fluctuates above and below the average concentration. Thus, although the drug was once at steady state, its concentration does not remain uniform; rather, it increases, peaks, and declines, although within a constant range.

For some drugs, the time required to reach therapeutic blood concentration may be too long. For example, when using digoxin, with a half-life of about 1.6 days, the physician would not be able to wait 8 days (1.6 days times five half-lives) to achieve steady-state blood concentration levels to control a life-threatening arrhythmia, such as atrial fibrillation. Therefore, an initial large dose, called a loading dose, would be administered to reach the desired therapeutic blood concentration level. Consequently, smaller maintenance doses would be given daily to replace the amount of drug eliminated since the last dose. These dosages maintain a therapeutic blood concentration in the body at all times.

Clearance

Drug clearance refers to the removal of a drug from the body. A drug with a slow clearance rate is removed from the body slowly; one with a high clearance rate is removed rapidly. A drug with a high clearance rate may require more frequent administration and higher doses than a comparable drug with a low clearance rate. A drug with a low clearance rate can accumulate to a toxic concentration in the body unless it is administered less frequently or at lower doses.

Onset, Peak, and Duration

Besides absorption, distribution, metabolism, and excretion, three other factors play an important role in a drug's pharmacokinetics:

1. Onset of action
2. Peak concentration
3. Duration of action

The **onset of action** refers to the time when the drug is sufficiently absorbed to reach an effective blood level and sufficiently distributed to its site of action to elicit a therapeutic response.

As the body absorbs more of the drug, the drug concentration in the blood rises, more drug reaches the site of action, and the therapeutic response increases. These occurrences characterize the **peak concentration** level for the drug dose administered.

As soon as the drug begins to circulate in the blood, it also begins to be eliminated. Eventually drug elimination exceeds its absorption rate because less of the drug dose remains to be absorbed. At this point, the drug concentration in the blood and the drug's effect begin to decline. When the blood concentration falls below the minimum needed to produce an effect, drug action ceases, although some drug remains in the blood. Therefore, the **duration of action** is the length of time that drug concentration is sufficient in the blood to produce a therapeutic response.

A drug's onset, peak, and duration are determined primarily by its bioavailability (the extent to which a drug's active ingredient is absorbed and transported to its site of action) and drug concentration in the blood.

PHARMACODYNAMICS

Pharmacodynamics is the study of the mechanisms by which specific drug dosages act to produce biochemical or physiological changes in the body.

Drugs can act in four different ways. They may bind to a receptor site, change the physical properties of cells, chemically combine with other chemicals, or alter a normal metabolic pathway. Each of these actions involves a physio-chemical interaction between the drug and a functionally important molecule in the body.

Mechanisms of Action

To understand pharmacodynamics, one must differentiate between drug action and drug effect. The interaction at the cellular level between a drug and cellular components, such as the complex proteins that make up the cell membrane, enzymes, or target receptors, represents *drug action*. The response resulting from drug action represents the *drug effect*, which may affect total body function. For example, when insulin is administered, the expected drug action is glucose transport across the cell membrane. The lowering of the blood glucose level represents the expected drug effect.

Drug Receptors

Once a drug has arrived at the target tissue, it must induce the desired biochemical or physiological response. Most drugs must bind to *drug receptors* to cause their desired response. Drug receptors are generally proteins present on the surface of the cell membrane. When a drug combines with the drug receptor, a physiological response occurs. Drug receptors are often compared with "locks," whereas drugs are the "keys" that fit these locks. Once the drug is bound to the receptor (that is, the "key" is inserted into the "lock"), biochemical actions begin that ultimately lead to the desired response.

A drug attracted to a receptor displays an *affinity* for that receptor. When a drug displays an affinity for a receptor and then enhances or stimulates the functional properties of the receptor, the drug acts as an *agonist.* A drug that is not an agonist can compete with an agonist for a receptor by occupying the receptor, thereby preventing the action of the agonist. Such a drug, called an *antagonist,* does not initiate an effect. Instead, the antagonist prevents a response from occurring.

There are two types of antagonists. The first, a competitive antagonist, competes with the agonist for receptor sites. For example, naloxone is a competitive antagonist with an affinity for opioid receptors. Because naloxone competes with opioids for these receptors, parenteral administration of naloxone reverses opioid-induced respiratory depression in 1 to 2 minutes, thereby reversing the effects of opioid overdose.

The second type of antagonist, the noncompetitive antagonist, inhibits agonist response regardless of agonist concentration. For example, the noncompetitive antagonist phenoxybenzamine protects the patient from the intermittent release of large amounts of catecholamines from adrenal tumors.

Classification of Receptors

Drug receptors usually are classified by the effects produced. However, a nonselective drug may interact with more than one receptor type, thereby causing multiple effects. Also, some receptors are classified further by their specific effects. For example, the beta-receptors usually produce increased heart rate and bronchial relaxation, besides other systemic effects.

Beta-receptors, however, can be subdivided into $beta_1$-receptors (which act primarily on cardiac tissue) and $beta_2$-receptors (which act primarily on smooth muscles and gland cells). $Beta_1$-receptors predominate in the heart; $beta_2$-receptors predominate in the lungs. Administering a nonselective beta antagonist, or beta-blocker, such as propranolol, to a patient with tachycardia decreases the heart rate. Unfortunately, the nonselectivity of propranolol also will block $beta_2$-receptors, which could precipitate an asthmatic attack in a susceptible patient. Administering a selective $beta_1$ antagonist, such as metoprolol or atenolol, reduces the risk of receptor nonselectivity and specifically decreases heart rate but should not affect pulmonary function.

Epinephrine is a nonselective beta agonist used to treat acute asthmatic disorders. Unfortunately, when administered subcutaneously, epinephrine interacts with $beta_1$- and $beta_2$-receptors and further increases the asthmatic patient's accelerated heart rate. Therefore, terbutaline administered parenterally is a preferred drug; it is more selective for $beta_2$-receptors.

Drug Potency and Efficacy

Drug potency refers to the relative amount of a drug required to produce the desired response. Comparing the drug potency of one drug with that of another drug can reveal which is the more potent drug. The power of a drug to produce a therapeutic effect is called the drug's *efficacy*. Drugs that are agonists have both affinity and efficacy. Drugs that are antagonists have affinity but not efficacy, because they do not produce a physiological response. Classic illustrations of this principle are the drugs epinephrine and propranolol (Inderal). Epinephrine, once administered, is transported to its various target tissues—namely, the heart, the lungs, and the peripheral blood vessels. Once at these target tissues, it finds and binds to its receptors, which are called *beta-receptors*. If the drug is able to bind to these beta-receptors, then the desired physiological response will be seen. Several drugs themselves are inactive but can bind to beta-receptors in much the same manner as epinephrine. These drugs are referred to as *beta-blockers*, and the prototype drug of this group is propranolol. If a beta-blocker has already bound to the receptor, then epinephrine cannot bind,

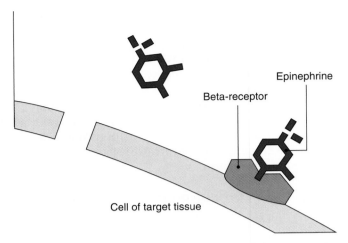

FIGURE 2–4 Epinephrine interacting with beta receptor.

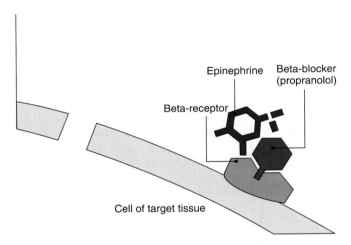

FIGURE 2–5 β receptor blocked by propranolol.

and the desired effect is effectively blocked (see Figures 2–4 and 2–5). A more detailed discussion of beta-receptors and beta-blockers can be found in Chapter 6.

Therapeutic Index

Once again, for a medication to be effective it must reach a certain concentration at the target tissue. The minimal concentration of a drug necessary to cause the desired response is referred to as the *therapeutic threshold*, or *minimum effective concentration*. A concentration below this therapeutic threshold will not induce a clinical response. There is also a point at which the drug concentration can get high enough to be toxic or even fatal. The general goal of drug therapy is to give the minimum concentration of a drug necessary to obtain the desired response (see Figure 2–6).

The difference between the minimum effective concentration and the toxic level varies significantly from drug to drug. The difference between these

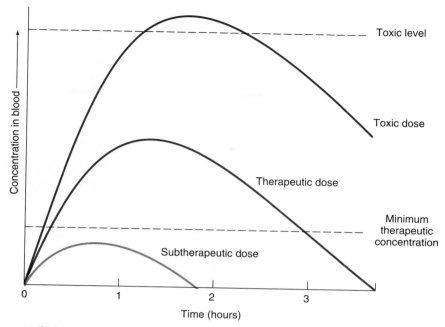

FIGURE 2–6 Comparison of blood levels following subtherapeutic, therapeutic and toxic doses of the same drug.

two concentrations is referred to as the *therapeutic index* and is usually obtained in the laboratory. Certain drugs, such as digitalis, have very little difference between the effective dose and the toxic dose. Such drugs are said to have a low therapeutic index. Drugs such as naloxone (Narcan), the narcotic antagonist, have a significant margin between the effective dose and the toxic dose and are said to have a high therapeutic index. Prehospital care providers should be familiar with the therapeutic indexes of the medications they use.

Special Considerations in Drug Therapy

Age, pregnancy, and lactation are important considerations in drug therapy. Both children and the elderly are particularly susceptible to the adverse effects of drugs. Consequently, drug dosages often must be modified for persons in these age groups. Likewise, special precautions must be taken when administering medications to a pregnant patient, because many medications will also affect the fetus. Certain drugs are excreted into the breast milk, which becomes a particular concern in mothers who are breast-feeding their infants. The following sections discuss these special considerations in drug therapy.

Pediatric Patients

Children are typically smaller than adults, and drug dosages must be reduced accordingly. Pediatric drug dosages are typically based on the child's body weight or body surface area (BSA). Thus, it is essential that prehospital personnel determine or approximate a child's weight before administering a medication. Often, the parents can provide an approximate weight from a recent doctor's visit. In emergencies the child's body weight can be estimated by determining the child's age and finding the average body weight for that age on a reference table.

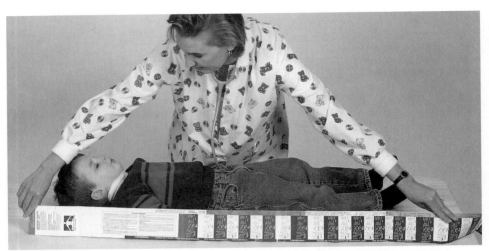

FIGURE 2–7 A Broselow Tape is useful for calculating drug dosages for pediatric patients.

Neonates (infants from birth to 4 weeks) are a special concern. Common sites of drug metabolism and elimination, such as the liver and kidneys, are not well developed in neonates. Thus both drug metabolism and excretion may be impaired. Drug dosages for neonates must often be modified to reflect these factors.

The American Heart Association (AHA) and the American Academy of Pediatrics (AAP) publish recommended drug dosages for most emergency medications. Often, the doses of common emergency drugs are listed on easy-to-use reference cards. To use these, prehospital care providers simply look up the child's age or weight. Below the age or weight are the recommended dosages for common emergency drugs.

Another popular device for determining pediatric drug dosages is the Broselow Tape (see Figure 2-7). The Broselow Tape is simply unfolded and placed alongside the supine child to measure the child from the top of the head to the bottom of the feet. The tape is divided into various color-coded drug dosage charts based on the child's length (which is directly related to the child's weight and body surface area). Prehospital care providers simply use the dosage chart that corresponds to the child's length. In addition to drug dosages, the Broselow Tape contains recommended endotracheal tube sizes, defibrillator settings, and other important emergency information.

Geriatric Patients

The elderly age group is the fastest growing segment of the U.S. population, and older adults are frequent users of the emergency medical services (EMS) system. The aging process begins at the cellular level and affects virtually every body system. Common physiological effects of aging include the following:

1. Decreased cardiac output
2. Decreased renal function
3. Decreased brain mass

Chapter 2 / Pharmacokinetics and Pharmacodynamics

4. Decreased total body water
5. Decreased body fat
6. Decreased serum albumin
7. Decreased respiratory capacity

These changes can lead to altered pharmacodynamics and pharmacokinetics for many medications. With aging, the rate of metabolism and the excretion of medications can be significantly decreased. In addition, there is often decreased protein binding because the level of serum albumin decreases. These factors combine to increase the relative potency of a drug. Consequently, the dosages of many medications must be reduced when administered to an elderly patient.

The elderly are more apt to suffer from more than one disease process at a time. In addition, they may be on chronic medications, which may affect the emergency medications paramedics need to administer in the prehospital setting. Multiple medical problems make drug dosing much more difficult. For example, treating a patient with congestive heart failure may be more difficult if the patient also has renal failure. In this case, the dosage of furosemide (Lasix) may need to be increased, and the dosage of morphine may need to be decreased. All factors must be considered before administering medications to the elderly.

Pregnancy and Lactation

Pregnancy presents two pharmacological problems. First, pregnancy causes a number of anatomical and physiological changes in the mother, including

1. Increased cardiac output
2. Increased heart rate
3. Increased blood volume (by up to 45 percent)
4. Decreased protein binding
5. Decreased hepatic metabolism
6. Decreased blood pressure

These anatomical and physiological changes must be considered prior to administering medications or fluids to a pregnant patient.

The second consideration associated with pregnancy is that any medication administered to the mother has the potential to cross the placenta and affect the fetus. Some drugs cross the placenta rapidly, but others do not. Thus, drugs should only be administered in pregnancy when the potential benefits outweigh the risks. The U.S. Food and Drug Administration (FDA) categorizes most drugs based on their safety in pregnancy (see Table 2–2).

As with pregnancy, drug therapy can affect a breast-feeding infant. Many medications are excreted readily into the breast milk. If the mother continues to breast-feed while receiving these medications, the medications can be excreted into the breast milk and be ingested by the baby. If a breast-feeding mother is to receive medications, she should be instructed to stop breast-feeding and pump her breasts. She should dispose of the expressed milk until it is certain that the drug has been cleared from her system. During the time she is pumping her breasts, she should switch the infant to a commercial formula.

TABLE 2–2

FDA Pregnancy Categories

Category	Description
A	Adequate studies in pregnant women have not demonstrated a risk to the fetus in the first trimester or later trimesters.
B	Animal studies have not demonstrated a risk to the fetus, but there are no adequate studies in pregnant women.
	OR
	Adequate studies in pregnant women have not demonstrated a risk to the fetus in the first trimester and there is no risk in the last trimester, but animal studies have demonstrated adverse effects.
C	Animal studies have demonstrated adverse effects, but there are no adequate studies in pregnant women; however, benefits may be acceptable despite the potential risk.
	OR
	No adequate animal studies or adequate studies of pregnant women have been done.
D	Fetal risk has been demonstrated. In certain circumstances, benefits could outweigh the risks.
X	Fetal risk has been demonstrated. This risk outweighs any possible benefit to the mother. Avoid using in pregnant or potentially pregnant patients.

SUMMARY

A basic understanding of pharmacokinetics and pharmacodynamics is essential for prehospital personnel to anticipate the desired therapeutic effects as well as any possible side effects of the medications they administer. Such factors as rate of absorption, elimination, minimum therapeutic concentration, and toxic levels should be considered in all drugs.

KEY WORDS

absorption. The process whereby a drug is moved from the site of application into the body and into the extracellular fluid compartment.

affinity. The tendency of a drug to combine with a specific drug receptor.

agonist. A drug or other substance that binds with a specific drug receptor and causes a physiological response.

albumin. Protein found in almost all animal tissue. It constitutes one of the major proteins in human blood.

antagonist. A drug or other substance that blocks a physiological response or that blocks the action of another drug or substance.

binding capacity. The degree to which a drug is bound to tissue or plasma proteins.

biotransformation. Biotransformation, also called metabolism, is the process of changing a drug into a different form, either active or inactive, by the body.

blood-brain barrier. Protective mechanism that selectively allows the entry of specific compounds into the brain. It is an effective boundary between the central nervous system and the peripheral nervous system.

cumulative effect. A phenomenon that occurs when a drug is administered in several doses, causing an increased effect. It is usually due to a buildup of a drug in the blood.

distribution.   The process whereby a drug is transported from the site of absorption to the site of action.

efficacy.   The power of a drug to produce a therapeutic effect.

elimination.   The process whereby a drug is removed from the body by excretion into the urine, feces, bile, saliva, sweat, breast milk, or expired air.

excretion.   The elimination of waste products from the body. *Excretion* is often used interchangeably with the term *elimination*.

globulin.   One of a broad category of simple proteins found in the body.

half-life.   The time required for a level of a drug in the blood to be reduced by 50 percent of its beginning level.

hemoglobin.   An iron-containing compound found within the blood cell that is responsible for the transport and delivery of oxygen to the body cells.

loading dose.   The initial dose of a drug given in a sufficient amount to achieve a therapeutic plasma level.

maintenance dose.   The dose of a drug necessary to maintain a constant therapeutic plasma level.

metabolism.   The sum total of all physical and chemical changes that occur within the body. In pharmacology it is often used interchangeably with the term *biotransformation*.

minimum effective concentration.   The minimum amount of drug needed in the bloodstream to cause the desired therapeutic effect.

onset of action.   The time interval between the administration of a drug and the first sign of its onset; onset of action is influenced by the physical and chemical properties of a drug as well as by its route of administration.

pH.   A scientific method of expressing the acidity or alkalinity of a solution, which is the logarithm of the hydrogen ion concentration divided by 1. The higher the pH, the more alkaline the solution; the lower the pH, the more acidic the solution.

pharmacodynamics.   The study of a drug's action on the body.

pharmacokinetics.   The study of how drugs enter the body, reach their site of action, and eventually are eliminated.

plasma (serum) level.   The amount of the drug present in the plasma. The peak plasma level refers to the highest concentration produced by a specific dose.

solubility.   The tendency of a drug to dissolve.

therapeutic index.   An index of the drug's safety profile, which is determined by calculating the difference between the drug's therapeutic threshold and toxic level. It is typically determined in the laboratory.

therapeutic range.   The difference between the minimal therapeutic and toxic concentrations of a drug. Drugs with a low therapeutic range present a higher risk of toxicity than do drugs with a high therapeutic range. The therapeutic range is also referred to as the margin of safety.

therapeutic threshold.   The minimum amount of drug needed in the bloodstream to cause a desired therapeutic effect.

toxicity.   The degree to which a substance is poisonous. At high doses drugs can produce toxic effects that are not seen at low doses.

toxic level.   The plasma level at which severe adverse reactions are expected or likely.

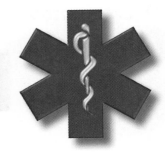

chapter 3

ADMINISTRATION OF DRUGS

OBJECTIVES

After completing this chapter, the reader should be able to

1. State the necessary components of a verbal or standing order.
2. Explain the six rights of drug administration.
3. Explain the advantages and disadvantages of alimentary versus parenteral administration.
4. List and explain three alimentary tract routes.
5. List and explain nine parenteral routes.
6. Briefly explain the following routes of drug administration:
   a. Subcutaneous route
   b. Intramuscular route
   c. Intravenous bolus
   d. Intravenous piggyback
   e. Via the endotracheal tube
   f. Via an intraosseous infusion
7. Describe the different methods of administering medications through inhalation therapy.
8. Describe the special considerations in administering medications to a pediatric patient.
9. Briefly explain the following pediatric routes of drug administration:
   a. Subcutaneous route
   b. Intramuscular route
   c. Rectal

INTRODUCTION

In the field of emergency medicine, medications must be administered promptly, in the correct dose, and by the correct route. Many drugs with a therapeutic value when given by the appropriate route can be fatal when given by an inappropriate route. Norepinephrine, for example, is a potent drug used to treat severe hypotension. It is designed to be given by slow, intravenous infusion. If given in an intravenous bolus, however, it may be fatal. This admonition applies to most medications used in emergency medicine.

The emergency scene is often hectic. Paramedics must often prepare and administer medications in the worst of environments. Consequently, it is essential that all prehospital personnel develop safe habits regarding drug preparation and drug administration. These safe habits serve to protect both the patient and the paramedic.

This chapter presents the procedures for medication preparation and administration of medications used in emergency medical practice.

PATIENT CARE USING MEDICATIONS

Paramedics are responsible for the standard of care for patients in their charge. They are, therefore, personally responsible—legally, morally, and ethically—for the safe and effective administration of medications. The following guidelines will help you to meet that responsibility:

- Know the precautions and contraindications for all medications you administer.
- Practice proper technique.
- Know how to observe and document drug effects.
- Maintain a current knowledge in pharmacology.
- Establish and maintain professional relationships with other health care providers.
- Understand the pharmacokinetics and pharmacodynamics.
- Have current medication references available.
- Take careful drug histories including:
  – Name, strength, and daily dose of prescribed drugs
  – Over-the-counter drugs
  – Vitamins
  – Herbal medications
  – Folk-medicine or folk-remedies
  – Allergies
- Evaluate the compliance, dosage, and adverse reactions.
- Consult with medical direction when appropriate.

THE MEDICATION ORDER

Prehospital personnel are responsible for preparing and administering many emergency drugs and fluids. The selection and administration of a particular medication depends on an accurate and complete patient assessment. The results of this assessment must be relayed to medical control or applied to prehospital treatment protocols or standing orders. An inaccurate or incomplete patient assessment may lead to administration of the wrong drug.

The first step in medication administration is the medication order. The order may be in the form of a direct verbal order or through written standing treatment orders. The order generally specifies the following:

1. Medication desired
2. Dose desired
3. Administration route
4. Administration rate

If possible, verbal medication orders should be written down as soon as they are received. After receiving the order, the paramedic should repeat the entire order back to the medical control physician. Doing so ensures that there is no misunderstanding related to the medication order. A typical medication order interchange is as follows:

Medical Control: Start an IV of lactated Ringer's solution at 125 mL per hour and administer 5 mg of diazepam intravenously over 1 minute.

Medic 1: Confirming an IV of lactated Ringer's solution at 125 mL per hour and 5 mg of diazepam intravenously over 1 minute.

Medical Control: Affirmative Medic 1.

In systems that utilize standing orders, paramedics first review the appropriate standing order. They then confirm the ordered medication, dosage, route, and rate of medication administration and, if possible, have another crew member review and double-check the standing order. Finally, paramedics prepare and administer the medication as detailed in the standing order.

It is essential to use good judgment regarding medication administration. Paramedics should always carefully evaluate the orders they receive. Occasionally, orders will be received that differ from accepted local prehospital protocols. In these cases, paramedics must contact the medical control physician and advise him or her of the discrepancy. If, after discussion of the discrepancy, the medical control physician does not change the order, paramedics should follow the order. The exceptions to this rule, of course, are orders that paramedics believe will harm the patient. If paramedics believe a particular medication or dose will harm the patient, they should notify the medical control physician that they are withholding the drug and give the reason for doing so. Paramedics must document well the circumstances surrounding the controversy and submit documentation to the system medical director for resolution. Although prehospital care providers are responsible to the medical control physician, they have a higher duty to protect the health and well-being of their patients.

SIX RIGHTS OF MEDICATION ADMINISTRATION

After paramedics have received the medication or fluid order, they should then administer the drug in question. In performing drug administration, prehospital care providers adhere to the *six rights of medication administration:*

1. Right patient
2. Right medication

3. Right dose
4. Right route
5. Right time
6. Right documentation

Right Patient

Ensuring that the right patient receives the right drug is usually not a problem in prehospital care because typically only one patient is being treated. However, in some circumstances more than one patient may be undergoing treatment, especially in multiple casualty incidents in which many patients are involved. In cases with multiple patients, it is prudent to use some label to distinguish patients. Some systems prefer to use the patient's last name. However, it is not uncommon for several members of one family to be involved in an emergency. Each family member usually has the same last name, and some have the same first name (e.g., William and William Jr.). In these cases, it is best to assign numbers (e.g., Patient 1 and Patient 2) or letters of the alphabet (e.g., Patient A and Patient B) to each patient to avoid confusion.

Confusion regarding multiple patients is more of a problem for medical control than for individual paramedics. A multiple casualty incident may utilize several ambulances, often with similar call signs. Personnel in each ambulance will contact medical control regarding the patient or patients they are transporting. Care should be taken to distinguish the patients and units to avoid confusion and possible medication error. Errors can be minimized by using effective scene management techniques such as the incident command system. In this system, each patient is designated with a number or letter at the time of triage. Radio communications, both initial and subsequent, should refer to the patient by this designation to help avoid confusion both in the field and at medical control.

Right Medication

A common error in prehospital drug administration is selection of the wrong medication. Most emergency medications are supplied in ampules, vials, or prefilled syringes. Many look very similar. To ensure that the right drug is selected, paramedics should carefully read the label. If the drug is supplied in a box, they should check the label on the box and compare it with the label on the vial or ampule itself after removing it from the box. Paramedics can never assume that a medication is correct simply because it is in the correct place in the drug box. They must always read and check the label three times.

Drug preparations and concentrations can vary. In addition to checking the drug name, paramedics should always check to ensure that the drug concentration is the one desired. This check is especially important for drugs that are carried in differing concentrations (e.g., epinephrine 1:1000 and epinephrine 1:10 000 or lidocaine 100 mg for intravenous bolus and lidocaine 1 g for intravenous infusion).

When following a physician's verbal order, repeat the order back to confirm that you both intend the same thing for the patient. Inspect the label on the drug at least three times before giving the medication to the patient: first as you remove the medication from the drug box or cabinet, second, as you draw the medication into the syringe and third, immediately before you administer the medication. The expiration date of a drug should always be checked prior to administration. The medication should be held up to the light and inspected for discoloration or particles in the solution. Expired and discoloured medications should be discarded. Routine (preferably daily) drug box inspections should detect any expired medications. However, paramedics should always double check the medication prior to administration.

Failure to confirm the medication name is one of the most common medication administration errors. If you have any question about a drug, do not administer it without confirmation. Showing the medication container to your partner and asking for confirmation is an easy way to further ensure that you are giving the right drug.

Right Dose

Administration of the correct drug dose is crucial. Errors in dosage occur in either calculating the correct dose or preparing the correct dose. Most drug orders are fairly straightforward, and many medications are supplied in unit-dose forms. In these cases, drug dosage calculation and drug preparation are easy. However, many medications, especially those administered by intravenous infusion, are much more difficult to dose. For these medications, paramedics should refer to standardized dosage charts to assist with preparation and administration of the desired dose.

Right Route

Most medications used in prehospital care are designed to be given by the intravenous route. However, certain medications can be given by other routes depending on the physician's orders. It is the paramedic's responsibility to know the various routes by which a particular drug can be administered. For example, the drugs hydroxyzine (Vistaril) and promethazine (Phenergan) are frequently used in the treatment of nausea. Promethazine can be administered both intravenously and intramuscularly. Hydroxyzine, in comparison, can be administered only by the intramuscular route.

Right Time

Most medication orders for prehospital care call for immediate ("stat") administration of the drug. These orders are generally one time orders. However, certain drugs may be administered repeatedly, especially in cardiac arrest situations, in which drugs are administered at specific time intervals.

An important consideration is the rate at which a drug should be administered. The rate is usually expressed as the period of time over which the drug in question should be administered. Many drugs can be administered rapidly as an intravenous bolus. Others must be administered at a specific rate. Diazepam, for example, should never be administered faster than 1 mL/min (5 mg/min). The rate of drug administration is particularly crucial for intravenous infusion medications (e.g., lidocaine, dopamine, and norepinephrine).

Right Documentation

The drugs you administer in the field do not stop affecting your patient when they enter the hospital. As a result, you must completely document all of your care, especially any drugs you have administered, so that long after you have gone on to your next call, other providers will know what drugs your patient has had.

GENERAL ADMINISTRATION ROUTES

The two primary channels for getting medications into the body are enteral (through the alimentary canal, or gastrointestinal (GI) tract,) and by parenteral routes. The GI tract provides a fairly safe but relatively slow-acting site for drug absorption. Oral, sublingual, and rectal preparations are given via the GI tract. Administration by the parenteral route can involve all routes other than the GI tract. This chapter deals primarily with medications given by injection. Paramedics use the parenteral route to provide a rapid onset of action and to ensure high blood levels of the drug. The parenteral route also is used when the GI route would inactivate the drug, in unconscious patients, and in unstable or seriously ill patients who require precise administration and monitoring. In acute care medicine, administration is almost always parenteral because the onset of action is much quicker and usually more predictable.

Table 3–1 compares the relative advantages and disadvantages of alimentary versus parenteral administration.

Enteral Tract Routes

The common enteral routes of administration used in general medical practice are as follows:

Oral (PO).   The best, and most convenient, way of administering drugs is by mouth. Most medical drugs are available in oral preparations. The effects of oral administration are often not seen until 30 to 45 minutes after administration.

TABLE 3–1

Comparison of Enteral vs Parenteral Routes

Enteral Route	
Advantages	*Disadvantages*
Simple Safe Generally less expensive Low potential for infection	Slow rate of onset Cannot be given to unconscious or nauseated patients Absorbed dosage may vary significantly because of actions of digestive enzymes and the condition of the intestinal tract
Parenteral Route	
Rapid onset Can be given to unconscious and nauseated patients Absorbed dosage and action are more predictable	Administration often difficult and painful Usually more expensive Side effects usually more severe Potential for infection

---

Orogastric/nasogstric tube (OG/NG). This route is generally used for oral medications when the patient already has the tube in place for other reasons.

Sublingual (SL). Some drugs can be administered sublingually (i.e., under the tongue). When administered in this fashion, the drug is placed under the tongue, where it quickly dissolves. The drug is then absorbed into the vast capillary network present in the mucous membranes. Nitroglycerin, a drug frequently used in the management of angina pectoris, is administered by this route.

Buccal. Absorption through this route between the cheek and gum is similar to sublingual absorption.

Rectal (PR). Rectal administration may have both local and systemic effects. It may be necessary to administer some medications rectally, especially if the patient is nauseated. The rectal route is frequently used in infants and children, who may not be able to swallow oral medications. Absorption of rectally administered drugs is generally somewhat slower than by the oral route.

Parenteral Routes

Any method of administration that does not involve passage through the digestive tract is termed parenteral. Parenteral routes include the following:

Topical. Certain drugs can be placed on the skin, where they are slowly absorbed into the capillary network underneath the skin. The rate of onset varies, but the duration of action is prolonged. This route is often used to administer nitroglycerin in the emergency setting.

Intradermal. Drugs can be injected into the dermal layer of the skin. The amount of medication that can be given via this route is limited, and systemic absorption (into the bloodstream) is very slow. Generally, this route is reserved for diagnostic skin tests, such as allergy testing.

Subcutaneous. With subcutaneous administration, medications are injected into fatty, subcutaneous tissue under the skin and overlying the muscle. The rate of absorption is slower than that seen with intramuscular and intravenous administration. Epinephrine 1:1000, which is used in the treatment of acute asthma and other respiratory emergencies, is almost always administered subcutaneously. A maximum of 2 mL of a drug can be given subcutaneously.

Intramuscular. The most commonly used route of parenteral medication administration is the intramuscular route. The drug is injected into muscle tissue, from which it is absorbed into the bloodstream. This method of administration has a predictable rate of absorption but is considerably slower than intravenous administration.

Intravenous. Most medications used in emergency medicine are designed to be administered intravenously. These can be in the form of an intravenous (IV) bolus or as a slow IV infusion, sometimes referred to as a piggyback infusion. The rate of absorption is rapid and predictable. Of all the routes frequently employed, however, IV administration of drugs has the most potential for causing adverse reactions.

Endotracheal. When an IV line cannot be started, it is sometimes possible to administer emergency medications down an endotracheal tube, which permits absorption into the capillaries of the lungs. It has been shown that this route has a rate of absorption as fast as the IV route. Drugs that can be administered endotracheally include epinephrine, lidocaine, naloxone, and atropine.

Sublingual injection.   In the rare instance in which neither an IV line can be started nor an endotracheal tube inserted, certain drugs can be injected into the vast capillary network immediately under the tongue. Lidocaine is the agent most frequently given by this route.

Intracardiac.   Injection of a medication directly into the ventricle of the heart is referred to as intracardiac administration. Because of the many complications associated with this procedure, it is reserved exclusively for life-threatening situations, such as cardiac arrest, when an IV line cannot be established nor an endotracheal tube placed. This is not a paramedic skill.

Intraosseous.   When an IV line cannot be started in children under 6 years of age, many emergency medications can be administered intraosseously. A needle can be placed in the anterior aspect of the proximal tibia, through which medications and fluids can be administered. The onset of action is similar to that for IV administration.

Inhalational.   Medications can be administered directly into the respiratory tree in cases of respiratory distress resulting from reversible airway disease including asthma and certain types of chronic obstructive pulmonary disease. These medications are usually nebulized into a water vapor and breathed with normal respiration.

Umbilical.   Both the umbilical vein and umbilical artery can provide an alternative to IV administration in newborns.

Vaginal.   Medications can be placed into the vagina, where they are absorbed into surrounding tissues. Most vaginal medications are supplied in creams or vaginal suppositories. The onset of action is slow, and the effects are generally limited to the lower female genital tract.

DRUG ADMINISTRATION AND PREPARATION

Preparation

Medications can be injected into several body spaces, and the type of injection depends on the body space that is used. The techniques and equipment used for each injection type vary. All injections require a liquid form of the prescribed drug and some type of syringe and needle, and the paramedic must know and use the correct type of needle and syringe for the different kinds of injections. For example, an intramuscular injection requires a long IM needle. A short subcutaneous needle would not reach the muscle, and pain or tissue damage could result.

Dead Space

Manufacturers calibrate syringes so that dead space compensation is not necessary.

Reconstitution and Withdrawal from a Vial

Liquid and powdered medications for parenteral administration are packaged in sterile vials. The paramedic can withdraw liquid medication into the syringe, but powdered forms must be reconstituted first. The paramedic must use sterile technique during all medication preparation and injection procedures to decrease the risk of infection.

Small air bubbles may adhere to the interior surface of the syringe when medication is withdrawn from a vial. This small amount of air would not harm the patient if injected, but it could change the dose of medication actually administered. Therefore, the paramedic should remove the air bubbles. To do so, he or she holds the syringe with the needle pointed upward, taps the side of the syringe until the bubbles accumulate at the hub, then slowly pushes the plunger until the air is expelled. If the amount of medication is not accurate after this procedure, the paramedic withdraws more of the drug to complete the prescribed dose.

Withdrawal from an Ampule

Liquid medications for parenteral administration also can be packaged in sterile ampules. Powdered ones rarely are packaged in ampules. Before administering medication from an ampule, the paramedic must withdraw it carefully.

Mixing Drugs

On occasion, the paramedic must mix drugs in one syringe. In prehospital care, mixing may be necessary to administer a narcotic, such as morphine, and an antiemetic, such as gravol.

Skin Preparation

After filling the syringe, the paramedic must prepare the patient's skin for injection. If the skin is soiled, it should be washed and dried thoroughly if possible. Then an alcohol swab is used to clean the skin. An iodine (Betadine) swab may be used as well. Alcohol swabs should only be used with patients allergic to iodine.

Care should be taken not to touch the patient's skin with anything except the sterile swab. When using a disinfectant, the paramedic should always begin at the point where the needle will be inserted and wipe in a spiral pattern from the center outward. Cleaning from the puncture site outward carries bacteria away from the site.

Before injecting the medication, the disinfected area should be allowed to dry for about 1 minute, if possible. Blowing on or fanning the area to hasten the drying process is discouraged because these activities increase the risk of contamination. Injecting while the skin is still moist can introduce alcohol or iodine into the tissues and causes irritation. Allowing the skin to dry before injection in many cases reduces injection pain.

MEDICAL DIRECTION

Paramedics do not practice autonomously. You will operate under the license of a medical director who is responsible for all of your actions; This responsibility extends to the administration of medication.

The medical director determines which medications you will use and the routes by which you will deliver them. Some states have a "state drug list" whereby the medications a service may carry is dictated by law or legislation or a regulatory agency. While some medications can be administered via off-line medical direction (written standing orders), you will need specific authorization for others after consulting on-line or direct medical direction. You must strictly abide by all of your medical director's guidelines.

Knowing all drug administration protocols is essential, especially which drugs to administer under standing orders and which to deliver only after authorization from medical direction. You can ill afford to waste valuable time looking up procedures and directives for the critical patient who requires immediate drug therapy. Furthermore, because inappropriate drug delivery can have serious consequences, you may face severe legal ramifications even if your patient suffers no harm.

Body Substance Isolation

Establishing routes for drug delivery presents the constant potential for exposure to blood and other body fluids. Always take appropriate body substance isolation (BSI) measures to decrease your risk of exposure. The type of BSI you use will vary according to the delivery route and your patient's condition. At a minimum, you should wear gloves. Optimally you will also wear goggles and a mask. Remarkably, the simplest form of BSI is often the most neglected; hand washing. Washing your hands before and after patient contact is one of the most effective ways to decrease your exposure to infectious material.

MEDICAL ASEPSIS

Medical asepsis describes a medical environment free of pathogens. Many paramedical procedures, especially those related to drug administration, place the patient at increased risk for inflection. The external environment is full of microorganisms, many of them pathogenic. Techniques such as intravenous access or endotracheal intubation can allow pathogens to enter the patient's body, where they may cause local of systemic complications.

Sterilization

The most aseptic environment is a sterile one. A sterile environment is free of all forms of life. Generally, environments are sterilized with extensive heat or chemicals. A sterile environment is difficult to attain in the prehospital setting. Consequently, you must practice medically clean techniques to minimize your patient's risk of infection. Medically clean techniques involve the careful handling of sterile equipment to prevent contamination. For example, much of the equipment used for drug administration is packaged sterilely. Once you open the package, you must use a medically clean technique to keep the equipment clean and uncontaminated until you use it. If you drop a piece of equipment on a dirty surface, you should discard it and obtain a new piece. Other medically clean techniques, including hand washing, glove changing and discarding equipment in opened packages help to prevent equipment and patient contamination. Remember, too, that many patients have lowered immunity levels or carry infectious diseases. Thus, keeping the ambulance and equipment clean is another essential medically clean procedure.

Disinfectants and Antiseptics

When administering medications you must use disinfectants and antiseptics to assure local cleanliness. Do not confuse disinfectants and antiseptics; the distinction is important. **Disinfectants** are toxic to living tissue. You will therefore use them only on non-living surfaces or objects such as the inside of an ambulance or laryngoscope blades after use. Never use disinfectants on living tissue.

Antiseptics are not toxic to living tissue. They destroy or inhibit pathogenic microorganisms already living on surfaces and are generally used to cleanse the local area before needle puncture. Common antiseptics include alcohol and iodine preparations used either alone or together. Frequently, antiseptics are diluted disinfectants.

DISPOSAL OF CONTAMINATED EQUIPMENT AND SHARPS

Blood and body fluid can harbor infectious material that endangers the health care provider, family, bystanders or the patient himself. Many times the patient is infected with pathogenic organisms long before signs and symptoms appear. Therefore, you must treat all blood and body fluids as potentially infectious.

Drug administration commonly involves needles in direct contact with the patient's blood and body fluid. Once used, a needle represents a significant risk. Inadvertent needle sticks, the most common accident in health care as a whole, can transmit diseases between the patient and paramedic. Properly handling needles and other sharps before and after patient use can prevent many of these accidental needle sticks. To minimize or eliminate the risk of an accidental needle stick, take these precautions.

- *Minimize the tasks you perform in a moving ambulance.* Use needles as sparingly as possible in the back of a moving ambulance. When appropriate, perform all interventions involving needles on scene. If en route, it may be occasionally necessary to have the driver pull the ambulance over to the side of the road and stop briefly.

- *Immediately dispose of used sharps in a sharps container.* You should dispose all sharps, including needles and prefilled syringes directly into the sharps container without removing or bending a needle. You should also dispose of items such as use ampoules in the sharps container. Avoid dropping sharps onto the floor for later disposal. In the heat of the moment, you may forget the sharp or misplace it.

- *Recap needles only as a last resort.* If you absolutely must recap a needle, never use two hands to do so. Place the sharp on a stationary surface and replace the cap with one hand. While the one-hand method is still hazardous, it at least reduces the chance for accidental needle stick.

MEDICATION ROUTES USED IN EMERGENCY MEDICINE

Emergency medications are often administered parenterally by either the subcutaneous, intramuscular, intravenous, endotracheal, intraosseous, or inhalational route. Paramedics must always use universal precautions in patient care, particularly with drug administration. This section outlines the procedure for administration by each of these routes. Prior to the administration of any medication, the following steps should be completed:

Administration of Medication

1. Identify any patient allergies prior to base hospital contact.
2. Take and record vital signs.
3. Determine if the order is consistent with training and scope of practice.
4. Confirm order by repeating:
   a. Medication
   b. Dosage, volume, and concentration
   c. Route of administration
5. Write down the order and time of order.
6. Select proper medication and check the name of the medication:
   a. When the medication is first selected
   b. When drawing up the medication
   c. Prior to administering to patient
   d. When replacing medication in storage or disposing of ampule
7. Check for cloudiness, particles, discoloration, and expiration date.
8. Confirm order and medication with partner.
9. Prior to administration of any medication, check the six rights:
   a. Right patient
   b. Right medication
   c. Right dose or amount
   d. Right route
   e. Right time
   f. Right documentation
10. Record drug, dose and volume, route, and time and check and record patient vital signs.

All drug administration skill checklists are in appendix G.

Transdermal Administration

Medications given by the transdermal route promote slow, steady absorption. Nitroglycerin, hormones and analgesics are commonly administered transdermally. Transdermal delivery can also produce localized effects, as with anti-inflammatories and other bacteriostatic and softening agents. Applying medication locally avoids passing larger quantities of the medication throughout the entire body, where it is not needed. Transdermal medications include lotions, ointments, creams, foams, wet dressings, adhesive backed applications and suppositories.

Sublingual

Sublingual drugs are absorbed through the mucous membranes beneath the tongue. The sublingual region is extremely vascular and permits rapid absorption with systemic delivery. These medications are generally dissolvable tablets or sprays. One commonly administered medication is nitroglycerin.

Subcutaneous Injection

Subcutaneous (SC) injections provide a slow, sustained release of medication and a longer duration of action and are used when the total volume injected is no more than 1 mL of liquid. Many medications, including insulin, heparin, and epinephrine, are given by the SC route.

SC injection sites, all areas relatively distant from bones and major blood vessels, include the area over the scapula, the lateral aspects of the upper arm and thigh, and the abdomen. At least 1 inch (2.5 cm) pinched fold of skin and tissue is necessary for administering SC injections. Burned, edematous, or scarred skin should not be used as a SC injection site, nor should the area 2 inches (5 cm) in diameter around the umbilicus or belt line.

Aspiration is not necessary with SC injection because subcutaneous tissue usually contains only small blood vessels. Therefore, the danger of unintended IV injection is minimal. In fact, aspirating SC injections may cause tissue damage that could affect drug absorption adversely.

Intramuscular Injection

Intramuscular (IM) injection is useful when drug action faster than that provided by SC injection is desired but rapid effects are not required. The onset of action usually occurs within 10 to 15 minutes after an IM injection. However, the blood flow to the injection site affects the absorption rate. The most common muscles into which drugs are administered are the deltoid and the gluteus. In general, 5 mL of fluid can be administered with an IM injection, but a maximum of 1 mL of medication can be given into the deltoid, whereas 10 mL can be given into the gluteus. Accurate identification of injection sites is important because major blood vessels and nerves traverse the muscle groups used for IM injections. Therefore, using an inappropriate injection site could result in permanent damage to the patient. The technique for administering an IM injection is the same for both adult and pediatric patients. The paramedic should use the Z-track method for IM injection.

It is important to note that, as a rule, patients presenting with a chief complaint of chest pain should not receive medications by the intramuscular route. Intramuscular injection of medication may cause an elevation of certain muscle enzymes that routinely circulate in the blood. In the emergency department these enzymes are frequently measured to determine whether the chest pain is of myocardial origin. An intramuscular injection in the prehospital phase of emergency medical care can cause a false elevation of these enzymes, which can subsequently confuse the emergency department physician as he or she attempts to determine the etiology of the chest pain. On some occasions, however, the medical control physician may permit intramuscular injections when no other immediate route is available and administration of the medication is essential.

Intravenous Administration

Medications are administered intravenously to obtain an immediate onset of action, to obtain the highest possible blood concentration of a drug, and to treat conditions that require the constant titration of medication. In many cases, life-threatening situations such as shock require such constant titration.

Sites used for IV administration include the veins on the hand and wrist, the forearm veins that traverse the antecubital fossa, the veins on the scalp and umbilical vessels (for infants), and the superficial veins of the leg and foot when other sites cannot be used.

As mentioned previously, there are two distinct methods of IV medication administration: (1) the IV bolus and (2) slow IV infusion (sometimes called "piggyback"). Emergency medications administered by the IV bolus technique are usually administered with prefilled syringes. Many medications, however, are still available only in ampule or vial form.

In all but a few cases, it is essential that an IV be established before administering medications intravenously. Establishing an IV line makes the repeated administration of medications less traumatic.

Endotracheal Administration

The endotracheal route is very effective and often forgotten in the emergency setting. When an IV cannot be established, and the patient is in dire need of lidocaine, naloxone, atropine, or epinephrine, which may be the case in cardiac arrest, these drugs may be instilled via the endotracheal tube. The rate of absorption is as fast as with IV administration. When administering a medication via the endotracheal tube, the dose should be increased to 2 to 2.5 times the intravenous dose.

A common situation follows: A patient is encountered in ventricular fibrillation and is immediately countershocked. The patient converts to an improved rhythm with a fair pulse. An IV line cannot be immediately established, however. The patient begins to have frequent multifocal premature ventricular contractions. Lidocaine can now be administered down the endotracheal tube to stabilize the rhythm until a peripheral line can be established.

Intraosseous Injection

It is often difficult to establish an IV line in children younger than 6 years of age. In instances in which an IV cannot be established and the child needs emergency medications or fluids, an intraosseous line can be established. A needle is placed into the proximal tibia, approximately 1 to 3 cm below the tibial tuberosity, on the anterior surface. The needle is advanced through the cortex of the bone into the bone marrow cavity. Entry into the marrow cavity is evidenced by a lack of resistance after penetrating the bony cortex, the needle standing upright without support, the ability to aspirate bone marrow into a syringe connected to the needle, or the free flow of the infusion without significant subcutaneous infiltration. Fluids and drugs administered into the marrow cavity quickly enter the circulatory system. The onset of action of drugs administered by this route is similar to that found with IV injection. Drugs that can be administered by this route include the catecholamines, lidocaine, atropine, and sodium bicarbonate, as well as fluids. Intraosseous infusion is only indicated in children younger than 6 years of age and only when an IV line cannot be established.

Inhalational Administration

Many medications used in the treatment of respiratory emergencies are administered by inhalation. The most common example is oxygen. In addition, some medications are designed to be administered into the respiratory tree. The most common of these are the bronchodilators, including metaproterenol (Alupent), racemic epinephrine, isoetharine (Bronkosol), ipratropium (Atrovent), and salbutamol (Ventolin). If these drugs are administered directly into the respiratory tree, they can quickly reach their site of action with minimal absorption delays. Following are three common methods for administering these medications:

Metered-dose inhalers.   Metered-dose inhalers are aerosolized forms of the medication in a small canister. Most bronchodilators are supplied in this form. Many patients have inhalers at home and use them routinely. The canister is attached to a mouthpiece. The patient places his or her lips around the mouthpiece, begins to inhale, and presses the canister. When the canister is pressed, a metered amount of the drug is delivered in aerosol form. The amount of drug delivered is accurate and limited. Metered-dose inhalers are designed for single-patient use (see Figure 3–1). Some metered-dose inhalers come equipped with a spacer. The spacer is a cylindrical canister between the inhaler and the mouthpiece. Prior to administration, the patient will depress the inhaler sending a measured dose of drug into the spacer. The patient will then breathe in and out of the spacer through the mouthpiece, thus inhaling the drug into the lungs. The system is particularly useful for patients who have a hard time operating and inhaling the metered-dose inhaler. This is common in

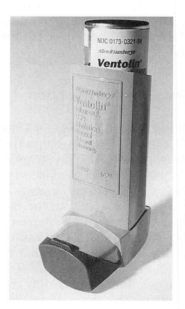

FIGURE 3–1   Metered-dose inhaler.

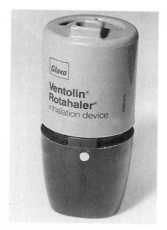

FIGURE 3–2   Spinhaler (Ventolin rotohaler).

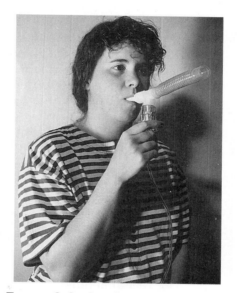

FIGURE 3–3   Small volume nebulizer.

the elderly and in young children. The spacer, when used in conjunction with a metered dose inhaler, is very effective.

Spinhaler, rotahaler.   These commercial devices are designed for patients who have difficulty operating the metered-dose inhalers. Special capsules are placed in the device. When inhaled, the capsules release medication that is delivered to the respiratory tree (see Figure 3–2).

Small-volume nebulizer.   Small-volume nebulizers, also called updraft or handheld nebulizers, are the most commonly used method of administering inhaled medications in the emergency setting. The nebulizer has a chamber into which a solution of the medication, usually diluted with 2 to 3 mL of sterile saline, is placed. Oxygen or compressed air is blown past the chamber, causing the medication to be aerosolized. The patient inhales the aerosolized medication with each breath. This method of bronchodilator administration is advantageous because it delivers supplemental oxygen, delivers the medication over a 5- to 10-minute interval, and is supplied in single-dose ampules (see Figure 3–3).

Administering drugs safely to a child requires special attention to the six rights because any medication error can have a much greater impact on a child than on an adult. For each route of administration, the paramedic must modify adult administration techniques for a pediatric patient. No matter which route is used, the paramedic should attempt to elicit the child's cooperation to make medication administration as easy as possible. If the child is unable to cooperate, the paramedic may need to ask a parent to assist and hold the child during administration.

Although absorption from the GI tract is less predictable than from other routes, oral administration may be used. In prehospital care, the administration of Tylenol may be required in febrile patients. Administering medications to a child may be a challenge.

If an infant or small child must be restrained for medication administration, the paramedic should use a syringe without a needle to administer small, controlled doses. To minimize the risk of choking or aspirating, the paramedic should hold the child's head upright or to the side.

The paramedic then slides the syringe into the child's mouth about halfway back between the gums and cheeks and squirts a small amount of medication. This administration technique offers several advantages. Placing the medication deep in the side of the mouth makes it difficult for the child to lose the medication by spitting or drooling. Although medication administration may take longer because the drug is given in small amounts, this technique reduces the risk of choking, coughing, and vomiting because it does not stimulate the gag reflex.

Intramuscular Injection

For an IM injection the paramedic should use the smallest-gauge needle appropriate for the medication, usually a needle that is 25 to 22 gauge. The needle length should not exceed 1 inch (2.5 cm), except in the adult-sized adolescent, who may require a 1 1/2 inch (3.8 cm) needle.

The recommended injection sites vary with age. The vastus lateralis and rectus femoris muscles are the recommended sites for an infant or toddler. For a child who has been walking for about 1 year, the paramedic can give the injection in the ventrogluteal or dorsogluteal area. Walking develops muscles and thus reduces the risk of sciatic nerve damage during an IM injection. For an older child, an injection site such as the deltoid, gluteus maximus, ventrogluteus, vastus lateralis, or rectus femoris may be used. The same injection technique used in an adult is used in a child. If necessary, the child's parent or the paramedic's partner may be asked to hold the child still during injection.

Subcutaneous Administration

Subcutaneous administration is the same in a child as in an adult. Injection sites include the abdomen and the middle third of the upper arm or thigh. The needle should be 27 to 23 gauge and 3/8 to 5/8 inch (1 to 1.5 cm) long.

Intravenous Administration

Pediatric IV administration poses several challenges for the paramedic. Pediatric IV administration is the same as for an adult, with the caution that any medication error can have a much greater impact on a child than on an adult.

Rectal Administration

Drug absorption from the rectum may be unpredictable. Nevertheless, medications may be administered rectally when oral administration or other routes are not available. For example, in a febrile patient having a seizure, administration of medications by other routes would be difficult. In this situation, the rectal administration of diazepam (Valium) or lorazepam (Ativan) may be indicated.

SUMMARY

It is essential that acute care personnel be competent with all of the medication routes used in emergency medicine. These skills can be developed only after repeated practice in the classroom and the clinical setting. It is important for paramedics to be familiar with all of the medications used in routine prehospital care in their system and the routes by which the medications are administered. If there is any doubt concerning an order or an administration route, the medical control physician or a drug reference source should be consulted. Each time a medication is administered, the paramedic should ensure he or she has met each of the six rights of medication administration: right patient, right medication, right dose, right route, right time, and right documentation.

This book is not a substitute for a rigorous classroom instruction session on medication administration. It is designed purely as a teaching aid for the student and as a reference source for others.

KEY WORDS

alimentary canal. The digestive tract.

antiseptic. Cleaning agent that is not toxic to living tissue.

asepsis. A condition free of pathogens.

bolus. A method of intravenous medication administration by which a drug is rapidly administered rather than infused over a period of time.

disinfectant. Cleansing agent that is toxic to living tissue.

endotracheal. A route of medication administration by which drugs are administered down an endotracheal tube.

inhalation. Entrance of a substance into the body through the respiratory tract.

intracardiac. Administration of medications directly into the heart. This route is not recommended for prehospital care.

intradermal. A parenteral route of medication administration by which a drug is injected into the dermal layer of the skin.

intramuscular injection. A common parenteral route of medication administration by which a drug is injected into the skeletal muscle.

intraosseous. A route of fluid and drug administration in which select medications or fluids are injected into the bone marrow. This route is considered an alternative to venous access in children under the age of 6 years.

intravenous. A commonly used parenteral route of medication administration by which a drug is injected directly into venous circulation.

intravenous infusion. A method of medication administration by which a drug or fluid is given over time.

local. Limited to one area of the body.

medically clean. Careful handing to prevent contamination.

metered-dose inhaler. A device for administering medication by inhalation; it consists of a canister containing a liquid that, when activated, delivers the medication via a fine mist.

piggyback. A method of administering a medication by slow IV infusion.

rectal. An enteral route of medication administration by which a drug is instilled in the rectum.

stat. Latin abbreviation meaning "immediately."

sterile. Free of all forms of life.

subcutaneous. A common parenteral route of medication administration by which a drug is injected into the loose connective tissue between the dermis and the muscle.

sublingual. A route of medication administration by which a drug is absorbed across the rich blood supply of the tongue.

systemic. Throughout the body.

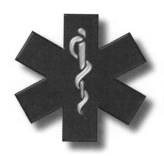

chapter 4

DRUG DOSAGE CALCULATIONS

OBJECTIVES

After completing this chapter, the reader should be able to

1. Define the metric system.
2. Identify and utilize the common metric prefixes, multiples, and submultiples.
3. Utilize the rules of the metric system.
4. Convert between units of the metric system.
5. Convert between units of the metric system and the customary or apothecary system.
6. Solve a basic order word problem using either the ratio and proportion, cross multiplication, or formula method.
7. Recognize an order based on patient's weight.
8. Solve an order problem based on patient weight using the simple three-step method.
9. Recognize the two basic types of concentration problems.
10. Define and recognize a weight/volume percentage solution.
11. Find the amount of solute in a weight/volume percentage solution using either the formula method or the ratio and proportion method.
12. Find the concentration of a solution using either the formula method or the ratio and proportion method.

13. Recognize an intravenous drip problem.

14. Organize the information from an intravenous drip problem.

15. Recognize and be familiar with the dimensional analysis method of solving intravenous drip problems.

16. Recognize and be familiar with the rule of fours method of solving intravenous drip problems.

17. Solve an intravenous drip problem using either the dimensional analysis or the intravenous rule of fours method.

18. Recognize an intravenous drip problem based on patient weight.

19. Organize the information from an intravenous drip problem that is based on patient weight.

20. Solve an intravenous drip problem based on patient weight using either the dimensional analysis or rule of fours method.

21. Recognize an intravenous order of milliliters per hour that needs to be converted to drops per minute.

22. Utilize the formula method to solve a conversion from milliliters per hour to drops per minute.

INTRODUCTION

Administration of the correct drug dosage is essential to proper prehospital medical care. This skill will be tested in written exams, practical skill stations, and on a daily basis in the prehospital environment. Medications used in emergency medicine are available from many different manufacturers. They also vary in concentration, volume, and packaging. The importance of being familiar with the common emergency drug preparations and calculating correct dosages cannot be overemphasized. All prehospital personnel should be able to prepare the correct medication dose quickly and accurately from available ampules, vials, pills, tablets, or other prepackaged medications regardless of drug concentration, volume, or packaging. This responsibility requires knowledge, skill, and practice. This chapter will help paramedics prepare to meet that responsibility.

Familiarity with the systems of measurement frequently used in medicine, especially the metric system, is essential to meet this responsibility. Conversion from one system to another is often required.

In this chapter a review of the metric system, common mathematical operations, and dosage calculations are presented. The practice problems at the end of this chapter provide an opportunity to hone the skills learned.

SECTION 1: THE METRIC SYSTEM

The International System of Units (SI), or the metric system, is an international system of measurement originating in France during the period of the French Revolution. It has been internationally developed and is approved for use in the United States with some minor modifications. The metric system is the standard system of weights and measures used worldwide in the sciences, including medicine and pharmacology. However, tradition has caused some apothecary and household weights and measures, known as the customary system, to endure in the United States.

The metric system is a decimal system based on multiples or submultiples of the number 10. All units are either 10 times larger or 1/10 as large as the next unit. Because the metric system is based on 10, the conversion from one unit to another is simple. To change from one multiple or submultiple to another requires moving only a decimal point. Greek prefixes are used to express these multiples and submultiples. Different prefixes produce units that are of an appropriate size for the application that is needed.

Units of the Metric System

There are many units in the metric system. The following units of the metric system are approved for use in the United States and are the units most commonly used in the prehospital environment:

- Meter (m) for length
- Degrees Celsius (°C) for temperature
- Gram (g) for mass
- Liter (L) for volume

The liter (L) is not an SI unit. That is why the abbreviation, or symbol, is capitalized. The SI unit for volume is the cubic meter (m^3). However, the liter (L) is an approved and preferred unit of volume in Europe, Canada, and the United States. Other nonmetric units that are acceptable to use in the United States include the minute, the hour, and the nautical mile.

Multiples, Submultiples, and Prefixes of the Metric System

Units are used like home bases. Very large numbers or very small numbers can be difficult to manage. The metric system answers this problem with an easy solution: Multiples or submultiples are used in a decimal system and each is given a prefix to attach to the base unit. Although Table 4–1 does not list all of them, it lists some of the common multiples, submultiples, and prefixes of the metric system. Symbols over 1 million are capitalized; all others are lowercase.

TABLE 4–1

Common Multiples, Submultiples, and Prefixes of the Metric System

Multiples and Submultiples	Prefix Name	Prefix Symbol
$1\ 000\ 000\ 000 = 10^9$	giga-	G
$1\ 000\ 000 = 10^6$	mega-	M
$1\ 000 = 10^3$	kilo-	k
$100 = 10^2$	hecto-	h
$10 = 10^1$	deka-	da
	Base unit	
$0.1 = 10^{-1}$	deci-	d
$0.01 = 10^{-2}$	centi-	c
$0.001 = 10^{-3}$	milli-	m
$0.000\ 001 = 10^{-6}$	micro-	μ
$0.000\ 000\ 001 = 10^{-9}$	nano-	n

Instead of using a large number of zeros, a person making metric conversions can simply change the prefix. A quantity of 1000 g of something is much easier to work with mathematically if it is converted to 1 kg.

Metric Conversions

Converting within the metric system is logical and simple. The most common multiples or prefixes used in the prehospital setting are the *kilo-*, the *milli-*, and the *micro-*. One can convert between these multiples by a factor of 1000 by either multiplying or dividing by 1000 depending on the need. Examples of common metric conversions follow:

$$
\begin{aligned}
1 \text{ kg} &= 1000 \text{ g} \\
1 \text{ g} &= 1000 \text{ mg} \\
1 \text{ mg} &= 1000 \text{ } \mu\text{g} \\
1 \text{ L} &= 1000 \text{ mL}
\end{aligned}
$$

Let us say we have 1 mg of a drug and we need to divide it up to work with it more effectively. Rather than deal with fractions, we can simply convert it to 1000 μg. Now, it will be easier to divide and work with.

Some conversions between the customary and the metric systems may still be necessary. Just ask anyone in the United States how much they weigh. What unit will they respond with? Pounds. Because prehospital medicine uses the metric system, common conversion factors between the two systems are provided in Table 4–2.

The following temperature conversion formulas may also prove helpful:

$$
°\text{C} = (°\text{F} - 32) \times \frac{5}{9}
$$

$$
°\text{F} = (°\text{C} \times \frac{9}{5}) + 32
$$

Rules of the Metric System

Units

The written names of all metric units start with lowercase letters unless they begin a sentence. The units *meter, gram, liter,* and so on begin with lowercase letters. The one exception, however, is degrees Celsius. The unit

TABLE 4–2

Common Conversion Factors between the Metric and Customary Systems

Metric		Customary
5 mL	=	1 tsp
15 mL	=	1 T (tablespoon)
30 mL	=	1 fl oz
950 mL	=	1 qt
3.8 L	=	1 gal
2.54 cm	=	1 inch
65 mg	=	1 gr
0.45 kg	=	1 lb
1 kg	=	2.2 lb

degrees is lowercase, but the word *Celsius* is capitalized. Normal body temperature would be written as

37 degrees Celsius

Symbols (Abbreviations)

Generally, the metric symbols or the abbreviations are written in lowercase letters. For example

km for kilometer
mg for milligram

The liter is not an SI unit, but it is approved for use in the United States and Europe. So, to set it apart, the symbol for liter is generally capitalized. Also, if a unit name is derived from a person's name, it is also capitalized.

L for liter
Pa for pascal
mL for milliliter

Plurals

The full written names of units (e.g., meter, gram, and liter) are only made plural when the numerical value that precedes them is more than 1. One exception to this rule is 0 degrees Celsius.

0 degrees Celsius
2 liters
0.25 liter *not* 0.25 liters

Symbols for units are not made plural:

50 mL = 50 milliliters
50 mL *not* 50 mL's

Spacing

A space is used between the number and the symbol (abbreviation) for which it refers.

5 km
10 mg
40° C

Hyphens

Hyphens between a number and a metric unit are not necessary when used as a one-thought modifier. If a hyphen is used, the name of the metric value should be written out. Hyphens should not be used with symbols (abbreviations).

1-liter bag *not* 1-L bag
5-kilometer run *not* 5-km run

Commas

Spaces are used in place of commas when writing metric values that contain five or more digits. For values with four digits, either a space or no space is acceptable. The spaces are added on either side of the decimal point.

1 234 567 km *not* 1,234,567 km

2000 mL or 2 000 mL

0.123 456 kg

Period

A period is not used with metric unit names and symbols (abbreviations) except at the end of a sentence.

50 cm *not* 50 cm.

Decimal Point

A period is used as a decimal point within numbers to designate decimal fractions. When the number is less than 1 (a decimal fraction), a 0 is written before the decimal point. This leading 0 is especially important in drug calculations because it draws attention to the decimal point and prevents drug dosage errors. Common fractions are not used in the metric system.

0.5 mg *not* .5 mg

SECTION 2: FIND THE ORDERED DOSE

The ordered dose is the most simple dosage calculation for the prehospital care provider. In this type of problem, the paramedic is given an order to administer a medication to a patient. There are three components to locate in this type of problem: the doctor's order, the concentration of the drug on hand, and what unit to administer.

The Doctor's Order

The order from the physician includes the amount of the medication and should also include the route of administration. The routes of administration include subcutaneous, intramuscular, intravenous (IV), endotracheal, sublingual, intraosseous, intralingual, transdermal, oral, and rectal. Orders can be verbal or written as a standing order or protocol. The order in the example that follows is known as a *basic order*.

Concentration

The second item to identify is the concentration or "what's on hand," as referred to by some texts. The paramedic is given the concentration of either a vial, an ampule, a prefilled syringe, or a tablet. Concentrations can be listed as common fractions, ratio percentages, percentage solutions, or by mass (e.g., grams and milligrams).

Unit to Administer

It is essential to look at the doctor's order and identify the unit of measurement that will be administered to the patient. Some texts refer to the unit to administer as "what you are looking for."

All three components can be identified in the following example.

EXAMPLE PROBLEM

A physician orders 2.5 mg of morphine to be administered IV to a patient with substernal chest pain. You have a 1 mL vial that contains 10 mg of morphine (10 mg/mL). How many milliliters are you going to have to draw into a syringe and push IV into your patient?

Note: Some problems may not ask, "How many milliliters?" They may simply ask, "How much are you going to administer?" You will have to deduce "milliliters" from the context of the problem.

To solve dosage calculation problems consistently and accurately you must be organized. Developing the habit of organization early will make drug dosage problems seem easier. So, before starting any calculations, write down all of the components to the problem.

Doctor's order	2.5 mg of morphine IV
Concentration	10 mg/mL or 10 mg per 1 mL
Unit to administer	mL

Now that you have identified the three components, you will need to solve the problem. There are three methods that can be used. The first two methods are basic algebraic equations and the third is a formula.

Ratio and Proportion Method

1. On the left side of the proportion, put the ratio that is known:

$$10 \text{ mg} : 1 \text{ mL} ::$$

2. On the right side of the proportion, put the ratio that is unknown (usually the ratio composed of the order). It is essential that you put the *units* on both sides of the equation in the same sequence:

$$10 \text{ mg} : 1 \text{ mL} :: 2.5 \text{ mg} : x \text{ mL}$$

3. Now put the proportion in the form of a basic algebraic equation. The extremes can be placed to the left of an equal sign and the means to the right.

$$10x = 2.5 \times 1$$

4. Multiply the right side:

$$10x = 2.5$$

5. Divide both sides by the number in front of x and check to see if the answer's unit matches what you are looking for:

$$x = 0.25 \text{ mL}$$

Cross Multiplication Method

The cross multiplication method is very similar to the ratio and proportion method. It simply sets up the problem using common fractions. The first fraction can be the concentration. The second fraction is the doctor's order over what is to be administered.

$$\frac{10 \text{ mg}}{1 \text{ mL}} = \frac{2.5 \text{ mg}}{x \text{ mL}}$$

Cross multiply the fractions by multiplying the numerators by the opposite denominators. The resulting algebraic equation is exactly the same as from the preceding equation:

$$10x = 2.5 \times 1$$
$$10x = 2.5$$
$$x = 0.25 \text{ mL}$$

In both methods, remember to place the unit to administer, or "what you are looking for," into the answer.

Formula Method

Some people prefer to memorize a formula to solve this type of problem. The following formula will be helpful if you prefer this method:

$$\text{Volume to be administered } (x) = \frac{\text{(Volume on hand) (Ordered dose)}}{\text{(Concentration on hand)}}$$

Using the preceding example, place each of the components in their proper places in the formula:

EXAMPLE PROBLEM

A physician orders 2.5 mg of morphine to be administered IV to a patient with substernal chest pain. You have a 1 mL vial that contains 10 mg of morphine (10 mg/mL). How many milliliters are you going to have to draw into a syringe and push IV into your patient?

1. Fill in the formula:

$$x = \frac{(1 \text{ mL}) (2.5 \text{ mg})}{10 \text{ mg}}$$

2. Cancel any like units (mg):

$$x = \frac{(1 \text{ mL}) (2.5 \text{ mg})}{10}$$

3. Work the algebra:

$$x = \frac{2.5}{10}\,\text{mL}$$

$$x = 0.25\,\text{mL}$$

SECTION 3: FIND THE UNITS PER KILOGRAM

Finding the units per kilogram adds a new dimension to the problems in the previous section. Instead of a basic order, the doctor will order a certain number of units (e.g., grams and milligrams) of a drug to be administered based on the patient's weight, almost always in kilograms. This is referred to as an order based on patient's weight. Look at the following example.

EXAMPLE PROBLEM

The doctor orders 5 mg/kg of bretylium IV to be administered to your patient. You have premixed syringes with 500 mg/10 mL. Your patient weights 220 lb. How many milliliters will you administer?

You can see that the order of 5 mg/kg of bretylium is a little different than a basic order. Start by writing down all of the key information. In this type of problem, add a patient weight category. Always begin with organizing the information:

Doctor's order	5 mg/kg bretylium IV
Concentration	500 mg/mL
Unit to administer	mL
Patient's weight	220 lb

Look at the order. It is directly tied to the patient's weight. Put another way, the order is saying, "For every kilogram of patient, give 5 mg of bretylium."

In the following three-step method, only step 2 is new. The other steps have been covered in previous sections.

Three-Step Method

1. Convert the patient's weight from pounds to kilograms.
2. Convert the ordered dose based on patient's weight to a basic order.
3. Find the ordered dose.

Step 1: Convert pounds to kilograms

$$220\,\text{lb} \div 2.2 = 100\,\text{kg}$$

or

$$220\,\text{lb} \times 0.45 = 99\,\text{kg}$$

Note: For ease of computation, 99 kg could then be approximated to 100 kg without compromising patient care.

Step 2: Converting the order by weight to a basic order
This step can be calculated by using a formula or by using the ratio and proportion method.

Formula Method

$$x = \frac{\text{Ordered dose} \times \text{Weight (kg)}}{1 \text{ kg}}$$

Set up the formula.

$$x = \frac{5 \text{ mg} \times 100 \text{ kg}}{1 \text{ kg}}$$

The unit of kilogram in the numerator cancels out the unit of kilogram in the denominator, leaving milligrams. Now, work the math:

$$x = 500 \text{ mg}$$

This is the basic ordered dose. You can now proceed to step 3 or look at the ratio and proportion method.

Ratio and Proportion Method

$$5 \text{ mg} : 1 \text{ kg} :: x \text{ mg} : 100 \text{ kg}$$
$$x = 5 \times 100$$
$$x = 500 \text{ mg}$$

Either way, this is now a basic order that can be worked with. Draw a line through the order based on patient weight and write in the new basic order of 500 mg over it. This habit will help keep information organized. Now, the ordered dose must be calculated.

Step 3: Find the ordered dose
Because you now have a basic order, find the ordered dose using the method that you prefer from Section 2.

Answer: 10 mL

SECTION 4: CONCENTRATION PROBLEMS

Prehospital care providers encounter two types of concentration problems. The first type of concentration problem, amount of solute problems, tests knowledge of the solutions that paramedics work with. The second type not only helps in finding the concentration in an IV bag but is also a major step used when solving IV drip problems (Section 5).

Amount of Solute

Concentration problems dealing with amount of solute are seen more often on tests than in practical applications. They involve searching for the amount of solute in a weight/volume percentage solution. Weight/volume percentage is a commonly used percentage concentration with prehospital solutions. It always expresses the number of grams of solute in a total of 100 mL of solution.

For example, 50 percent dextrose in water, or $D_{50}W$, is a common pre-hospital drug. This expression means that there are 50 g of dextrose in every 100 mL of solution. The fraction expression of the weight/volume percentage solution is as follows:

$$\frac{50 \text{ g}}{100 \text{ mL}} \text{ of dextrose in water}$$

Knowing this, it is obvious that when there are 50 mL of this solution, there are 25 g of dextrose. Following are a couple of examples of how this type of problem could be worded.

EXAMPLE PROBLEM

You have a 250 mL bag of D_5W. How many grams of dextrose are in the bag?

Formula Method

Number of grams (x) = Percentage of solution $\times$ Volume of solution

Filling in the formula and working the problem solves the preceding example:

$$x = \frac{5 \text{ g}}{100 \text{ mL}} \times 250 \text{ mL}$$

$$x = \frac{1250}{100} \text{ g}$$

$$x = 12.5 \text{ g}$$

Hint: If the problem had asked for answers in milligrams, the grams would need to be converted to milligrams to find the correct answer.

Ratio and Proportion or Cross Multiplication Method

This problem could also be worked using either the ratio and proportion or cross multiplication methods:

$$5 \text{ g} : 100 \text{ mL} :: x \text{ g} : 250 \text{ mL} \qquad or \qquad \frac{5 \text{ g}}{100 \text{ mL}} = \frac{x \text{ g}}{250 \text{ mL}}$$

$$100x = 5 \times 250$$

$$100x = 1250$$

$$x = 12.5 \text{ g}$$

These same types of problems can be twisted around. What if the number of grams to be administered and the percentage were given and the amount to be infused was the unknown? Look at the following example.

EXAMPLE PROBLEM

The doctor orders 12.5 g of 5 percent dextrose to be infused. How many milliliters will be infused?

A formula, the ratio and proportion method, or cross multiplication may be used to solve this type of problem.

Formula Method

$$\text{Volume } (x) = \frac{\text{Amount ordered (g)}}{\text{Percentage}}$$

$$x = \frac{12.5 \text{ g}}{5 \text{ percent}}$$

or mathematically the same:

$$x = 12.5 \text{ g} \times \frac{5 \text{ g}}{100 \text{ mL}}$$

$$x = 12.5 \text{ g} \times \frac{100 \text{ mL}}{5 \text{ g}}$$

$$x = \frac{1250}{5} \text{ mL}$$

$$x = 250 \text{ mL}$$

Ratio and Proportion Method

Still using the preceding example, we can use the ratio and proportion method to find out the answer:

$$5 \text{ g} : 100 \text{ mL} :: 12.5 \text{ g} : x \text{ mL}$$

$$5x = 1250$$

$$x = 250 \text{ mL}$$

Find the Concentration of a Solution

In most facilities and EMS systems, the pharmacy or drug manufacturer prepares solutions for IV use. However, in small hospitals, rural EMS systems, and other settings (such as testing sites), paramedics are required to measure, prepare, and administer these solutions.

The second type of concentration problem is used to find the concentration of a particular premixed IV solution (or syringe, vial, or the like). It is also used as a major step in solving IV drip problems. It is important to know the answer to the question, What do they mean by concentration? The usual answer is how many milligrams or micrograms of a drug are contained per 1 mL of a given solution. There are other ways to express concentration, but when prehospital care workers are referring to an IV solution's concentration they usually mean a per milliliter concentration.

EXAMPLE PROBLEM

One gram of lidocaine has been added to a 250 mL bag of D_5W. What is the concentration?

Formula Method

A standard formula is used to express concentration. Once it is set up, it is simply a matter of reducing the fraction to a denominator of 1.

$$x = \frac{\text{Solute (grams or milligrams of drug)}}{\text{Solvent (liters or milliliters of volume)}}$$

Set up the formula:

$$x = \frac{1 \text{ g lidocaine}}{250 \text{ mL } D_5W}$$

Convert grams to milligrams (lidocaine is ordered in milligrams):

$$x = \frac{1000 \text{ mg lidocaine}}{250 \text{ mL } D_5W}$$

Reduce the fraction to a denominator of 1:

$$x = \frac{1000 \text{ mg lidocaine}}{250 \text{ mL } D_5W} \div \frac{250}{250}$$

$$x = \frac{4 \text{ mg lidocaine}}{1 \text{ mL } D_5W}$$

This result can be expressed verbally as, "The concentration is 4 milligrams per milliliter" or "4 to 1." This is the per milliliter concentration.

Ratio and Proportion Method

$$1000 \text{ mg} : 250 \text{ mL} :: x \text{ mg} : 1 \text{ mL}$$

$$250x = 1000$$

$$x = 4 \text{ mg/mL}$$

Both of these methods can be used to find the per milliliter concentration of any solution.

SECTION 5: CALCULATE AN IV DRIP

Calculating IV drips has been a quandary for many prehospital care providers for a long time. Asking any paramedic, nurse, or doctor to set up an IV drip without a calculator, reference, electric pump, or computerized device will likely produce all kinds of moans and excuses. But that is exactly what paramedics are expected to do at test stations and in the prehospital environment. There is an easy way to solve drip problems. This section will examine both the dimensional analysis and the rule of fours methods. Paramedics may choose the method that works best for them.

IV Drip

In some cases, patients require medication to be infused on a continual basis. Paramedics will receive orders to administer a certain number of units (usually milligrams or micrograms) of a medication per minute to a patient through an IV. Known as an infusion, it is also referred to as an IV drip because it involves calculating the number of drops that "drip" and are delivered intravenously each minute to deliver the amount of drug the doctor is ordering.

Even though most of these IV infusions are commercially available already premixed, paramedics will be tested on mixing the medication and starting the infusion correctly. If an occasion occurs in which paramedics do not have a premixed bag, they will know what to do. This process involves drawing medication from a vial or ampule into a syringe and mixing it into an IV bag. Then, paramedics will be required to set a drip rate based on the doctor's order and the administration set that is available. The solution is the number of drops that fall each minute (gtt/min).

Formula Method (Dimensional Analysis)

If paramedics have a chemistry or algebra background, they will understand the formula method and probably prefer it. It very systematically and mathematically calculates the IV drip rate. If they do not like math or chemistry, they may not like this method. They do need to understand it, however. This method shows how a drip rate is calculated and answers a lot of questions that may arise later. Organization of the material is still the key to success.

EXAMPLE PROBLEM

A doctor orders 2 mg/min of lidocaine to be administered to a patient who was experiencing an arrhythmia. You have a vial that contains 1 g of lidocaine in 5 mL. Your ambulance carries only 250 mL bags of D_5W. Your administration set is a microdrip set (60 gtt/mL). At how many drops per minute will you adjust your administration set to drip?

Before starting any calculations, organize the information just as you were doing in Section 2. There are a couple of new categories in this type of problem.

Order	2 mg lidocaine IV
On hand	1 g lidocaine/5 mL
Bag	250 mL D_5W
Administration set	60 gtt/mL
Unit to administer	gtt/min

Formula (Dimensional Analysis) Method

$$x = \frac{\text{IV bag volume (mL)}}{\text{Amount of drug in bag}} \times \frac{\text{Unit ordered}}{1 \text{ min}} \times \frac{\text{Administration set (gtt)}}{1 \text{ mL}}$$

1. Fill in the formula:

$$x = \frac{250 \text{ mL}}{1 \text{ g}} \times \frac{2 \text{ mg}}{1 \text{ min}} \times \frac{60 \text{ gtt}}{1 \text{ mL}}$$

Note: The 5 mL in the vial on hand is not figured into the equation.

2. Convert the grams in the bag to match the milligrams in the doctor's order:

$$x = \frac{250 \text{ mL}}{1000 \text{ mg}} \times \frac{2 \text{ mg}}{1 \text{ min}} \times \frac{60 \text{ gtt}}{1 \text{ mL}}$$

3. Cancel out like units and zeros. Confirm that the remaining units are what you are looking for:

$$x = \frac{25}{10} \times \frac{2}{1\ \text{min}} \times \frac{6\ \text{gtt}}{1}$$

4. Multiply and reduce the fraction:

$$x = \frac{300\ \text{gtt}}{10\ \text{min}}$$

$$x = \frac{30\ \text{gtt}}{1\ \text{min}} \quad \text{or} \quad 30\ \text{gtt/min}$$

You can now set your drip rate on the IV administration set. Remember, in most ambulances and test centers, an electric or computerized IV pump will not be available and you will have to set the rate by hand.

Rule of Fours Method

This method is called the rule of fours because it is based on multiples of the number 4. This is also known as the "easy" way. Many people find it far simpler than the formula method or dimensional analysis. It requires the memorization of a process, not a formula, and requires only simple logic and very little math. Look at the same example problem from earlier:

EXAMPLE PROBLEM

A doctor orders 2 mg/min of lidocaine to be administered to a patient who was experiencing an arrhythmia. You have a vial that contains 1 g of lidocaine in 5 mL. Your ambulance carries only 250 mL bags of D$_5$W. Your administration set is a microdrip set (60 gtt/mL). At how many drops per minute will you adjust your administration set to drip?

We begin by organizing the information from the problem similarly to how it was done in the previous example. However, this time we add a new category: the concentration of the IV solution (1 g into 250 mL).

Note: Finding the concentration in the bag is the *key* to solving IV drip problems when using this method. Refer to Section 4 to review this process.

Order	2 mg lidocaine IV
On hand	1 g lidocaine/5 mL
Bag	250 mL D$_5$W
Concentration	4 mg/mL
Administration set	60 gtt/mL
Unit to administer	gtt/min

1. *Compare.* Now that the information is organized, a logical comparison can be made between the concentration and the administration set. Looking at the concentration we could say that in every 1 mL there are 4 mg of lidocaine. We could also say that there are 60 drops in each milliliter. Therefore, in every 60 drops there are 4 mg or 60 gtt/4 mL.

2. *Set up.* Set up the rule of fours "clock" based on step 1. Drops go on the inside of the clock, and milligrams go on the outside. The relationship between the 4 mg and the 60 gtt becomes the 12 o'clock position. Halfway around the clock is the logical half of that relationship. So, 30 gtt equals 2 mg and so on around the clock.

$$4 \text{ mg/mL CLOCK}$$

1 gram into 250 mL yields 4 mg/mL

3. *Look.* Find the doctor's order on the outside of the "clock" and compare it with the drops per minute on the inside. This is the rate at which the administration set is to drip.

$$x = 30 \text{ gtt/min}$$

It is that easy. Different "clocks" can be set up depending on the concentration in the IV bag and/or the administration set available. These parameters can change. The process of setting up the "clock" will be the same and work every time. You will find that there are just a few "clocks" that you will use regularly.

SECTION 6: CALCULATE AN IV DRIP BASED ON PATIENT WEIGHT

This section takes the calculation in the previous section just one step further. It adds the dimension of patient weight. IV drip medication orders can be based on patient weight just as basic orders can.

EXAMPLE PROBLEM

An order is received to administer 10 μg/kg/min of dopamine IV. You have a vial that contains 200 mg of dopamine in 10 mL (200 mg/10 mL). You also have 250 mL bags of D_5W with a microdrip administration set. Your patient weighs 176 pounds. At how many drops per minute will you adjust your administration set to drip?

Organize the material as before. This time the category of patient weight is added. Remember that finding the concentration in the bag is still the key to solving drip problems.

Order	10 mg/kg/min
On hand	200 mg dopamine/10 mL
Bag	250 mL D_5W
Administration set	60 gtt/mL
Concentration	800 μg/mL
Patient's weight	176 lb
Unit to administer	gtt/min

1. Convert the patient's weight to kilograms.
   176 lb ÷ 2.2 = 80 kg

2. Convert the doctor's order from micrograms per kilogram per minute to micrograms per minute.
   10 mg × 80 kg = 800 mg/min

3. You now have the ordered dose. Find the concentration in the bag and use the "clock" or use the dimensional analysis method to solve.

800 mg/mL CLOCK

200 milligrams into 500 mL yields 800 mg/mL

Answer: 60 gtt/min

The dimensional analysis method may also be used to solve this type of problem. After converting the patient's weight and the doctor's order, use the formula from Section 5.

SECTION 7: MILLILITERS PER HOUR TO DROPS PER MINUTE

Sometimes, doctors order IVs to be infused in milliliters per hour or over a specific period of time. To set an IV's administration set, the order must be converted to drops per minute. This section shows how to convert that type of order. A simple conversion formula is all that is needed.

EXAMPLE PROBLEM

The doctor orders you to start an IV of normal saline to run at 100 mL/hr. You have a macrodrip set of 15 gtt/mL. At how many drips per minute will you set your administration set to drip?

Note: Macrodrip administration sets can vary in size.

Formula Method

$$x = \frac{\text{Order amount (mL)}}{\text{Order time (min)}} \times \frac{\text{Administration set (gtt)}}{1 \text{ mL}}$$

1. Fill in the formula. Convert the doctor's order in hours to minutes when you enter the ordered time:

$$x = \frac{100 \text{ mL}}{60 \text{ min}} \times \frac{15 \text{ gtt}}{1 \text{ mL}}$$

2. Cancel units, zeros, and multiply:

$$x = \frac{150 \text{ mL}}{6 \text{ min}}$$

3. Simplify the fraction:

$$x = \frac{25 \text{ gtt}}{1 \text{ min}} \qquad \text{or} \qquad 25 \text{ gtt/min}$$

PRACTICE PROBLEMS

Section 1

Solve the following conversion problems. Answers may be found in Appendix F.

1. 1 g = _____ mg
2. 1 mg = _____ µg
3. 1 mg = _____ g
4. 0.8 mg = _____ µg
5. 1.5 L = _____ mL
6. 400 000 mg = _____ g
7. 800 mg = _____ g
8. 500 mL = _____ L
9. 37 °C = _____ °F
10. 104 °F = _____ °C
11. 1/4 gr = _____ mg
12. 2 Tbsp = _____ mL
13. 180 lb = _____ kg
14. 7 lb = _____ kg
15. 25 kg = _____ lb

Section 2

Solve the following dosage calculation problems. Answers may be found in Appendix F.

1. The doctor orders 1 mg of epinephrine IV for a pulseless and apneic patient in ventricular fibrillation. Epinephrine is supplied as 0.1 mg/mL. How many milliliters will you give?

2. Medical control orders 200 mg of lidocaine IV for your patient in ventricular tachycardia. The prefilled syringe reads 50 mg/mL. How many milliliters will you administer?

3. Your patient meets the criteria for the standing order of 0.5 mg of atropine IV. It comes supplied in your ambulance as 1 mg/10 mL. How many milliliters will you give?

4. You receive an order in the emergency center to administer 100 mEq of sodium bicarbonate IV. Your prefilled syringe label reads 50 mEq/50 mL. How many milliliters will you administer?

5. A radio order is received from medical control to administer 10 mg of Valium IV push to your patient experiencing seizures; 5 mg/mL is printed on the vial of Valium. How many milliliters will you administer?

6. You are assessing a patient in severe congestive heart failure and medical control orders 5 mg of morphine IV. The prefilled syringe reads 15 mg/mL. How many milliliters will you administer?

7. Your patient is bradycardic and you are ordered to administer 0.6 mg of atropine IV. The prefilled syringe reads 0.4 mg/mL. How many milliliters will you administer?

8. Your patient is exhibiting paroxysmal supraventricular tachycardia (PSVT). Vagal maneuvers are ineffective and medical control orders 6 mg of adenosine rapid IV push. The vial reads 3 mg/mL. How many milliliters will you administer?

9. A patient's ventricular fibrillation (v-fib) is refractory to lidocaine and defibrillation attempts. Medical control orders 400 mg of bretylium over 1 minute IV. The prefilled syringe reads 50 mg/mL, 10 mL total volume. How many milliliters will you administer?

10. A patient's Dextro-stix reads approximately 40 mg/dL and she is unconscious. Medical control orders 25 g of dextrose IV bolus. The prefilled syringe reads 0.5 g/mL. How many milliliters will you administer?

Section 3

Solve the following dosage calculation problems. Answers may be found in Appendix F.

1. Your 150 lb patient is experiencing multifocal PVCs and complains of chest pain. Your standing orders state to administer 1 mg/kg of lidocaine. The vial reads 100 mg/5 mL. How many milliliters will you administer?

2. Your patient from problem 1 does not respond to the lidocaine, and medical control orders 5 mg/kg of bretylium IV. Bretylium is supplied in prefilled syringes containing 500 mg/10 mL. How many milliliters will you administer?

3. The doctor orders 0.01 mg/kg of atropine IV for your bradycardic patient who weighs 130 lb. The atropine in your ambulance reads 1 mg/mL. How many milliliters will you administer?

4. You are ordered to administer sodium bicarbonate at 1 mEq/kg to a patient who weighs 160 lb. It is supplied by the emergency center's medication cabinet in prefilled syringes that read 50 mEq/50 mL. How many milliliters will you administer?

5. A severely bradycardic 44 lb pediatric patient does not respond to your initial treatments. Standing orders tell you to administer 0.01 mg/kg epinephrine IV. Your ampule reads 10 mg/10 mL. How many milliliters will you administer?

Section 4

Solve the following concentration problems. Answers may be found in Appendix F.

1. The doctor orders 200 mg of dopamine to be added to a 250 mL bag of D_5W. What is the per milliliter concentration? *Hint:* Dopamine is ordered in micrograms.

2. How many grams of sodium chloride are in a 1000 mL bag of 0.9 percent normal saline?

3. The doctor orders 0.5 g of aminophylline to be placed in a 100 mL bag of D_5W for an IV piggyback. What is the per milliliter concentration?

4. There is a prefilled syringe of 1 percent lidocaine in your ambulance. It contains 5 mL. How many milligrams does it contain?

5. There is another prefilled syringe in your ambulance. It contains 2 percent lidocaine. It also contains 5 mL. How many milligrams does it contain?

6. You are ordered to prepare a lidocaine drip; 1 g is ordered to be placed into a 250 mL bag of D_5W. What is the per milliliter concentration?

7. You are reading the label on a 250 mL bag in the ICU. The label reads 400 mg dopamine added. The bag now has 150 mL left in it. What is the per milliliter concentration in the bag now?

8. Your patient has accidentally overdosed on Cardizem. The doctor orders 300 mg of a 10 percent solution of calcium chloride IV. How many milliliters will you administer?

9. 1 mg of epinephrine has been added to a 250 mL bag of D_5W. What is the per milliliter concentration?

10. The label on a 500 mL bag hanging in the ICU reads 1 g lidocaine added. What is the per milliliter concentration?

Section 5

Solve the following IV drip problems. Answers may be found in Appendix F.

1. The doctor orders 400 μg/min of dopamine to be administered IV. You have a vial that contains 200 mg of dopamine in 10 mL (200 mg/10 mL). Your ambulance has 250 mL bags of D_5W, and you choose a microdrip administration set (60 gtt/mL). At how many drops per minute will you adjust your administration set to drip?

2. You are ordered to administer an Isuprel drip at 4 μg/min. You are ordered to place 1 mg into a 250 mL bag of D_5W. At what rate will you set your microdrip (60 gtt/mL) administration set?

3. Your patient's blood pressure is critically low following conversion from ventricular fibrillation. Medical control orders you to mix 400 mg of dopamine into a 250 mL bag of D_5W and infuse it at 800 μg/min. What is the drip rate with a microdrip administration set (60 gtt/mL)?

4. The doctor orders a starting dose of 2 μg/min of epinephrine. Your assistant has mixed 1 mg of epinephrine into a 250 mL bag of normal saline. What is the drip rate with a microdrip administration set (60 gtt/mL)?

5. You are ordered to administer a lidocaine drip at 2 mg/min. You have 2 g of lidocaine added to a 500 mL bag. What is the drip rate with a microdrip administration set (60 gtt/mL)?

6. Solve problem 5 using a macrodrip administration set (10 gtt/mL).

7. You receive orders to initiate a Bretylol drip following conversion of multifocal Premature Ventricular Contractors (PVCs). The order is for 1 mg/min. You have 1 g of Bretylol added to a 250 mL bag of D_5W and a microdrip administration set (60 gtt/mL). What is the drip rate?

8. You receive an order to start a dopamine drip at 600 μg/min. You place 800 mg of dopamine into a 500 mL bag of normal saline. What is the drip rate with a microdrip administration set (60 gtt/mL)?

9. Solve problem 5 using a macrodrip administration set (15 gtt/mL).

10. You have an order to administer lidocaine at 4 mg/min. The 1 L bag of normal saline has had 4 g of lidocaine added. What is the drip rate with a microdrip administration set (60 gtt/mL)?

Section 6

Solve the following IV drip problems based on patient weight. Answers may be found in Appendix F.

1. You receive an order to administer dopamine to a 176 lb patient at 5 μg/kg/min; 200 mg of dopamine have been added to a 250 mL bag of D_5W. What is the drip rate with a microdrip administration set (60 gtt/mL)?

2. A 22 lb pediatric patient requires an epinephrine drip at 0.1 μg/kg/min. You place 1 mg of epinephrine in a 250 mL bag of D_5W. What is the drip rate with a microdrip administration set (60 gtt/mL)?

3. Your patient in problem 2 does not significantly improve and the doctor doubles the order to 0.2 μg/kg/min. What is the drip rate?

4. A 132 lb cardiac patient is in cardiogenic shock. The doctor orders a dopamine drip at 10 μg/kg/min. Your partner has just placed 400 mg of Intropin into a 500 mL bag of normal saline. At how many drops per minute will you adjust your microdrip administration set to drip?

5. You are transporting a 66 lb pediatric patient with a congenital heart defect. The doctor orders 20 μg/kg/min of lidocaine to be infused. Your partner hands you a 250 mL bag of D_5W that she has labeled "200 mg lidocaine added." What is the drip rate with a microdrip administration set (60 gtt/mL)?

6. The patient in problem 5 does not significantly improve. You are told to increase the current infusion to 40 μg/kg/min. Now what is the drip rate?

7. Your cardiac patient is exhibiting the signs and symptoms of cardiogenic shock. Among other procedures, standing orders call for a dopamine drip at 3 μg/kg/min. The patient's wife states that her husband weighs 150 lb. The vial of dopamine

to be added is labeled 200 mg/5 mL. You have a 250 mL bag of D_5W and a microdrip set. What is the drip rate to be?

8. You are setting up an Isuprel drip for your 75 lb pediatric patient suffering from refractory bronchospasm. The doctor has ordered 0.1 μg/kg/min. The vial is labeled 1 mg/5 mL. You have a 250 mL bag of D_5W and a microdrip set (60 gtt/mL). What is the drip rate to be?

9. You are completing your report after delivering a patient to the emergency center, and you notice that the dopamine dose ordered by medical control is missing from your notes. To avoid any problems, you decide to determine the ordered dose based on the information available. The patient weighs 176 lb and the IV infusion is flowing through a microdrip administration set at 30 gtt/min. The label you put on the 500 mL bag of normal saline reads "800 mg dopamine added." What was the doctor's original dose per kilogram per minute order?

10. You are in the same situation as you were in problem 9. The patient weighs 220 lb. The infusion set is a microdrip set and is flowing at 30 gtt/min. The label on the 250 mL bag of D_5W reads "200 mg dopamine added." What was the doctor's original dose per kilogram per minute order?

Section 7

Solve the following problems of converting milliliters per hour to drops per minute. Answers may be found in Appendix F.

1. The doctor orders you to start an IV of normal saline to run at 100 mL/hr. You have a microdrip administration set (60 gtt/min). What is the drip rate?

2. While doing internship hours at the emergency center, you are asked to start an IV of D_5W to run at 200 mL/hr. You have a macrodrip set (15 gtt/mL). What is the drip rate?

3. Your standing order is to start an IV of normal saline to run at 90 mL/hr. Now you have a macrodrip administration set of 10 gtt/mL. What is the drip rate?

4. A 6-week-old pediatric patient is admitted to the emergency center severely dehydrated. The order reads to infuse 100 mL of 0.45 percent sodium chloride in 2.5 percent D_5W over 1 hour. This is to be followed with 200 mL/hr of the same fluid over 8 hours. What are the two drip rates using a microdrip set?

5. The order on the patient's chart in a busy emergency center reads 1500 mL Plasmanate IV over 10 hours. You choose a 15 gtt/mL administration set. What is the drip rate?

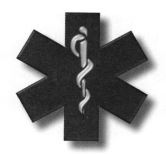

chapter 5

FLUIDS, ELECTROLYTES, AND INTRAVENOUS THERAPY

OBJECTIVES

After completing this chapter, the reader should be able to

1. Identify the body's major fluid compartments and the proportion of total body water they contain.

2. List the major electrolytes and discuss the role they play in maintaining a fluid balance within the human body.

3. Define the following terms and explain the role each process plays in human fluid dynamics:

   a. Diffusion

   b. Osmosis

   c. Active transport

   d. Facilitated diffusion

4. Identify the major elements of blood and describe their purposes.

5. List the various fluid replacement products and describe the advantages and disadvantages of field use.

6. Define hypotonic, hypertonic, and isotonic solutions.

7. State the size of intravenous catheter to be used for particular applications.

8. State the type of intravenous catheter to be used for particular applications.

9. Explain the different types of intravenous fluids that can be used.

10. State which intravenous administration sets should be used and in what circumstances.

11. List the possible sites an intravenous tube can be inserted and the rationale for each.

12. Demonstrate the procedure for inserting an intravenous tube.

13. Describe the procedure for collecting blood samples from an intravenous tube.

INTRODUCTION

One of the most important aspects of prehospital care is the administration of intravenous (IV) fluids and electrolytes. There are two major reasons for administering intravenous fluids during the prehospital phase of emergency medical care. The first is to immediately replace intravascular blood volume, and the second is to provide an easily accessible route for the administration of lifesaving emergency drugs.

FLUIDS

Water is the most abundant substance in the human body. Approximately 60 percent of the total body weight is water, which is located within two fluid compartments, or spaces. The largest of these fluid compartments is the *intracellular fluid (ICF) compartment*, which includes all fluids found within the cells. Three-fourths of all body water is within the intracellular compartment. The remaining water can be found outside of the cell membrane in the *extracellular fluid (ECF) compartment*. There are two major components of the ECF: *intravascular fluid*, which is found within the blood vessels and outside of the cell membranes; and the *interstitial fluid*, that fluid found outside the cell membrane yet not within any defined blood vessels. The relationship of the various fluid compartments is illustrated as follows:

Extracellular Fluid   15 percent of total body weight
   (Interstitial fluid 10.5 percent of total body weight)
   (Intravascular fluid 4.5 percent of total body weight)
Intracellular Fluid   45 percent of total body weight
Total Body Water   60 percent of total body weight

Internal Environment

The internal environment is the extracellular fluid, which bathes each body cell. An important balance must be maintained regarding the internal environment. Whenever one aspect of the internal environment deviates from normal, as frequently occurs in injury and illness, the body immediately responds and returns to normal. The body's tendency to maintain all of its physiological activities in proper balance, including the internal environment, is called *homeostasis*.

ELECTROLYTES

In addition to the body fluids, some important chemicals are also required for life. These chemicals are divided into two main classes: *electrolytes* and *nonelectrolytes*. Chemicals that take on an electrical charge when placed in water are called electrolytes; chemicals that do not take on an electrical charge are called nonelectrolytes. All electrolytes are measured in quantities called *milliequivalents (mEq)*. Sodium bicarbonate, a common emergency drug, is an electrolyte. When placed in water, it quickly divides into charged particles, or ions. All dosages of sodium bicarbonate are calculated in milliequivalents. Certain electrolytes, when dissolved in water, take on a positive charge. These are called *cations*. The major cations—sodium (Na^+), calcium (Ca^{2+}) potassium (K^+), and magnesium (Mg^{2+})—have a special significance. Sodium (Na^+) and calcium (Ca^{2+}) have their greatest concentration in the extracellular fluid, and potassium (K^+) and magnesium (Mg^{2+}) are more concentrated in intracellular space. Imbalances in any one of these electrolytes can result in major problems.

Sodium (Na^+)

Sodium is the most abundant extracellular cation and is especially important in the regulation of body water. Sodium is also important in nerve impulse transmission and in the transfer of calcium into the cell. The most common source of sodium is sodium chloride, or table salt. Sodium is often found in conjunction with chloride (Cl) or bicarbonate, (HCO^{3-}).

Regulation of sodium occurs in the kidney, primarily through reabsorption in the tubules. Aldosterone is the hormonal regulator. Secreted by the kidney, aldosterone increases renal absorption of sodium. Because of sodium's high attraction for water, alterations in sodium and water balance are closely related. An imbalance in one leads to an imbalance in the other. Hypernatremia, or too much sodium, may be due to either an acute gain in sodium or a loss of water without corresponding loss of sodium.

Calcium (Ca^{2+})

Calcium is necessary for the structure of bone and teeth. It also functions as an enzyme cofactor for blood clotting and is required for hormone secretion, membrane stability and permeability, and muscle contraction. One common source of calcium is dairy products.

Most calcium in the body is located in bone tissue, with the remainder found in the plasma and body cells. Inside the cells, calcium is necessary for energy used by muscle fibers to contract. The strength of the contraction is directly related to the concentration of calcium. Calcium is often found in conjunction with phosphate (HPO_4).

Blood levels of calcium are closely regulated by parathyroid hormone (PTH), vitamin D, and calcitonin (from the thyroid gland). Renal regulation of calcium requires PTH, which is secreted in response to low plasma levels.

Potassium (K^+)

Potassium is necessary in the transmission and conduction of nerve impulses, maintenance of normal cardiac rhythms, and skeletal smooth muscle contraction. It is also required for glycogen deposits in the liver and skeletal muscles. In this capacity, potassium works closely with sodium, momentarily trading places with sodium across the cellular membranes to maintain electrical neutrality. This action conducts nerve impulses from one end of the cell to the other. It becomes extremely important in the conduction of cardiac rhythms and the movement of calcium into the cell for muscle contraction.

Magnesium (Mg^{2+})

Approximately 40 to 60 percent of magnesium is stored in muscle and bone. Most of the remainder is stored intracellulary and appears to be related to potassium and calcium. Magnesium activates the enzyme (ATPase) that is essential for normal cell membrane function and is the energy source for the sodium-potassium pump. Physiological effects include relaxing smooth muscle and increasing the stability of cardiac cells, thus reducing the potential for dysrhythmias.

Electrolytes that take on a negative charge are called *anions*. Examples of anions found within the body include chlorine (Cl^-), bicarbonate (HCO_3^-), phosphate (HPO_4^-), and most of the organic (carbon-based) molecules. In addition to the fluid balance mentioned earlier, electrical neutrality must be carefully maintained between cations and anions.

CELL PHYSIOLOGY

To maintain physiological homeostasis, there must be an exchange of electrolytes and water materials across the membrane of the cell. The cell membrane is very complex. It is said to be *semipermeable*, meaning that it allows certain compounds to pass readily across it while restricting the passage of others. Many materials must pass across the cell membrane including oxygen, carbon dioxide, nutrients, fluids, and electrolytes. There are three major ways to move substances across the cell membrane: *diffusion, facilitated diffusion,* and *active transport.* Diffusion is a passive process, whereas facilitated diffusion and active transport require energy expenditure by the cell (see Figure 5–1).

Diffusion

Diffusion occurs when concentrations of various substances become higher on one side of the semipermeable cell membrane. When this difference occurs, an *osmotic gradient* is created. The side of the cell membrane with the higher concentration is said to be *hypertonic* with respect to the other side. Conversely, the side of the membrane with the lower concentration is said

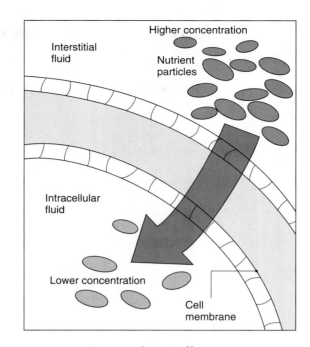

FIGURE 5-1 Diffusion.

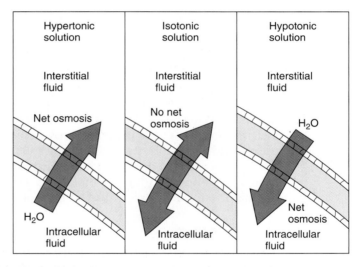

FIGURE 5-2 Relationships and effects of hypotonic, isotonic and hypertonic
solutions.

to be *hypotonic* in relation to the other (see Figure 5–2). When both sides of
the cell membrane have an equal concentration of the substance in question, the system is said to be *isotonic*. These concepts underpin the rationale for IV therapy. IV fluids with a solute concentration less than that of
blood are said to be hypotonic solutions. An example of a hypotonic solution is 0.45 percent sodium chloride (one-half normal saline).

Substances that have a solute concentration equal to that of blood are
said to be isotonic. Lactated Ringer's solution and 0.9 percent sodium chloride are examples of isotonic fluids. An example of a hypertonic solution is

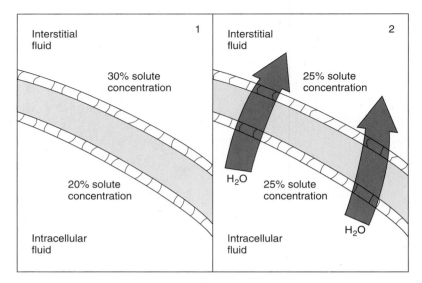

FIGURE 5–3 Osmosis.

50 percent dextrose in water. Although not a classical IV fluid, it plays a major role in prehospital care. One of the most important substances that passes across the cell membrane is water. Water diffuses readily across the cell membrane from an area of higher water concentration to an area of lesser water concentration. The diffusion of water in this manner is called *osmosis* (see Figure 5–3).

Facilitated Diffusion

Certain molecules can move across the cell membrane by a process known as *facilitated diffusion.* Glucose is an example of such a molecule. Facilitated diffusion requires the assistance of "helper proteins" on the surface of the cell membrane. These proteins, once activated, bind to the glucose molecule. After binding, the protein changes its configuration and transports the glucose molecule into the cell, where it is released. The transport protein is then ready for another glucose molecule. Depending on the substance being transported, facilitated diffusion may or may not require energy.

Active Transport

Sometimes it is desirable for the body to maintain a gradient along a cell membrane. This is especially true regarding the ions sodium (Na^+) and potassium (K^+). To sustain life, the concentration of sodium outside the cell membrane must be significantly higher than that inside the cell. Also, the concentration of potassium must be maintained at a much higher level within the cell. To maintain the gradient, the sodium must be pumped out of the cell and potassium must be pumped into the cell. Both of these processes require energy. This is an example of active transport.

BLOOD

One of the most important aspects of the extracellular fluid, and thus the internal environment, is blood. Blood is the main element involved in the oxygenation of body cells, transport of nutrients, transport of control main-

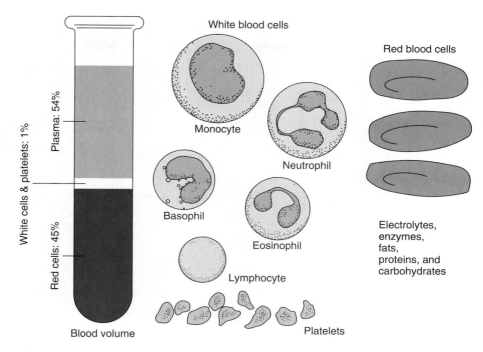

FIGURE 5–4 Various components of blood.

tenance factors (hormones), waste removal, and temperature regulation. Blood is a complex substance divided into two basic components: plasma and formed elements.

Plasma

Plasma is the complex fluid portion of blood. Plasma communicates continually through pores in the capillaries with the fluid that is circulating between the cells (interstitial fluid). Plasma is approximately 92 percent water and contains a number of formed elements (see Figure 5–4).

Formed Elements

Formed elements consist of plasma proteins, plasma lipids, electrolytes, nutrients, and cellular elements such as red blood cells, white blood cells, and platelets. The formed elements make up approximately 45 to 50 percent of blood volume. The continuous movement of blood keeps the formed elements dispersed throughout the plasma, where they are available to carry out the following functions:

1. Respiratory: Delivery of oxygen to the cells and exchange of carbon dioxide
2. Nutritional: Delivery of other substances needed for cellular metabolism (glucose and other carbohydrates, amino acids, fatty acids, vitamins, minerals, and trace elements)

Blood

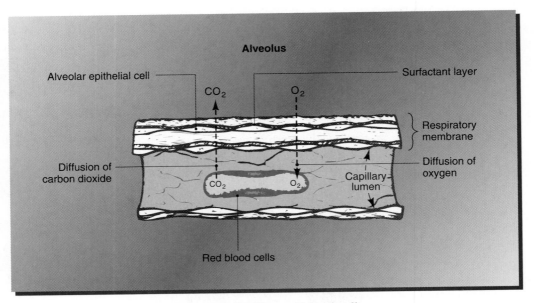

FIGURE 5-5 The red blood cell.

3. Regulatory: Delivery of substances such as electrolytes and hormones

4. Excretory: Removal of cellular debris and waste products such as those of cellular metabolism (carbon dioxide, water, and acids)

5. Protective: Defense against injury and invading microorganisms

There are three major classes of blood cells. The first are the red blood cells, or *erythrocytes* (see Figure 5–5). Erythrocytes have an important iron-containing protein called *hemoglobin.* Hemoglobin is responsible for the transport of oxygen and carbon dioxide. A significant percentage of blood, approximately 45 percent, is red blood cells. The percentage of red blood cells present is referred to as the *hematocrit.* White blood cells, or *leukocytes,* are the second type of cells found in the blood. The leukocytes are responsible for combating infection. The last type of blood cells present is platelets, or *thrombocytes,* responsible for blood clotting.

Blood Types

An antigen is the protein identifier in most cells. The presence or absence of a particular antigen identifies that cell as either "self" or "foreign." Once a cell is identified as foreign, specific antibodies to that cell are formed. Subsequently, all antigens (cells with that specific foreign identifier) are attacked and destroyed. This is termed an antigen-antibody reaction. When the reaction occurs because two types of blood are mixed, it is called "transfusion reaction." At least two commonly occurring antigens, each of which can trigger antigen-antibody reaction, have been found in human blood cells, especially on the cell membrane surfaces. There are two types of antigens in the blood that are more likely than others to cause reactions: the ABO system of antigens and the Rh system.

TABLE 5-1

ABO Blood Types

Blood Types	Antibodies	Can Receive	Can Donate to
Type A	B antibodies	Type A or O	Type A, AB
Type B	A antibodies	Type B or O	Type B, AB
Type AB	No antibodies	Type AB, A, B, O	Type A, B, AB
Type O	A and B antibodies	Type O	Type A, B, AB, O

ABO Types

The ABO group consists of two major antigens, labeled A and B, that are found on the surfaces of red blood cells (RBCs). These antigens can appear by themselves or together or be entirely absent. The result of their presence or absence is one of the four blood types:

Type A. Individuals with blood type A carry the A antigen on the RBCs.

Type B. Individuals with blood type B carry the B antigen on the RBCs.

Type AB. Individuals with blood type AB carry the A and B antigens on the RBCs.

Type O. Individuals with blood type O carry neither antigen on the RBCs.

In the ABO system, the body spontaneously develops antibodies to the other blood types. This system determines which blood type or types each person can receive without triggering a transfusion reaction (see Table 5–1).

Rh Factor

The second important system in blood transfusion is the Rh system. The Rh antigen, type D, is widely prevalent. People with this type of antigen are said to be Rh positive; those without the type D antigen are said to be Rh negative. Approximately 85 to 95 percent of Americans are Rh positive.

Antibodies to the Rh factor do not occur naturally and must be acquired through exposure to Rh-positive blood. This process is most evident in Rh-positive babies born to Rh-negative mothers. The mother must be given a vaccine after each birth to prevent the formation of antibodies to any subsequent Rh-positive fetuses. In adult Rh-negative patients, a similar but delayed reaction can occur if Rh-positive blood is received. On receiving the second Rh-positive transfusion, a severe and potentially life-threatening reaction may occur in the patient.

IV THERAPY

As mentioned earlier, there are two major indications for IV therapy. The first is to replace fluid losses, which may occur as a result of hemorrhage caused by trauma or from severe diarrhea, vomiting, heat exhaustion, or burns. It is best to replace the fluid losses with intravenous fluids of similar isotonicity. The second is to provide a route for the administration of drugs.

There are two major classes of IV fluids: colloids and crystalloids. *Colloids* contain compounds of high molecular weight, usually proteins, which do not readily diffuse across the cell membrane. In addition, they exert *colloid osmotic pressure*, which means they tend to attract water into the intravascular space. Thus, a small amount of a colloid can be administered to a patient with a greater than expected increase in intravascular volume. This is because the colloid will draw water from the interstitial space and the intracellular compartment to increase the intravascular volume. Common examples of colloids include the following:

Plasma protein fraction (Plasmanate).   Plasmanate is a protein-containing colloid. The principal protein present is albumin, which is suspended, along with other proteins, in a saline solvent.

Salt-poor albumin.   Salt-poor albumin contains only human albumin. Each gram of albumin holds approximately 18 mL of water in the bloodstream.

Dextran.   Dextran is not a protein but a large sugar molecule with osmotic properties similar to those of albumin. It comes in two molecular weights (40,000 and 70,000 Da). Dextran 40 has 2 to 2.5 times the colloid osmotic pressure of albumin.

Hetastarch (Hespan).   Hetastarch, like dextran, is a sugar molecule with osmotic properties similar to those of protein. It does not appear to share many of dextran's side effects.

Colloid replacement therapy, at present, does not have a role in prehospital care except under rare circumstances. Colloid products are expensive and have a short shelf life.

Crystalloids contain only water and electrolytes. These substances all readily diffuse across the cell membrane. Crystalloids are the primary solutions used in prehospital intravenous fluid therapy. Because there are multiple fluid preparations, it is often helpful to classify them according to the *tonicity* related to plasma:

Isotonic solutions.   Isotonic solutions have electrolyte composition similar to that of blood plasma. When placed into a normally hydrated patient, they do not cause a significant fluid or electrolyte shift.

Hypertonic solutions.   Hypertonic solutions have a higher solute concentration than does plasma. These fluids tend to cause a fluid shift out of the intracellular compartment into the extracellular compartment when administered to a normally hydrated patient. Later, there is a diffusion of solutes in the opposite direction.

Hypotonic solutions.   Hypotonic solutions have less of a solute concentration than does plasma. When administered to a normally hydrated patient, they cause a movement of fluid from the extracellular compartment into the intracellular compartment. Later, solutes move in an opposite direction.

Paramedics choose replacement fluids based on patient needs and the patient's underlying problem. As a rule, hemorrhage occurs so fast that there is not time for a significant fluid shift between the extracellular and intracellular space. Consequently, replacement fluids are most commonly isotonic; lactated Ringer's solution and normal saline are used most often. If the patient is dehydrated because of fluid loss from diarrhea or fever, then there is a greater deficit of water than sodium. In this case, the paramedic may be asked to use hypotonic fluids such as one-half normal saline.

Some replacement fluids contain a single element, such as sodium chloride or dextrose, whereas others contain multiple elements. Solutions such as lactated Ringer's are designed so that the concentration of electrolytes is very similar to that of the plasma; they are thus referred to as *balanced salt solutions.*

Three of the most commonly used solutions in prehospital care are lactated Ringer's solution, 0.9 percent sodium chloride (normal saline), and 5 percent dextrose in water (D_5W).

Lactated Ringer's solution. Lactated Ringer's solution is an isotonic electrolyte solution. It contains sodium chloride, potassium chloride, calcium chloride, and sodium lactate in water.

Normal saline. Normal saline is an electrolyte solution containing sodium chloride in water that is isotonic with extracellular fluid.

5 percent dextrose in water. D_5W is a hypotonic glucose solution used to keep a vein open and to supply the calories necessary for cell metabolism. Although it has an initial effect of increasing the circulatory volume, glucose molecules rapidly move across the vascular membrane. The resultant free water follows almost immediately, leaving little effect on circulating blood volume.

Both lactated Ringer's solution and normal saline are used to replace fluid volume because their administration causes an immediate expansion of the circulatory volume. However, as was noted earlier, due to the movement of the electrolytes and water, two-thirds of either of these solutions is lost to the interstitial space within 1 hour. Lactated Ringer's solution is a better IV fluid than normal saline for the patient who is losing blood. However, it is not compatible with whole blood, which will most likely be given when the patient arrives at the emergency department. In aggressive fluid resuscitation, it is recommended that paramedics initiate two IV lines, one with lactated Ringer's solution and one with normal saline.

The second reason for initiating an IV infusion in the field is to provide a route for the administration of drugs. The following IV fluids are most frequently used in prehospital emergency care (see Table 5–2).

PLASMA PROTEIN FRACTION (PLASMANATE)

Class: Natural colloid

Description

Plasma protein fraction is a protein-containing colloid that is suspended in a saline solvent. The principal protein in plasma protein fraction is serum human albumin. Other proteins present include globulin and gamma globulin. Plasma protein fraction is prepared from large pools of human plasma. It is quite expensive and has a very short shelf life. Although rarely used in the prehospital phase of emergency medical care, plasma protein fraction is preferred by some emergency specialists in the management of hypovolemic states, especially burn shock. After a patient sustains a severe burn, fluid is lost from the blood into the surrounding tissue. Plasma protein fraction, because it remains in the circulating

TABLE 5–2

Approximate Ionic Concentrations (mEq/l) and Calories per Liter

	Ionic Concentrations (mEq/l)					Calories per liter	Osmolarity[a] (mOsm/l)	pH Range[b]
	Sodium	Potassium	Calcium	Chloride	Lactate			
5% Dextrose Injection, USP	0	0		0	0	170	252	3.5–6.5
10% Dextrose Injection, USP	0	0	0	0	0	340	505	3.5–6.5
0.9% Sodium Chloride Injection, USP	154	0	0	154		0	308	4.5–7.0
Sodium Lactate Injection, USP (M/6 Sodium Lactate)	167	0	0	0	167	54	334	6.0–7.3
2.5% Dextrose & 0.45% Sodium Chloride Injection, USP	77	0	0	77	0	85	280	3.5–6.0
5% Dextrose & 0.2% Sodium Chloride Injection, USP	34	0	0	34	0	170	321	3.5–6.0
5% Dextrose & 0.33% Sodium Chloride Injection, USP	56	0	0	56	0	170	365	3.5–6.0
5% Dextrose & 0.45% Sodium Chloride Injection, USP	77	0	0	77	0	170	406	3.5–6.0
5% Dextrose & 0.9% Sodium Chloride Injection, USP	154	0	0	154	0	170	560	3.5–6.0
10% Dextrose & 0.9% Sodium Chloride Injection, USP	154	0	0	154	0	340	813	3.5–6.0
Ringer's Injection, USP	147.5	4	4.5	156	0	0	309	5.0–7.5
Lactated Ringer's Injection	130	4	3	109	28	9	273	6.0–7.5
5% Dextrose in Ringer's Injection	147.5	4	4.5	156	0	170	561	3.5–6.5
Lactated Ringer's with 5% Dextrose	130	4	3	109	28	180	525	4.0–6.5

[a]Normal physiological isotonicity range is approximately 280–310 mOsm/l. Administration of substantially hypotonic solutions may cause hemolysis, and administration of substantially hypertonic solutions may cause vein damage.

[b]pH ranges are USP for applicable solution, corporate specification for non-USP solutions.

blood volume, is effective in maintaining adequate blood volume and blood pressure. It is usually used in combination with lactated Ringer's solution or normal saline.

Mechanism of Action

Plasmanate is a protein-containing colloid that remains in the intravascular compartment. It increases intravascular volume by attracting water from other fluid compartments by virtue of its colloid osmotic pressure.

Indications

Hypovolemic shock, especially burn shock
Hypoproteinemia (low protein states)

Contraindications

There are no major contraindications to plasma protein fraction when used in the treatment of life-threatening hypovolemic states.

Precautions

It is important to monitor constantly the response of the patient and adjust the rate of infusion accordingly. The patient should be monitored for elevated blood pressure and pulmonary edema during and following plasmanate administration.

Side Effects

Chills, fever, urticaria (hives), nausea, and vomiting have all been reported with plasma protein fraction use.

Dosage

The plasma protein fraction infusion rate should be titrated according to the patient's hemodynamic response. In the management of shock secondary to burns, the physician's orders regarding the rate of administration must be closely followed. Standard formulas for IV fluid administration have been developed. The medical control physician will use these formulas in judging the correct rate of intravenous administration.

Interactions

Solutions should not be mixed with or administered through the same administration sets as other intravenous fluids.

Route

Intravenous infusion

How Supplied

Plasma protein fraction is supplied in 250 and 500 bottles of a 5 percent solution. An administration set is usually attached.

DEXTRAN

Class: Artificial colloid

Description

Dextran is a colloid that differs significantly from plasma protein fraction. Instead of proteins, dextran contains chains of sugars that are approximately the same molecular weight as serum albumin. Thus, because of their large molecular size, they remain within the circulating blood volume for an extended period. Although not as effective as plasma protein fraction, dextran has proved effective as an adjunctive aid in the management of hypovolemic shock. Dextran is supplied in two molecular weights. Dextran 40 has an average molecular weight of approximately 40,000 Da. Dextran 40 is secreted by the kidneys much more readily than the higher molecular weight form, dextran 70 (molecular weight of 70,000 Da). The higher molecular weight form tends to be broken down into glucose instead of being secreted in the dextran form, as occurs with dextran 40. The decision on which type of dextran to use in prehospital care rests with the system medical director. Because dextran is excreted through the urine, urine output is usually maintained with the administration of dextran.

Mechanism of Action

Dextran is a sugar-containing colloid used as an intravascular volume expander. It remains in the intravascular compartment for approximately 12 hours. It increases intravascular volume by attracting water from other fluid compartments by virtue of its colloid osmotic pressure.

Indication

Hypovolemic shock

Contraindications

Dextran should not be administered to patients who have a known hypersensitivity to the drug. It should not be administered to patients with congestive heart failure, renal failure, or known bleeding disorders.

Precautions

A major drawback to the use of dextran is that it coats the red blood cells, thus preventing accurate blood typing and possibly hindering administration of whole blood if required. A tube of blood should be drawn before administering dextran for blood typing at the hospital.

Allergic reactions, ranging from mild to severe anaphylaxis, have been known to occur following the administration of dextran. If these occur, therapy should be immediately discontinued. In the case of mild reactions, the patient should be closely monitored, and emergency resuscitative drugs should be readily available. Severe allergic reactions may require the administration of epinephrine, diphenhydramine (Benadryl), and possibly corticosteroids. It is usually preferable to use crystalloid solutions, such as lactated Ringer's solution, rather than dextran, in the management of profound hypovolemic shock.

Side Effects

Rash, itching, dyspnea, chest tightness, and mild hypotension have all been reported with dextran use. The incidence of these side effects is very low, however, and reactions are generally mild.

Increased bleeding time has also been reported with dextran use due to its interference with platelet function.

Interactions

Dextran should not be administered to patients who are receiving anticoagulants because it significantly retards blood clotting.

Dosage

The dosage of dextran is titrated according to the patient's physiological response. In the management of burn shock, it is especially important to follow standard fluid resuscitation regimens to prevent possible circulatory overload.

Route

Intravenous infusion

How Supplied

Dextran 40 and dextran 70 are supplied in 250 and 500 mL bottles.

HETASTARCH (HESPAN)

Class: Artificial colloid

Description

Hetastarch is an artificial colloid differing from both plasma protein fraction and dextran. Hetastarch is derived from amylopectin and chemically resembles glycogen. The average molecular weight is approximately 450,000 Da, which gives it colloidal properties similar to those of human albumin. Intravenous infusion of hetastarch results in plasma volume expansion slightly greater than the amount infused.

Because the colloidal properties of hetastarch are quite similar to those of human albumin, it has proved effective in the management of hypovolemic shock, especially burn shock. It does not appear to share the blood-typing problems seen with dextran.

Mechanism of Action

Hetastarch is a starch-containing colloid used as an intravascular volume expander. Following administration, the plasma volume is expanded slightly in excess of the volume of hetastarch administered. This effect has been observed for up to 24 to 36 hours. Hetastarch increases intravascular volume by virtue of its colloid osmotic pressure.

Indications

Hypovolemic shock, especially burn shock
Septic shock

Contraindications

There are no major contraindications to hetastarch when used in the management of life-threatening hypovolemic states.

Precautions

It is important to constantly monitor the response of the patient and adjust the rate of infusion accordingly. The patient should be monitored for signs of pulmonary edema and elevated blood pressure during and following hetastarch administration.

Large volumes of hetastarch may alter the body's coagulation mechanism. Hetastarch should be used with caution in patients who are receiving anticoagulants.

Side Effects

Nausea, vomiting, mild febrile reactions, chills, itching, and urticaria (hives) have been reported with hetastarch administration. Severe anaphylactic reactions have been rarely reported.

Interactions

Hetastarch should not be administered to patients who are receiving anticoagulants.

Dosage

The hetastarch infusion rate should be titrated according to the patient's hemodynamic response. In the management of burn shock, the physician's orders regarding the rate of administration must be closely followed. Standard formulas for colloid administration to burn patients have been developed. It is important to remember that a fall in blood pressure in burn shock occurs much later than with hemorrhagic causes.

Route

Intravenous infusion

How Supplied

Sterile 6 percent hetastarch in 0.9 percent sodium chloride is supplied in 500 mL bottles.

LACTATED RINGER'S SOLUTION (HARTMANN'S SOLUTION)

Class: Isotonic crystalloid solution

Description

Lactated Ringer's solution is one of the most frequently used IV fluids in the management of hypovolemic shock. It is an isotonic crystalloid solution containing electrolytes in the following concentrations:

Sodium (Na^+) 130 mEq/L
Potassium (K^+) 4 mEq/L
Calcium (Ca^{2+}) 3 mEq/L
Chloride (Cl^-) 109 mEq/L

In addition to the electrolytes mentioned earlier, lactated Ringer's solution contains 28 mEq of lactate (lactic acid), which acts as a buffer.

Mechanism of Action

Lactated Ringer's solution replaces water and electrolytes.

Indications

Hypovolemic shock
Keep open IV

Contraindications

Lactated Ringer's solution should not be used in patients with congestive heart failure or renal failure.

Precautions

Patients receiving lactated Ringer's solution should be monitored to prevent circulatory overload.

Side Effects

Rare in therapeutic dosages

Interactions

Few in the emergency setting

Dosage

Crystalloids, such as lactated Ringer's solution, diffuse out of the intravascular space and into the surrounding tissues in less than an hour. Thus, it is often necessary to replace 1 L of lost blood with 3 to 4 L of lactated Ringer's solution.

In severe hypovolemic shock, lactated Ringer's solution should be infused through large-bore (14- or 16-gauge) IV cannulas. These infusions should be administered "wide open" until a systolic blood pressure of approximately 100 mm Hg is achieved. When this blood pressure is attained, the infusion should be reduced to about 100 mL/hr. If the blood pressure falls again, then the infusion rate should be increased and adjusted accordingly. Adjunctive devices, such as the pneumatic anti-shock garment (PASG) and extremity elevation, may be used in the management of severe hypovolemic shock.

Route

Intravenous infusion

How Supplied

Lactated Ringer's solution is supplied in 250, 500, and 1000 mL bags and bottles.

 ## 5 PERCENT DEXTROSE IN WATER (D₅W)

Class: Hypotonic dextrose-containing solution

Description

When vigorous fluid replacement is not indicated, 5 percent dextrose in water (D_5W) may be used. D_5W can be used for the administration of intravenous drugs. D_5W is hypotonic, which prevents circulatory overload in patients with congestive heart failure.

Mechanism of Action

D_5W provides nutrients in the form of dextrose as well as free water.

Indications

IV access for emergency drugs
For dilution of concentrated drugs for intravenous infusion

Contraindications

D_5W should not be used as a fluid replacement for hypovolemic states.

Precautions

Dextrose-containing solutions are acidic and may produce local venous irritation. Subcutaneous administration from extravasation may result in tissue necrosis.

As with any IV fluid, it is important to watch for signs of circulatory overload when administering D_5W.

When treating hypoglycemia, it is imperative that a tube of blood be drawn before administering D_5W or 50 percent dextrose ($D_{50}W$).

Side Effects

Rare in therapeutic dosages

Interactions

D_5W should not be used with phenytoin (Dilantin) or amrinone (Inocor).

Dosage

D_5W is usually administered through a minidrip (60 drops/mL) set at a rate of "to keep open" (TKO).

Route

Intravenous infusion

How Supplied

D_5W is supplied in bags and bottles of 50, 100, 150, 250, 500, and 1000 mL.

10 PERCENT DEXTROSE IN WATER ($D_{10}W$)

Class: Hypertonic dextrose-containing solution

Description

Ten percent dextrose in water ($D_{10}W$) is a hypertonic solution. Like D_5W, $D_{10}W$ is used only when vigorous fluid replacement is not indicated. $D_{10}W$ has twice as much carbohydrate as does D_5W, which makes it of use in the management of hypoglycemia.

Mechanism of Action

$D_{10}W$ provides nutrients in the form of dextrose as well as free water.

Indications

Neonatal resuscitation
Hypoglycemia

Contraindications

$D_{10}W$ should not be used as a fluid replacement for hypovolemic states.

Precautions

Dextrose-containing solutions are acidic and may produce local venous irritation. Subcutaneous administration from extravasation may result in tissue necrosis.
As with any IV fluid, it is important to be alert for signs of circulatory overload.
When treating hypoglycemia, it is imperative that a tube of blood be drawn before administering $D_{10}W$ or 50 percent dextrose ($D_{50}W$).

Side Effects

Rare in therapeutic dosages

Interactions

$D_{10}W$ should not be used with phenytoin (Dilantin) or amrinone (Inocor).

Dosage

The administration rate of $D_{10}W$ usually depends on the patient's condition.

Route

Intravenous infusion

How Supplied

$D_{10}W$ is supplied in bottles and bags of 50, 100, 150, 250, 500, and 1000 mL.

 # 0.9 PERCENT SODIUM CHLORIDE (NORMAL SALINE)

Class: Isotonic crystalloid solution

Description

The use of 0.9 percent sodium chloride, or normal saline (as it is often called), has several applications in emergency medicine. Normal saline contains 154 mEq/L of sodium ions (Na^+) and approximately 154 mEq/L of chloride (Cl^-) ions. Because the concentration of sodium is near that of blood, the solution is considered isotonic. Normal saline is especially useful in heat stroke, heat exhaustion, and diabetic ketoacidosis.

Mechanism of Action

Normal saline replaces water and electrolytes.

Indications

Heat-related problems (heat exhaustion, heat stroke)
Freshwater drowning
Hypovolemia
Diabetic ketoacidosis
Keep open IV

Contraindications

The use of 0.9 percent sodium chloride should not be considered in patients with congestive heart failure because circulatory overload can be easily induced.

Precautions

Normal saline contains only sodium and chloride. When large amounts of normal saline are administered, it is quite possible for other important physiological electrolytes to become depleted. In cases in which large amounts of fluids may have to be administered, it might be prudent to use lactated Ringer's solution.

Side Effects

Rare in therapeutic dosages

Interactions

Few in the emergency setting

Dosage

The specific situation being treated dictates the rate at which normal saline is administered. In severe heat stroke, diabetic ketoacidosis, and freshwater drowning, it is quite likely that paramedics will be called on to administer the fluid quite rapidly. In other cases, it is advisable to administer the fluid at a moderate rate (e.g., 100 mL/hr).

Route

Intravenous infusion

How Supplied

Normal saline is supplied in 250, 500, and 1000 mL bags and bottles. Sterile normal saline for irrigation should not be confused with that designed for intravenous administration.

 ## 0.45 PERCENT SODIUM CHLORIDE (ONE-HALF NORMAL SALINE)

Class: Hypotonic crystalloid solution

Description

One-half normal saline (0.45 percent sodium chloride) solution is a hypotonic crystalloid solution containing approximately one-half the concentration of sodium and chloride as does blood plasma.

Mechanism of Action

One-half normal saline replaces free water and electrolytes.

Indication

Patients with diminished renal or cardiovascular function for whom rapid rehydration is not indicated

Contraindications

Cases in which rapid rehydration is indicated

Precautions

One-half normal saline contains only sodium and chloride. When large amounts of one-half normal saline are administered, it is possible for other important physiological electrolytes to become depleted. In cases in which large amounts of fluids must be administered, it might be prudent to use lactated Ringer's solution.

Side Effects

Rare in therapeutic dosages

Interactions

Few in the emergency setting

Dosage

The specific situation and patient condition dictate the rate at which one-half normal saline is administered.

Route

Intravenous infusion

How Supplied

One-half normal saline is supplied in 250, 500, and 1000 mL bags and bottles.

5 PERCENT DEXTROSE IN 0.45 PERCENT SODIUM CHLORIDE (D$_5$1/2NS)

Class: Hypertonic dextrose-containing crystalloid solution

Description

Five percent dextrose in 0.45 percent sodium chloride (D$_5$1/2NS) is a versatile fluid. It contains the same amount of sodium and chloride as does one-half normal saline. Dextrose has been added for its nutrient properties, providing 80 calories per liter.

Mechanism of Action

D$_5$1/2NS replaces free water and electrolytes and provides nutrients in the form of dextrose.

Indications

Heat exhaustion
Diabetic disorders
For use as a TKO solution in patients with impaired renal or cardiovascular function

Contraindication

D$_5$1/2NS should not be used when rapid fluid resuscitation is indicated.

Precautions

Dextrose-containing solutions are acidic and may produce local venous irritation. Subcutaneous administration from extravasation may result in tissue necrosis.

As with any IV fluid, it is important to watch for signs of circulatory overload when administering D$_5$1/2NS.

When treating hypoglycemia, it is imperative that a tube of blood be drawn before administering D$_5$1/2NS or 50 percent dextrose (D$_{50}$W).

Side Effects

Rare in therapeutic dosages

Interactions

D$_5$1/2NS should not be used with phenytoin (Dilantin) or amrinone (Inocor).

Dosage

The specific situation and patient condition dictate the rate at which D$_5$1/2NS should be administered.

Route

Intravenous infusion

How Supplied

D$_5$1/2NS is supplied in bottles and bags containing 250, 500, and 1000 mL of the fluid.

5 PERCENT DEXTROSE IN 0.9 PERCENT SODIUM CHLORIDE (D$_5$NS)

Class: Hypertonic dextrose-containing crystalloid solution

Description

Five percent dextrose in 0.9 percent normal saline is a hypertonic crystalloid to which 5 g of dextrose per 100 mL of fluid has been added for its nutrient properties.

Mechanism of Action

D$_5$NS replaces free water and electrolytes and provides nutrients in the form of dextrose.

Indications

Heat-related disorders
Freshwater drowning
Hypovolemia
Peritonitis

Contraindications

D$_5$NS should not be administered to patients with impaired cardiac or renal function.

Precautions

Dextrose-containing solutions are acidic and may produce local venous irritation. Subcutaneous administration from extravasation may result in tissue necrosis.

D$_5$NS contains only the electrolytes sodium and chloride. When large amounts of fluids must be administered, it might be prudent to use lactated Ringer's solution to prevent depletion of the other physiological electrolytes.

When treating hypoglycemia, it is imperative that a tube of blood be drawn before administering D$_5$NS or 50 percent dextrose (D$_{50}$W).

Side Effects

Rare in therapeutic dosages

Interactions

D_5NS should not be used with phenytoin (Dilantin) or amrinone (Inocor).

Dosage

The specific situation and patient condition dictate the rate at which D_5NS is given.

Route

Intravenous infusion

How Supplied

D_5NS is supplied in bags and bottles containing 250, 500, and 1000 mL of the solution.

 ## 5 PERCENT DEXTROSE IN LACTATED RINGER'S SOLUTION (D_5LR)

Class: Hypertonic dextrose-containing crystalloid solution

Description

Five percent dextrose in lactated Ringer's solution (D_5LR) contains the same concentration of electrolytes as does lactated Ringer's solution. In addition to the electrolytes, however, 5 g of dextrose per 100 mL of fluid has been added for nutrient properties. This added dextrose causes the solution to be hypertonic.

Mechanism of Action

D_5LR replaces water and electrolytes and provides nutrients in the form of dextrose.

Indications

Hypovolemic shock
Hemorrhagic shock
Certain cases of acidosis

Contraindications

D_5LR should not be administered to patients with decreased renal or cardiovascular function.

Precautions

Patients receiving D_5LR should be constantly monitored for signs of circulatory overload. It is essential that a blood sample be drawn before administering D_5LR to patients with hypoglycemia.

Dextrose-containing solutions are acidic and may produce local venous irritation. Subcutaneous administration from extravasation may result in tissue necrosis.

Side Effects

Rare in therapeutic dosages

Interactions

D_5LR should not be used with phenytoin (Dilantin) or amrinone (Inocor).

Dosage

In severe hypovolemic shock, D_5LR should be infused through a large-bore catheter (14 or 16 gauge). This infusion should be administered "wide open" until a blood pressure of 100 mm Hg is achieved. When the blood pressure is attained, the infusions should be reduced to 100 mL/hr. In other cases, the specific situation and patient condition dictate the rate of administration.

Route

Intravenous infusion

How Supplied

D_5LR is supplied in bags and bottles containing 250, 500, and 1000 mL of the fluid.

INSERTION OF INDWELLING IV CATHETER

One of the earliest stages in the management of an acutely ill or injured patient is the placement of an IV catheter. In trauma cases an IV catheter provides access for fluid resuscitation, whereas in medical disorders it provides a route for drugs that must be given intravenously.

Before inserting an IV catheter, several decisions must be made to ensure the best possible care for the patient. They are as follows:

1. What Size Catheter Should Be Inserted?

When managing patients with trauma who require rapid fluid administration, it is imperative that a large catheter, 16 gauge, be inserted. It is important to remember that patients who are likely to need whole blood on arrival at the hospital require a large-bore catheter. (18 gauge or larger). Medical patients may receive an 18 or 20 gauge catheter.

2. What Type of IV Catheter Should Be Inserted?

As a rule, an over-the-needle catheter is all that should be used in the prehospital setting. Butterfly catheters are usually too small to administer large amounts of fluids rapidly. Butterfly catheters should be carried for use in children, however. Occasionally, an adult with exceptionally small veins may be encountered, and, in this case, a butterfly catheter may be inserted if one of the other types of catheters cannot be placed.

3. What Type of IV Fluid Should Be Used?

Usually, the decision of what type of IV fluid to use is left up to the base station physician or written in the protocols. It is important to be familiar with the types of fluids that have been discussed in this chapter.

4. What Type of Administration Set Should Be Used?

There are two general types of IV administration sets. The macrodrip, or standard, set delivers in the neighborhood of 10 to 20 gtt/mL, depending on the manufacturer. Minidrip, or microdrip, sets deliver anywhere from 50 to 60 gtt/mL, depending on the manufacturer. If a large quantity of fluids will be administered, then a macrodrip set should be used. Whenever a paramedic is going to administer a drug, he or she should use a minidrip set. This is especially true for piggyback drug infusions. Many systems also use Buretrol or Volutrol sets for administering aminophylline and similar drugs. If these sets are used, paramedics should remember them when preparing to administer drugs such as aminophylline.

5. Where Should the IV Be Inserted?

Routinely, IV infusions should be started in the larger veins of the forearm. These are usually the most accessible and the least painful for the patient. When these veins are not available, as often occurs in shock and trauma, then any of the other peripheral sites should be attempted.

The veins of the leg and the external jugular in the neck are considered peripheral veins. When treating medical or traumatic emergencies, the rule of thumb for starting an intravenous infusion is "any port in a storm." In a cardiac/traumatic arrest, the antecubital vein is a preferred site.

Procedure for Intravenous Cannulation

Once these five decisions have been made, then the actual procedure of inserting the IV can begin. The procedure is as follows:

1. Observe body substance isolation precautions.
2. Receive the order.
3. Confirm the order and write it down.
4. Prepare the equipment and don gloves and protective eyewear:
   a. Appropriate IV fluid
   b. Appropriate administration set
   c. Appropriate indwelling catheter
   d. Extension IV tubing
   e. Tourniquet
   f. Antibiotic swab

g. 2 × 2 gauze pad

h. 1-inch tape

i. Antibiotic ointment

j. Short arm board

5. Remove the envelope from the IV fluid.

6. Inspect the fluid, making sure that it is not discolored and does not contain any particulate matter; check that it contains the amount of fluid it should have. Do not administer if discolored, if particles are present, or if less than the indicated quantity of fluid is present.

7. Open and inspect the IV tubing.

8. Attach the extension tubing.

9. Close the clamp on the tubing.

10. Remove the sterile cover from the IV fluid and the administration set.

11. Insert the administration set into the IV fluid.

12. Squeeze the drip chamber to fill it with fluid.

13. Bleed all of the air out of the IV tubing.

14. Hang the bag on an IV pole (or have a bystander hold it) at the appropriate height.

15. Place the tourniquet on the patient to occlude venous flow only.

16. Select a suitable vein and palpate it (see Figures 5–6 and 5–7).

17. Prepare the site by cleansing it with an antibiotic swab.

18. Make the puncture using appropriate sterile technique, enter the vein, observe flashback, and advance the catheter (see Figures 5–8 through 5–10).

19. Connect the IV tubing and remove tourniquet.

20. Slowly open the valve.

21. Confirm that the fluid is flowing appropriately without any evidence of infiltration.

22. Apply an antibiotic ointment over the puncture and cover with a sterile 2 × 2 gauze pad or adhesive bandage.

23. Securely tape the IV catheter and tubing down.

24. Adjust the flow rate.

25. Apply a short arm board.

26. Label the IV bag with the patient's name, date, time the IV was initiated, gauge of the catheter, and your initials.

27. Confirm with medical control the successful completion of the IV.

28. Monitor the patient for the desired effects and any undesired ones as well.

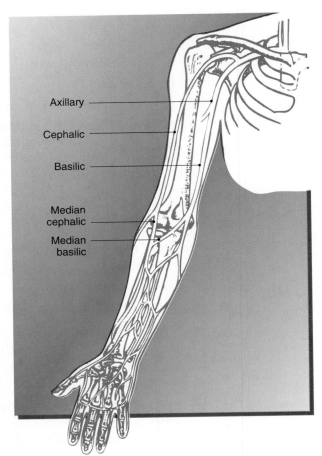

Axillary ————

Cephalic ————

Basilic ————

Median
cephalic ————

Median
basilic ————

FIGURE 5–6 Veins of the arm.

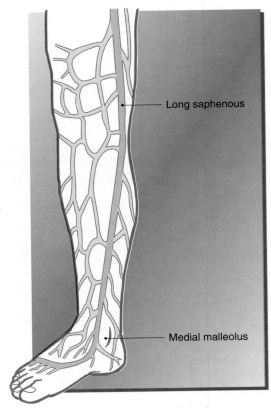

Long saphenous

Medial malleolus

FIGURE 5–7 Veins of the leg.

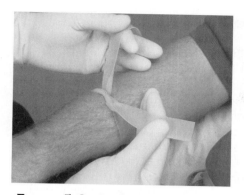

FIGURE 5-8 Apply the tourniquet.

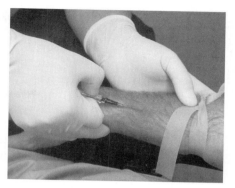

FIGURE 5-9 Puncture the skin.

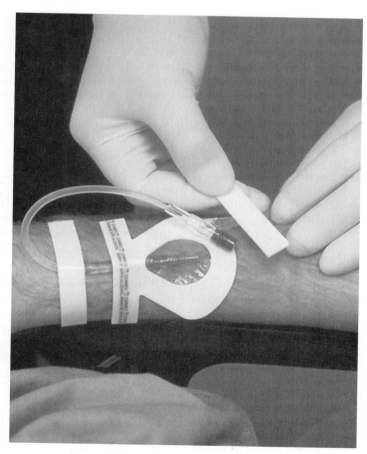

FIGURE 5-10 Securing the catheter.

COLLECTION OF BLOOD SAMPLES FOR LABORATORY ANALYSIS

Prehospital personnel may be required to obtain blood samples in the field for later laboratory analysis. Although this practice was more common in the past, there are still instances in which this practice is important. There are several advantages to obtaining blood samples in the field.

First, it provides the emergency department physician with information about the patient before medical intervention. This information is especially important in cases of suspected hypoglycemia when 50 percent dextrose is administered (although electronic glucometers are very accurate and thus the need for blood samples prior to glucose administration is diminishing). In situations in which a patient may be trapped or transport to the hospital is otherwise delayed, blood samples can be taken to the hospital before the patient so that blood can be typed, cross-matched, and ready when the patient eventually arrives in the emergency department. Whenever a prehospital intervention might affect the subsequent care of the patient (e.g., administering dextran, which may inhibit blood typing), the paramedic should always draw a blood sample according to local protocol.

Most commonly, blood samples are taken when an IV is started. The paramedic should always follow universal precautions when caring for a patient and especially when handling a blood sample. Gloves and goggles should be worn. After placing the IV catheter and before connecting the IV line, a 10 mL syringe can be attached to the catheter and blood gently withdrawn from the vein. The syringe can be removed and the IV line connected. It is important to withdraw the blood from the syringe slowly. Withdrawing it rapidly can damage the blood cells, causing them to rupture and leak their contents, which in turn can erroneously alter the blood chemistries and render the sample useless.

Once blood is withdrawn from a patient, it is usually placed into evacuated blood collection tubes (Vacutainer). These tubes have a vacuum that allows the tube to fill with a predetermined amount of blood. Most tubes contain a chemical to keep the blood from clotting. Each tube has a different colored rubber top, depending on its use and contents. The type of tube a paramedic may be asked to draw may vary from region to region. After withdrawing the blood as described earlier, an 18-gauge needle is placed on the syringe. The needle is inserted into the rubber top and the tube is allowed to fill with blood. The paramedic should not attempt to overfill the tube or press on the plunger of the syringe, but allow the vacuum to fill the vial.

After the vials are filled, they should be inverted several times to mix the blood and the anticoagulant. The patient's name, date, time drawn, paramedic's name, and incident number (if any) are immediately written on the vial. The tubes are given to the appropriate emergency department personnel on arrival. The paramedic documents on the patient report form the time the blood was drawn and to whom it was given. At critical scenes, labelling tubes may be difficult. As an alternative until tubes can be labelled, tape the tubes to the IV bag.

BLOOD TRANSFUSIONS

When mismatched blood is transfused, the donor's antibodies can bind to antigens on the recipient's red blood cells (RBCs). This reaction, known as a transfusion reaction, causes clumping of RBCs in the blood (agglutination) and subsequent hemolysis (RBCs breaking apart). Transfusion reaction can only be prevented by complete and careful type matching between donor and recipient.

Paramedics occasionally transport a patient receiving blood. These patients need careful monitoring for signs and symptoms of transfusion reaction. The severity of the reaction depends on the degree of incompatibility, the amount of blood given, and the rate of administration. Onset is usually rapid, either during or immediately after a transfusion. More rarely, it occurs later. Signs and symptoms include anxiety; facial flushing; pain in the neck, chest, and lumbar area; tachycardia; cold, clammy skin; hypotension; nausea or vomiting; dizziness; hives; headaches; and fever.

When signs and symptoms of transfusion reaction appear, the transfusion should be discontinued immediately. A physician should be consulted as soon as possible and a crystalloid infusion for drug administrations maintained. A diuretic such as mannitol (Osmitrol) and an antihistamine such as diphenhydramine (Benadryl) may be indicated. One of the most lethal effects of transfusion reaction is kidney shutdown, which can begin within a few minutes to a few hours and may progress to lethal renal failure.

SUMMARY

As with the skills of medication administration, the insertion of an IV requires vigorous mannequin, classroom, and clinical training under the supervision of a qualified instructor.

KEY WORDS

colloid. A substance of high molecular weight, such as plasma proteins. Colloids tend to remain in the intravascular space, as opposed to crystalloids, which tend to diffuse out.

crystalloid. A solution containing crystalline substances, such as normal saline.

diffusion. The movement of solute (substances dissolved in a solution) from an area of greater concentration to an area of lesser concentration.

electrolytes. A chemical substance that dissociates into charged particles when placed in water.

erythrocytes. Red blood cells; responsible for transport of oxygen.

extracellular. The space outside the cell membrane.

hematocrit. A measure of the number of red blood cells found in the blood, stated as a percentage of the total blood volume.

homeostasis. The body's natural tendency to keep the natural environment constant.

hypertonic. A state in which a solution has a higher solute concentration on one side of a semipermeable membrane than on the other side.

hypotonic. A state in which a solution has a lower solute concentration on one side of a semipermeable membrane than on the other side.

intracellular. The space and materials within the cell membrane.

intravascular. The space within the blood vessels.

isotonic. A state in which solutions on opposite sides of a semipermeable membrane are equal in concentration.

leukocytes. White blood cells; responsible for fighting infection.

osmosis. The movement of a solvent (water) across a semipermeable membrane from an area of lesser (solute) concentration to an area of greater (solute) concentration; osmosis is a form of diffusion.

semipermeable membrane. A specialized biological membrane, such as that which encloses the body's cells, that allows passage of certain substances and restricts the passage of others.

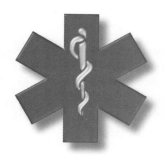

chapter 6

THE AUTONOMIC NERVOUS SYSTEM

OBJECTIVES

After completing this chapter, the reader should be able to

1. Describe the anatomy and physiology of the autonomic nervous system.
2. Compare sympathetic and parasympathetic actions.
3. Explain the function of the sympathetic nervous system.
4. List the four adrenergic receptors and explain the effect of each one on body organs.
5. Explain the function of the parasympathetic nervous system.

INTRODUCTION

The autonomic nervous system is a part of the peripheral nervous system and is responsible for control of involuntary, or visceral, bodily functions. It controls crucial cardiovascular, respiratory, digestive, urinary, and reproductive functions. It also plays a key role in the body's response to stress.

Many of the medications used in emergency care act directly or indirectly on the autonomic nervous system. Thus, it is essential that prehospital personnel have a good understanding of the structure and function of the autonomic nervous system. This chapter discusses the anatomy and physiology of the autonomic nervous system as it applies to emergency pharmacological therapy.

The *nervous system* is the body's principal control system. It regulates virtually all bodily functions via electrical impulses transmitted through nerves. Closely related to the nervous system is the *endocrine system*. Like the nervous system, the endocrine system is an important control system. However, unlike the nervous system, it exerts its effect on the body through the release of specialized chemical substances called *hormones*.

The nervous system is customarily divided into the central nervous system and the peripheral nervous system. The *central nervous system (CNS)* consists of the brain and spinal cord. In contrast, the *peripheral nervous system (PNS)* is composed of the cranial nerves and the peripheral nerves. The peripheral nervous system can be further divided into the somatic nervous system and the autonomic nervous system. The *somatic nervous system (SNS)* controls voluntary motor functions such as movement. The *autonomic nervous system (ANS)* controls involuntary automatic functions (see Figure 6–1).

The two functional divisions of the autonomic nervous system are the sympathetic nervous system and the parasympathetic nervous system. The *sympathetic nervous system* allows the body to function under stress. It is often referred to as the *fight-or-flight* aspect of the nervous system. The *parasympathetic nervous system*, on the other hand, primarily controls vegetative functions such as digestion of food. It is often referred to as the *feed-or-breed* or *rest-and-repose* aspect of the autonomic nervous system. The parasympathetic nervous system is in constant opposition to the sympathetic nervous system (see Table 6–1).

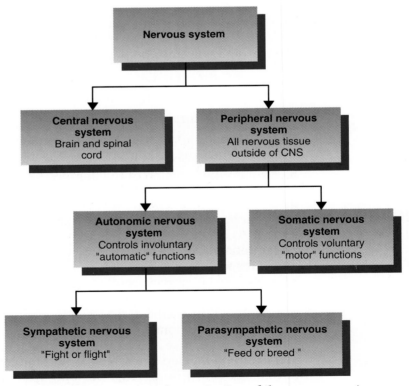

FIGURE 6–1 Functional organization of the nervous system.

TABLE 6–1

Comparison of Sympathetic and Parasympathetic Actions

Organ	Sympathetic stimulation	Parasympathetic stimulation
Heart	Increased rate	Decreased rate
	Increased contractile force	Decreased contractile force
Lungs	Bronchodilation	Bronchoconstriction
Kidneys	Decreased output	No change
Systemic blood vessels		
Abdominal	Constricted	None
Muscle	Constricted α	None
	Dilated β	None
Skin	Constricted	None
Liver	Glucose release	Slight glycogen synthesis
Blood glucose	Increased	None
Pupils	Dilated	Constricted
Sweat glands	Copious sweating	None
Basal metabolism	Increased up to 100%	None
Skeletal muscle	Increased strength	None

Autonomic Nervous System Anatomy and Physiology

The autonomic nervous system arises from the central nervous system. The nerves of the autonomic nervous system exit the central nervous system and subsequently enter specialized structures called *autonomic ganglia*. In the autonomic ganglia, the nerve fibers from the central nervous system interact with nerve fibers that extend from the ganglia to the various target organs. Autonomic nerve fibers that exit the central nervous system and terminate in the autonomic ganglia are called *preganglionic nerves*. Autonomic nerve fibers that exit the ganglia and terminate in the various target tissues are called *postganglionic nerves*. The ganglia of the sympathetic nervous system are located close to the spinal cord, whereas the ganglia of the parasympathetic nervous system are located close to the target organs (see Figure 6–2).

No actual physical connection exists between two nerve cells or between a nerve cell and the organ it innervates. Instead, there is a space between nerve cells called a *synapse*. The space between a nerve cell and the target organ is called a *neuroeffector junction*. Specialized chemicals called *neurotransmitters* are used to conduct the nervous impulse between nerve cells or between a nerve cell and its target organ. Neurotransmitters are released from presynaptic neurons and subsequently act on postsynaptic neurons or on the designated target organ. When released by the nerve ending, the neurotransmitter travels across the synapse and activates membrane receptors on the adjoining nerve or target tissue. The neurotransmitter is then either deactivated or taken back up into the presynaptic neuron. The primary neurotransmitters of the autonomic nervous system are *acetylcholine* and *norepinephrine*. Acetylcholine is utilized in the preganglionic nerves of the sympathetic nervous system and in both the preganglionic and postganglionic nerves of the parasympathetic nervous system. Norepinephrine is the primary postganglionic neurotransmitter of the sympathetic nervous system. Synapses that use acetylcholine as the neurotransmitter are called *cholinergic* synapses. Synapses that use norepinephrine as the neurotransmitter are called *adrenergic* synapses.

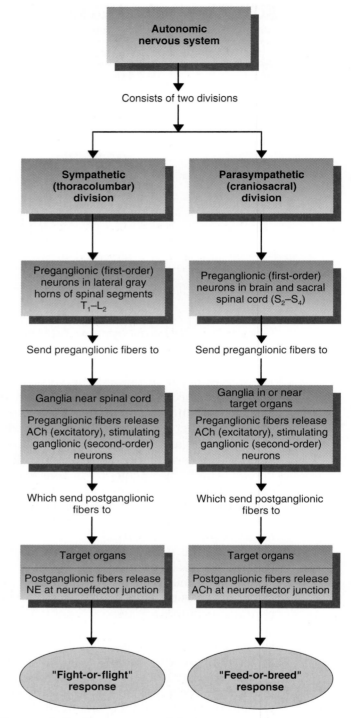

FIGURE 6-2 Components of the autonomic nervous system.

The Sympathetic Nervous System

The sympathetic nervous system arises from the thoracic and lumbar region of the spinal cord. Preganglionic nerves leave the spinal cord through the spinal nerves and end in the sympathetic ganglia. There are two types of sympathetic ganglia: sympathetic chain ganglia and collateral ganglia (see Figure 6–3). In addition, special preganglionic sympathetic nerve fibers innervate the adrenal medulla. Postganglionic nerves that exit the *sympathetic chain ganglia* extend to several peripheral target tissues of the sympathetic nervous system. When stimulated, these fibers have several effects, including the following:

- Stimulation of secretion by sweat glands
- Constriction of blood vessels in the skin
- Increase in blood flow to skeletal muscles
- Increase in heart rate and in the force of cardiac contractions
- Bronchodilation
- Stimulation of energy production

The *collateral ganglia* are located in the abdominal cavity. Nerves leaving the collateral ganglia innervate many of the organs of the abdomen. Stimulation of these fibers causes the following:

- Reduction of blood flow to abdominal organs
- Decreased digestive activity
- Relaxation of smooth muscle in the wall of the urinary bladder
- Release of glucose stores from the liver

Sympathetic nervous system stimulation also results in direct stimulation of the *adrenal medulla*. The adrenal medulla in turn releases the hormones *norepinephrine* (noradrenalin) and *epinephrine* (adrenalin) into the circulatory system. Approximately 80 percent of the hormones released by the adrenal medulla are epinephrine, with norepinephrine constituting the remaining 20 percent. Once released, these hormones are carried throughout the body, where they cause their intended effects by acting on hormone receptors. The release of norepinephrine and epinephrine by the adrenal medulla stimulates tissues that are not innervated by sympathetic nerves. In addition, it prolongs the effects of direct sympathetic stimulation. All of these effects serve to prepare the body to deal with stressful and potentially dangerous situations.

Adrenergic Receptors

Sympathetic stimulation ultimately results in the release of norepinephrine from postganglionic nerves. It subsequently crosses the synapse and interacts with adrenergic receptors. Shortly thereafter, the norepinephrine is taken up by the presynaptic neuron for reuse or is broken down by enzymes present within the synapse (see Figure 6–4). Sympathetic stimulation also results in the release of epinephrine and norepinephrine from the adrenal medulla. Both epinephrine and norepinephrine also interact with specialized receptors on the membranes of the target organs. These receptors, called *adrenergic receptors,* are located throughout the body. Once

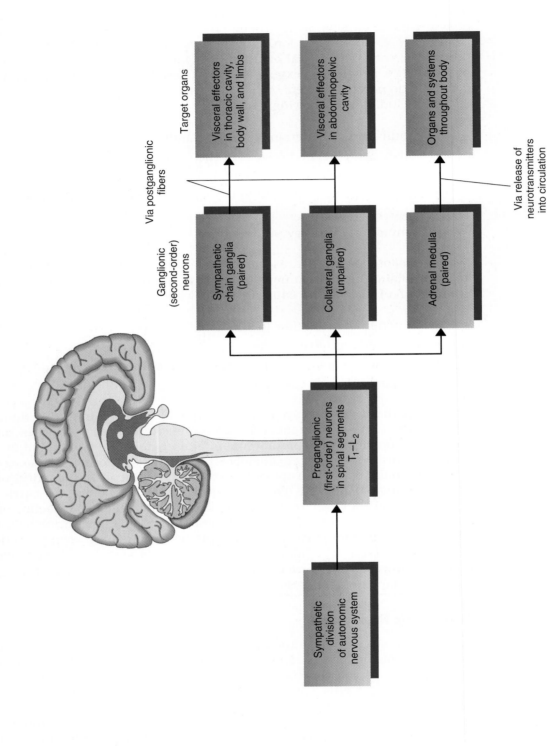

FIGURE 6–3 Organization of the sympathetic division of the autonomic nervous system.

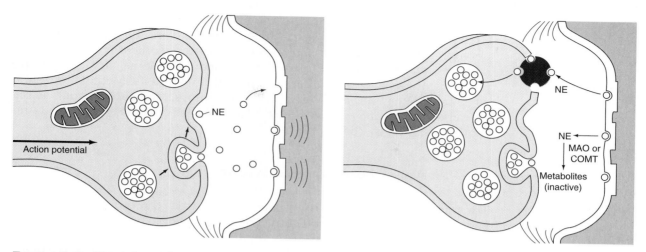

FIGURE 6–4 Physiology of an adrenergic synapse. Norepinephrine is released from the presynaptic nerve and stimulates receptors on the postsynaptic nerve. Subsequently, the norepinephrine is either taken up by the presynaptic nerve or deactivated by enzymes present in the synapse.

stimulated by the appropriate hormone, they cause a response in the organ or organs they control.

The two known types of sympathetic receptors are the adrenergic receptors and the dopaminergic receptors. The adrenergic receptors are generally divided into four types. These four receptors are designated *alpha₁* (α_1), *alpha₂* (α_2), *beta₁* (β_1), and *beta₂* (β_2). The α_1-receptors cause peripheral vasoconstriction, mild bronchoconstriction, and stimulation of metabolism. The α_2-receptors are found on the *presynaptic* surfaces of sympathetic neuroeffector junctions. Stimulation of α_2-receptors is inhibitory. They serve to prevent overrelease of norepinephrine in the synapse. When the level of norepinephrine in the synapse gets high enough, the α_2-receptors are stimulated and norepinephrine release is inhibited. Stimulation of β_1-receptors causes an increase in heart rate, cardiac contractile force, and cardiac automaticity and conduction. Stimulation of β_2-receptors causes vasodilation and bronchodilation (see Table 6–2). *Dopaminergic receptors*, although not fully understood, are believed to cause dilation of the renal, coronary, and cerebral arteries.

TABLE 6–2

Actions of the Adrenergic Receptors

Receptor	Actions
alpha₁ (α_1)	Peripheral vasoconstriction
	Increased contractile force (positive inotropic effect)
	Decreased heart rate (negative chronotropic effect)
alpha₂ (α_2)	Peripheral vasoconstriction (by limiting norepinephrine release)
beta₁ (β_1)	Increased heart rate (positive chronotropic effect)
	Increased contractile force (positive inotropic effect)
	Increased automaticity (positive dromotropic effect)
beta₂ (β_2)	Peripheral vasodilation
	Bronchodilation
	Uterine smooth muscle relaxation
	Gastrointestinal smooth muscle relaxation
Dopaminergic	Renal vasodilation
	Mesenteric vasodilation

Medications that stimulate the sympathetic nervous system are referred to as *sympathomimetics*. Medications that inhibit the sympathetic nervous system are called *sympatholytics*. Some medications are pure α-*agonists*, whereas others are pure α-*antagonists*. Some medications are pure β-agonists, whereas others are pure β-antagonists. Medications such as epinephrine stimulate both α- and β-receptors. Medications such as the bronchodilators are termed β selective, because they act more on β_2-receptors than on β_1-receptors.

The Parasympathetic Nervous System

The parasympathetic nervous system arises from the brain stem and the sacral segments of the spinal cord. The preganglionic neurons are typically much longer than those of the sympathetic nervous system because the ganglia are located close to the target tissues. Parasympathetic nerve fibers that leave the brain stem travel within four of the cranial nerves including the oculomotor nerve (III), the facial nerve (VII), the glossopharyngeal nerve (IX), and the vagus nerve (X). These fibers synapse in the *parasympathetic ganglia* with short postganglionic fibers, which then continue to their target tissues. Postsynaptic fibers innervate much of the body including the intrinsic eye muscles, the salivary glands, the heart, the lungs, and most of the organs of the abdominal cavity. The sacral segment of the parasympathetic nervous system forms distinct pelvic nerves that innervate ganglia in the kidneys, bladder, sex organs, and terminal portions of the large intestine (see Figure 6–5). Stimulation of the parasympathetic nervous system results in the following:

- Pupillary constriction
- Secretion by digestive glands
- Increased smooth muscle activity along the digestive tract
- Bronchoconstriction
- Reduction in heart rate and cardiac contractile force

Through these and other functions, the processing of food, energy absorption, relaxation, and reproduction are facilitated.

All preganglionic and postganglionic parasympathetic nerve fibers use *acetylcholine* as a neurotransmitter. Acetylcholine, when released by presynaptic neurons, crosses the synaptic cleft and activates receptors on the postsynaptic neuron or on the neuroeffector junction. Acetylcholine is also the neurotransmitter for the somatic nervous system and is present in the *neuromuscular junction*. Acetylcholine is very short-lived. Within a fraction of a second after its release, acetylcholine is deactivated by another chemical called *acetylcholinesterase*. *Acetic acid* and *choline*, which are produced when acetylcholine is deactivated, are taken back up by the presynaptic neuron (see Figure 6–6).

The emergency medication atropine is an antagonist to the parasympathetic nervous system and is used to increase heart rate. Atropine binds with acetylcholine receptors, thus preventing acetylcholine from exerting its effect. Medications such as atropine, which block the actions of the parasympathetic nervous system, are referred to as *parasympatholytics* or anticholinergics. Medications that stimulate the parasympathetic nervous system are referred to as *parasympathomimetics*.

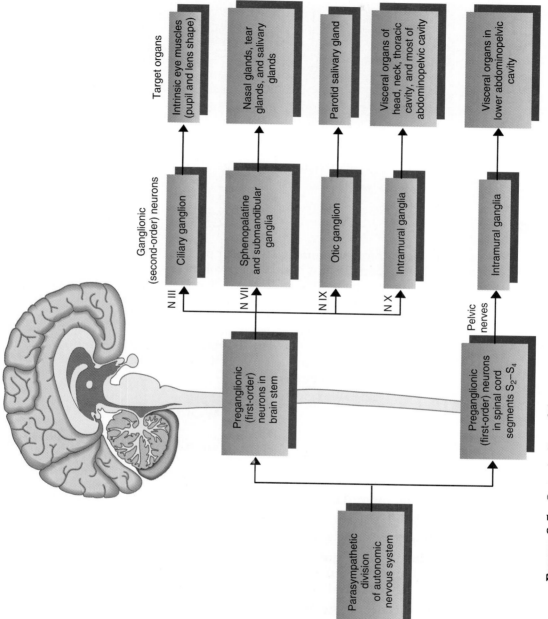

FIGURE 6-5 Organization of the parasympathetic division of the autonomic nervous system.

123

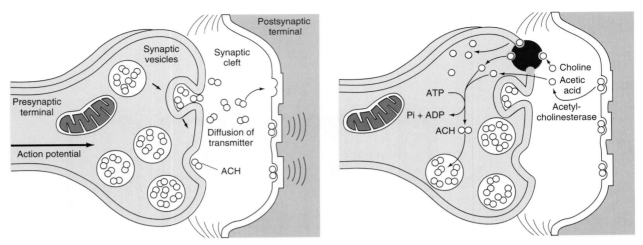

FIGURE 6-6 Physiology of a cholinergic synapse. Acetylcholine is released from the presynaptic nerve and stimulates receptors on the postsynaptic nerve. Subsequently, the acetylcholine is broken down by acetylcholinesterase and the products are taken up by the presynaptic nerve fiber.

SUMMARY

The autonomic nervous system is a part of the peripheral nervous system and is responsible for control of involuntary, or visceral, bodily functions. It maintains the body's internal environment by controlling crucial cardiovascular, respiratory, digestive, urinary, and reproductive functions. It also plays a key role in the body's response to stress.

Because many of the medications used in prehospital care act directly or indirectly on the autonomic nervous system, it is essential that prehospital personnel have a good understanding of the structure and function of the autonomic nervous system.

KEY WORDS

acetylcholine (ach).   Chemical neurotransmitter found in all autonomic preganglionic synapses and in parasympathetic postganglionic synapses.

adrenal medulla.   An endocrine gland, located atop the kidney, that manufactures and secretes epinephrine and norepinephrine.

adrenergic.   Related to or pertaining to the sympathetic nervous system.

alpha$_1$ adrenergic receptor.   A type of adrenergic receptor that, when stimulated, causes peripheral vasoconstriction, mild bronchoconstriction, and stimulation of metabolism.

alpha$_2$ adrenergic receptor.   A type of adrenergic receptor that, when stimulated, inhibits parts of the sympathetic nervous system. It serves to prevent the overrelease of norepinephrine in the synapse.

autonomic nervous system (ANS).   Part of the peripheral nervous system responsible for control of involuntary, or visceral, bodily functions.

beta$_1$ adrenergic receptor.   A type of adrenergic receptor that, when stimulated, causes an increase in heart rate, cardiac contractile force, and cardiac automaticity and conduction.

beta$_2$ adrenergic receptor. A type of adrenergic receptor that, when stimulated, causes vasodilation and bronchodilation.

bronchodilator. A drug that helps to improve breathing by relaxing the smooth muscle of the bronchioles, causing bronchodilation.

central nervous system (CNS). The central portion of the nervous system, consisting of the brain and spinal cord.

cholinergic. Related to or pertaining to the parasympathetic nervous system.

chronotrope. A drug or other substance that affects heart rate.

dromotrope. A drug or other substance that affects nerve conduction.

epinephrine. A naturally occurring hormone that stimulates the adrenal glands, increases cardiac output, and causes bronchodilation.

ganglia. A mass of nerve cells.

inotrope. A drug or other substance that affects the strength of the cardiac contraction.

neurotransmitter. A substance that is released from the axon terminal of a presynaptic neuron. On excitation it travels across the synaptic cleft to either excite or inhibit the target cell. Examples include acetylcholine, norepinephrine, and dopamine.

norepinephrine. A naturally occurring hormone that also serves as a sympathetic neurotransmitter. It is found in most postganglionic synapses.

parasympathetic nervous system. The division of the autonomic nervous system that is responsible for controlling vegetative functions.

peripheral nervous system. The portion of the nervous system outside the brain and spinal cord. It is composed of the cranial nerves and peripheral nerves.

somatic nervous system (SNS). The portion of the nervous system that controls voluntary motor functions such as movement.

sympathetic nervous system. The division of the autonomic nervous system that prepares the body for stressful situations.

sympatholytic (or antiadrenergic). Drugs that block beta adrenergic receptors and slow the heart rate.

sympathomimetic. A drug or other substance that causes effects such as those of the sympathetic nervous system (also called adrenergic).

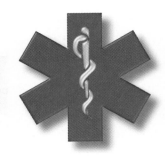

chapter 7

Drugs Used in the Treatment of Cardiovascular Emergencies

7. Describe digitalis and list the indications, contraindications, and dosages for its use.

8. Discuss the use of thrombolytics and aspirin in the treatment of myocardial infarction.

9. Describe and list the indications, contraindications, and dosages for aspirin and the thrombolytic agents streptokinase, anistreplase, and tissue plasminogen activator.

10. List the indications, contraindications, and dosages for sodium bicarbonate.

11. Explain the indications, contraindications, and dosages for morphine and nitrous oxide in the treatment of cardiac chest pain.

12. Discuss the use of diuretics in the management of congestive heart failure.

13. List the indications, contraindications, and dosages for the diuretics furosemide and bumetanide.

14. Describe the action of nitroglycerin in cardiac chest pain.

15. List the indications, contraindications, and dosages for the antianginal agents nitroglycerin, nitroglycerin spray, and nitroglycerin paste.

16. Define and explain a hypertensive crisis.

17. List the indications, contraindications, and dosages for the antihypertensives nifedipine, sodium nitroprusside, diazoxide, and hydralazine.

18. List the indications, contraindications, and dosages for calcium chloride.

INTRODUCTION

Most prehospital emergency drugs are used in the treatment of cardiac emergencies. These drugs, because of the nature of their actions, may be accompanied by many side effects. Some general classifications follow for our discussion of the emergency cardiovascular drugs:

Gases

Oxygen

Sympathomimetics

Epinephrine

Norepinephrine (Levophed)

Isoproterenol (Isuprel)

Dopamine (Intropin)

Dobutamine (Dobutrex)

Metaraminol (Aramine)

Amrinone (Inocor)

Sympathetic Blockers

Propranolol (Inderal)

Metoprolol (Lopressor)

Labetalol (Trandate, Normodyne)

Esmolol (Brevibloc)

Antiarrhythmics
Lidocaine (Xylocaine)
Procainamide (Pronestyl)
Bretylium tosylate (Bretylol)
Adenosine (Adenocard)
Verapamil (Isoptin, Calan)
Diltiazem (Cardizem)
Amiodarone (Cordarone)
Phenytoin (Dilantin)
Edrophonium chloride (Tensilon)
Magnesium sulfate
Propranolol (Inderal)

Parasympatholytics
Atropine sulfate

Cardiac Glycosides
Digoxin (Lanoxin)

Platelet Aggregation Inhibitors
Aspirin

Thrombolytics
Streptokinase (Streptase)
Anistreplase (Eminase)
Alteplase, tissue plasminogen activator (TPA) (Activase)

Alkalinizing Agents
Sodium bicarbonate

Analgesics
Morphine sulfate
Nitrous oxide (Nitronox)

Diuretics
Furosemide (Lasix)
Bumetanide (Bumex)

Antianginal Agents
Nitroglycerin (Nitrostat)
Nitroglycerin paste (Nitro-Bid Ointment)
Nitroglycerin spray (Nitrolingual Spray)

Antihypertensives
Nifedipine (Procardia)
Sodium nitroprusside (Nipride)
Hydralazine (Apresoline)
Diazoxide (Hyperstat)

Other Cardiovascular Drugs
Calcium chloride

OXYGEN

Oxygen is one of the most important drugs used in prehospital care. It is required by the body's cells to facilitate the breakdown of glucose into usable energy forms. Without oxygen, the breakdown of glucose is ineffective and incomplete. This breakdown without oxygen is termed *anaerobic metabolism*. Anaerobic metabolism yields *lactic acid*, a strong acid, as its end product. This acid, in conjunction with an increased carbon dioxide level, leads to systemic acidosis.

Oxygen is an odorless, tasteless, colorless gas that vigorously supports combustion. It is present in room air at a concentration of approximately 21 percent. This concentration is adequate for our daily activities. In injury and illness, however, the body needs increased levels of oxygen to maintain homeostasis.

℞ OXYGEN

Class: Gas

Description

Oxygen is an odorless, tasteless, colorless gas necessary for life.

Mechanism of Action

Oxygen enters the body through the respiratory system and is transported to the cells by hemoglobin, found in the red blood cells. Oxygen is required for the efficient breakdown of glucose into a usable energy form. Its onset of action following administration is immediate. The administration of enriched oxygen increases the oxygen concentration in the alveoli, which subsequently increases the oxygen saturation of available hemoglobin.

Indication

Hypoxia. Oxygen is indicated whenever hypoxia is suspected or possible, including for all forms of trauma, medical emergencies, chest pain that may be due to cardiac ischemia, any respiratory difficulty, during labor and delivery, and in any critical patient.

Contraindications

There are no contraindications to oxygen. *Hypoxic patients should never be deprived of oxygen for fear of respiratory depression.*

Precautions

Oxygen should be used cautiously in patients with chronic obstructive pulmonary disease (COPD). In these patients respirations are often regulated by the level of oxygen in the blood (hypoxic drive) instead of carbon dioxide. In some cases COPD patients may suffer respiratory depression if high concentrations of oxygen are delivered. The administration of high concentrations of oxygen to neonates for a prolonged period of time can damage the infant's eyes (retrolental fibroplasia). Although this is rarely a problem in prehospital care, it is a consideration in long-distance and prolonged transport. Oxygen delivered at a flow rate of 6 L/min or greater should be humidified to prevent drying of the mucous membranes of the upper respiratory system. When possible, oxygen administration should be monitored by use of pulse oximetry. Pulse oximetry is a noninvasive device that accurately measures the oxygen saturation of hemoglobin. It is relatively inexpensive, easy to apply, and quite accurate in detecting oxygen delivery problems.

Side Effects

There are few, if any, side effects associated with oxygen administration. Prolonged administration of high-flow, nonhumidified oxygen may cause drying of the mucous membranes, resulting in irritation and possibly nosebleeds.

Interactions

There are no interactions associated with oxygen administration. However, oxygen may increase the toxicity of certain herbicides (e.g., paraquat and diaquat) in patients who have ingested these poisons. These chemicals are sometimes sprayed on illicit agricultural products such as marijuana. Poisoning by these agents is uncommon.

Dosage

The dosage of oxygen is based on the patient's underlying problems. In the prehospital setting oxygen should be administered at the highest concentration available (see Table 7–1). Pulse oximetry, if available, should be used to guide care. General guidelines follow:

Cardiac arrest and other critical patients—100 percent oxygen concentration

Chronic obstructive pulmonary disease—35 percent oxygen concentration (increase as needed)

How Supplied

Oxygen is supplied in pressurized cylinders of varying size (see Table 7–2). Liquid oxygen is becoming more common in prehospital care. The sizes and types of liquid oxygen containers vary.

TABLE 7–1

Oxygen Delivery by Device

Oxygen delivery device	Flow rate (L/min)	Percentage delivered
Nasal cannula	1–6	24–44
Simple face mask	8–10	40–60
Venturi mask	4–12	24–50
Partial rebreathing mask	6–10	35–60
Nonrebreathing mask	6–10	60–95
Bag, valve, and mask with reservoir	10–15	40–90
Demand valve	10–15	100

TABLE 7–2

Capacity of Common Oxygen Cylinders

Cylinder name	Volume (L)
D	400
E	660
M	3000

Chapter 7 / Drugs Used in the Treatment of Cardiovascular Emergencies

The term *sympathomimetic* means to mimic the actions of the sympathetic nervous system. Drugs in this group do exactly that. They either act directly on receptors of the sympathetic nervous system or act indirectly by stimulating the release of *endogenous* catecholamines. *Catecholamine* is the name used to describe several drugs that are chemically similar. These drugs are epinephrine, norepinephrine (Levophed), dopamine (Intropin), isoproterenol (Isuprel), and dobutamine (Dobutrex). All of these agents, except isoproterenol and dobutamine, can be found naturally in the body. Isoproterenol and dobutamine are synthetic catecholamines. All sympathomimetics, monoamine oxidase inhibitors (MAOIs), and tricyclic antidepressants (TCAs) may increase blood pressure. To understand and appreciate the actions and roles of the sympathomimetics fully, it is essential to first review the sympathetic nervous system.

Sympathetic Nervous System

The *sympathetic nervous system* is sometimes called the fight-or-flight system. It is this part of the nervous system that prepares the body to deal with various stresses, whether real or imagined. Sometimes it is referred to as the *adrenergic system*. Both it and the other aspect of the autonomic nervous system, the parasympathetic nervous system, functionally oppose each other to maintain *homeostasis*. The *parasympathetic system* is sometimes called the *cholinergic system*.

As indicated by Table 7–3, the sympathetic nervous system tends to stimulate those organs needed to deal with stressful situations. It also tends to inhibit the use of organs not needed, such as the digestive tract.

The sympathetic nervous system uses the hormone *norepinephrine* to transmit impulses from the nerve to the effector cell. Chemicals that propagate the nervous impulse, such as norepinephrine, are called *neurotransmitters*. In emergency situations the norepinephrine released by the nerve endings may be augmented with epinephrine and norepinephrine secreted

TABLE 7–3

Comparison of Sympathetic and Parasympathetic Actions

Organ	Sympathetic stimulation	Parasympathetic stimulation
Heart	Increased rate	Decreased rate
	Increased contractile force	Decreased contractile force
Lungs	Bronchodilation	Bronchoconstriction
Kidneys	Decreased output	No change
Systemic blood vessels		
Abdominal	Constricted	None
Muscle	Constricted (α)	None
	Dilated (β)	None
Skin	Constricted	None
Liver	Glucose release	Slight glycogen synthesis
Blood glucose	Increased	None
Pupils	Dilated	Constricted
Sweat glands	Copious sweating	None
Basal metabolism	Increased up to 100%	None
Skeletal muscle	Increased strength	None

from the adrenal medulla. Like the adrenergic nerves, the adrenal medulla secretes norepinephrine. About 20 percent of the catecholamines secreted by the adrenals are in the form of norepinephrine. The remaining 80 percent are in the form of epinephrine (adrenalin).

When released, norepinephrine acts on specialized chemical receptors. These receptors are located at various points throughout the body. Once stimulated by the appropriate catecholamine, they cause a response in the organ or organs they control. There are two types of receptors, the *adrenergic receptors* and the *dopaminergic receptors*. The adrenergic receptors are further divided into four different types. These four types of receptors are designated *alpha$_1$* (α_1), *alpha$_2$* (α_2), *beta$_1$* (β_1), and *beta$_2$* (β_2). The α_1-receptors cause peripheral vasoconstriction and occasionally mild bronchoconstriction. The α_2-receptors, when stimulated, inhibit the release of norepinephrine. This effect is antagonistic to the actions of ; α_1-receptors and over time can cause peripheral vasodilation. The β_1-receptors, once stimulated, cause an increase in cardiac rate, cardiac force, and cardiac automaticity and conduction. The β_2-receptors cause vasodilation and bronchodilation. Dopaminergic receptors, though not totally understood, are believed to cause dilatation of the renal, coronary, and cerebral arteries. See Chapter 6 for a more detailed discussion of the autonomic nervous system.

Catecholamines

Certain drugs stimulate certain receptors to one degree or another. Norepinephrine, for example, has an effect on both α- and β-receptors. However, its effects are considerably stronger on α-receptors than on β-receptors. Consequently, norepinephrine is primarily regarded as an α-receptor-stimulating agent. Epinephrine, like norepinephrine, acts on both α- and β-receptors. However, unlike norepinephrine, epinephrine has a much greater effect on β-receptors and is considered a β-receptor-stimulating agent. Isoproterenol, the synthetic catecholamine occasionally used in emergency medicine, acts entirely on β-receptors with no α effects noted. Dopamine acts on both α- and β-receptors depending on the dosage. In addition, when used in certain doses, it acts on the dopaminergic receptors. This dopaminergic effect is quite useful because it tends to keep blood flowing to the renal arteries, even in emergency situations. One of the long-term major complications of severe medical emergencies such as cardiac arrest is renal failure. Using such agents as dopamine, which will maintain renal perfusion, helps in the long-term survival of the patient.

Drugs that cause an increase in the cardiac rate are called *positive chronotropic agents*. Drugs that cause an increase in cardiac force are referred to as *positive inotropic agents*. Drugs that cause an increase in contractility are referred to as *positive dromotropic agents*.

The primary use of the sympathomimetics in emergency medicine is to increase the blood pressure in cardiogenic shock. These drugs raise the blood pressure by one of two different methods. Drugs that stimulate α-receptors elevate blood pressure merely by peripheral vasoconstriction. Vasoconstriction reduces the size of the vascular pool, thus increasing the blood pressure. Drugs that act on β-receptors elevate blood pressure by causing an increase in cardiac output. Cardiac output can be defined as follows:

$$\text{Cardiac output} = \text{Stroke volume} \times \text{Heart rate}$$

TABLE 7–4

Comparison of Effects of α- and β-Adrenergic Receptor Activity on Selected Organs

Organ	α-adrenergic receptors	β-adrenergic receptors
Heart	No cardiac effect	Increased heart rate (β_1) Increased contractile force (β_1) Increased automaticity (β_1)
Systemic blood vessels	Vasoconstriction	Vasodilation (β_2)
Lungs	Mild bronchoconstriction	Bronchodilation (β_2)

TABLE 7–5

Listing of Sympathomimetic Drugs with Adrenergic Actions

Drug	Adrenergic effects		Arrhythmia potential
	α	β	
Epinephrine			
Low dose	+	+ +	+ + +
High dose	+ +	+ + +	+ + +
Norepinephrine			
Low dose	+ +	+	+ +
High dose	+ + +	+ +	+ +
Dopamine			
Low dose	+	+	+ +
High dose	+ + +	+ +	+ +
Isoproterenol	0	+ + +	+ + +
Dobutamine	0	+ + +	+
Amrinone	0	0	+

Thus,

$$\text{Blood pressure} = \text{Cardiac output} \times \text{Peripheral resistance}$$

The β-receptor-stimulating drugs, including epinephrine and dopamine, cause an increase in both heart rate (positive chronotropic) and stroke volume (positive inotropic). The different receptor effects are summarized in Table 7–4. Table 7–5 lists many of the sympathomimetic drugs used in emergency care, including their adrenergic effects and arrhythmia potential.

EPINEPHRINE 1:10 000

Class: Sympathetic agonist

Description

Epinephrine is a naturally occurring catecholamine. It is a potent α- and β-adrenergic stimulant; however, its effect on β-receptors is more profound.

Mechanism of Action

Epinephrine acts directly on α- and β-adrenergic receptors. Its effect on β-receptors is much more profound than its effect on α-receptors. The effects of epinephrine include the following:

Increased heart rate
Increased cardiac contractile force
Increased electrical activity in the myocardium
Increased systemic vascular resistance
Increased blood pressure
Increased automaticity

Epinephrine can stimulate spontaneous firing of myocardial conductive cells. In the emergency setting it is used to convert fine ventricular fibrillation to coarse ventricular fibrillation. This change significantly increases the chances of successful electrical defibrillation. In asystole it is used to initiate electrical activity in the myocardium. Once initiated, electrical defibrillation may be attempted.

Epinephrine's effects usually appear within 90 seconds of administration, and they are usually of short duration. Therefore, it must be administered every 3 to 5 minutes to maintain therapeutic levels.

Indications

Epinephrine is used in cardiac arrest (asystole, ventricular fibrillation, pulseless ventricular tachycardia, pulseless electrical activity), severe anaphylaxis, and severe reactive airway disease.

Contraindications

Epinephrine 1:10 000 is contraindicated in patients who do not require extensive cardiopulmonary resuscitative efforts. With simple allergic reactions and asthma, the 1:1000 dilution should be used and is administered subcutaneously.

Precautions

Epinephrine, like all catecholamines, should be protected from light. It can be deactivated by alkaline solutions such as sodium bicarbonate. Thus, it is essential that the intravenous (IV) line be adequately flushed between administrations of epinephrine and sodium bicarbonate.

Side Effects

Epinephrine can cause palpitations, anxiety, tremulousness, headache, dizziness, nausea, and vomiting. Because of its strong inotropic and chronotropic properties, epinephrine increases myocardial oxygen demand. Even in low doses it can cause myocardial ischemia. When administering epinephrine in the emergency setting, these effects should be kept in mind. Like most of the other drugs used in emergency medicine, epinephrine is only effective when the myocardium is adequately oxygenated.

Interactions

Epinephrine is pH dependent and can be deactivated when administered with highly alkaline solutions such as sodium bicarbonate. The effects of epinephrine can be intensified in patients who are taking antidepressants.

Dosage

Epinephrine 1:10 000 can be administered intravenously, intraosseously, or endotracheally. Common doses include the following:

Cardiac arrest (adults).   The dose of epinephrine in cardiac arrest is 1.0 mg of a 1:10 000 solution intravenously. This can be repeated every 3 to 5 minutes as required. Higher dosages may be ordered by medical control and are potentially helpful in the cardiac arrest setting. If an IV cannot be started, epinephrine can be administered endotracheally. The endotracheal dose should be increased at least 2 to 2.5 times the intravenous dose.

Cardiac arrest (children).   The initial dose of epinephrine in pediatric cardiac arrest is 0.01 mg/kg of a 1:10 000 solution intravenously (0.1 mL/kg). Second and subsequent doses should be 0.1 mg/kg of a 1:1000 solution intravenously (0.1 mL/kg). The total volume of drug administered remains the same because epinephrine 1:1000 is used instead of epinephrine 1:10 000.

Severe anaphylaxis or severe asthma (adults).   Intravenous epinephrine should only be used for life-threatening, severe anaphylaxis and severe asthma. Less-severe cases should be treated with epinephrine 1:1000 subcutaneously or with another β-agonist. In severe anaphylaxis or asthma the initial dose should be 0.3 to 0.5 mg intravenously. The dose may be repeated every 5 to 15 minutes as required. An epinephrine drip may be required in severe cases.

Severe anaphylaxis or severe asthma (children).   Intravenous epinephrine should only be used for life-threatening, severe anaphylaxis and severe asthma. Less-severe cases should be treated with epinephrine 1:1000 subcutaneously or with another β-agonist. In severe anaphylaxis or asthma the initial dose should be 0.01 mg/kg intravenously. The dose may be repeated every 5 to 15 minutes as required. An epinephrine drip may be required in severe cases.

How Supplied

Epinephrine 1:10 000 comes in prefilled syringes containing 1 mg of the drug in 10 mL of solvent.

NOREPINEPHRINE (LEVOPHED)

Class: Sympathetic agonist

Description

Norepinephrine is a naturally occurring catecholamine. It acts on both α- and β-adrenergic receptors. However, its action on α-receptors is more profound.

Mechanism of Action

Because of its action on α-receptors, norepinephrine is a potent peripheral vasoconstrictor. This vasoconstriction serves to increase blood pressure in cardiogenic shock and other hypotensive emergencies. Because norepinephrine also tends to constrict the renal and mesenteric blood vessels, it is reserved for emergencies in which dopamine may not be effective. As a rule, dopamine, which maintains renal and mesenteric perfusion, is the preferred vasopressor for treating cardiogenic shock.

Indications

Norepinephrine is used in hypotension (systolic blood pressure <70 mm Hg) refractory to other sympathomimetics and not related to hypovolemia, and in neurogenic shock.

Contraindications

Norepinephrine should not be given to patients who are hypotensive from hypovolemia.

Precautions

Because of the powerful effects of norepinephrine, it is essential to measure the blood pressure every 5 to 10 minutes to prevent dangerously high blood pressures. Fluid replacement should be initiated prior to administration of norepinephrine. Norepinephrine should be given through the largest vein readily available because it may cause local tissue necrosis if it extravasates. Phentolamine (Regitine) can be diluted in saline and infiltrated into the area of extravasation to help minimize necrosis and sloughing. Like the other sympathomimetics, norepinephrine can increase myocardial oxygen demand. It should be used with caution in persons with cardiac ischemia.

Side Effects

Norepinephrine can cause anxiety, tremulousness, headache, dizziness, nausea, and vomiting. It can also cause bradycardia as a reflex response to increased peripheral vasoconstriction. Because of its inotropic and chronotropic properties, norepinephrine increases myocardial oxygen demand. Even in low doses it can cause myocardial ischemia. When administering norepinephrine in the emergency setting, these effects should be kept in mind.

Interactions

Norepinephrine can be deactivated by alkaline solutions such as sodium bicarbonate. Concomitant administration with beta-blockers can result in markedly elevated blood pressure.

Dosage

The current dosage recommended by the American Heart Association for norepinephrine is 0.5 to 30 μg/min. Higher doses may be required to maintain adequate blood pressure. The best dilution is obtained by placing 8 mg in 500 mL of D_5W. This will give a concentration of 16 μg/mL. The same concentration can be attained by placing 4 mg in 250 mL of D_5W (see Figure 7–1).

Chapter 7 / Drugs Used in the Treatment of Cardiovascular Emergencies

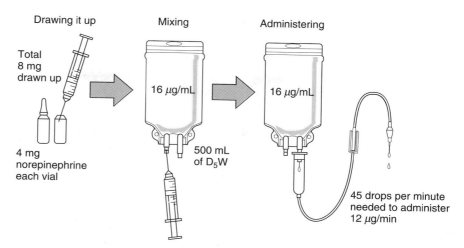

Total
8 mg
drawn up

Drawing it up

4 mg
norepinephrine
each vial

Mixing

16 μg/mL

500 mL
of D₅W

Administering

16 μg/mL

45 drops per minute
needed to administer
12 μg/min

FIGURE 7–1 Preparation of norepinephrine infusion.

Because of its potency, norepinephrine is given only in extremely diluted IV infusions. To control its administration, it should be piggybacked into an already established IV line.

How Supplied

Norepinephrine is supplied in 4 mL ampules containing 4 mg of the drug.

ISOPROTERENOL (ISUPREL)

Class: Sympathetic agonist

Description

Isoproterenol is a synthetic catecholamine. It primarily acts on β-adrenergic receptors.

Mechanism of Action

Isoproterenol is a potent, synthetic catecholamine that acts almost exclusively on β-receptors. Because it has no significant α-receptor-stimulating capabilities, its actions are primarily on the heart and lungs. In cardiac emergencies it may be used to increase heart rate in bradycardias that are refractory to atropine. With the advent of transcutaneous pacing, isoproterenol is seldom used by paramedics.

Indications

Isoproterenol is used in bradycardias refractory to atropine (when transcutaneous pacing is unavailable), bradycardias resulting from high-degree heart blocks (i.e., second-degree Mobitz II and third-degree blocks) when transcutaneous pacing is unavailable, and severe status asthmaticus.

Contraindications

Isoproterenol is not used to increase blood pressure in cardiogenic shock. It should only be used in shock resulting from bradycardias. Other sympathomimetics, such as dopamine and norepinephrine, should be used in cases of cardiogenic shock.

Precautions

When administering isoproterenol, the patient must be monitored for signs of ventricular irritability. These signs may take the form of premature ventricular contractions, ventricular tachycardia, or even ventricular fibrillation. Lidocaine should be readily available whenever isoproterenol is administered. It is important to be careful when administering isoproterenol. Like epinephrine, it significantly increases myocardial oxygen demand. The increase in myocardial oxygen uptake may increase myocardial infarction size. In patients who have not suffered a myocardial infarction, isoproterenol may cause myocardial ischemia. External pacing, if available, should be used instead of isoproterenol.

Side Effects

Isoproterenol can cause nervousness, headache, tremor, dysrhythmias, hypertension, angina, nausea, and vomiting. Many of these side effects are dose related.

Interactions

Isoproterenol can be deactivated by alkaline solutions such as sodium bicarbonate. It should be used with caution in patients with digitalis toxicity because it may aggravate tachydysrhythmias.

Dosage

The usual dosage of isoproterenol is 1 mg diluted in 500 mL of D_5W; this will give a concentration of 2 µg/mL. It should be titrated until the desired heart rate is attained or until signs of ventricular irritability, such as premature ventricular contractions, occur. The recommended infusion rate is 2 to 10 µg/min. Because of its potency, isoproterenol should only be given by IV infusion. An established IV line, into which the isoproterenol is piggybacked, should be maintained.

How Supplied

Isoproterenol is supplied in ampules containing 1 mg in either 1 or 5 mL of solvent. Prefilled syringes designed especially for IV infusion preparation are available.

 DOPAMINE HYDROCHLORIDE (INTROPIN)

Class: Sympathetic agonist

Description

Dopamine is a naturally occurring catecholamine. It is a chemical precursor of norepinephrine. It acts on α, β_1, and dopaminergic adrenergic receptors. Its effect on α-receptors is dose dependent.

Mechanism of Action

Dopamine is one of the most frequently used agents in the treatment of hypotension associated with cardiogenic shock. It is chemically related to both epinephrine and norepinephrine and increases blood pressure by acting on both α- and β_1-adrenergic receptors. Dopamine's effect on β_1-receptors causes a positive inotropic effect on the heart. It does not increase myocardial oxygen demand as much as isoproterenol and epinephrine do and does not have the same powerful chronotropic effects. Dopamine also acts on α-adrenergic receptors, causing peripheral vasoconstriction. Unlike norepinephrine, when used in therapeutic dosages dopamine maintains renal and mesenteric blood flow because of its effect on the dopaminergic receptors. For these reasons, dopamine is the most commonly used vasopressor. Dopamine increases both the systolic blood pressure and the pulse pressure (the difference between the systolic and diastolic blood pressures), but, as a rule, there is usually less effect on the diastolic pressure.

Indications

Dopamine is used in hemodynamically significant hypotension (systolic blood pressure of 70 to 100 mm Hg) not resulting from hypovolemia, and in cardiogenic shock.

Contraindications

Dopamine should not be used as the sole agent in the management of hypovolemic shock unless fluid resuscitation is well under way. Dopamine should not be used in patients with known pheochromocytoma (a tumor of the adrenal gland).

Precautions

Dopamine increases the heart rate and can induce or worsen supraventricular and ventricular arrhythmias. Whenever the dosage of dopamine surpasses 20 μg/kg/min, its α effects predominate and it functions very much like norepinephrine. Dopamine, like the other catecholamines, should not be administered in the presence of tachyarrhythmias or ventricular fibrillation.

Side Effects

Dopamine can cause nervousness, headache, dysrhythmias, palpitations, chest pain, dyspnea, nausea, and vomiting. Many of these side effects are dose related.

Interactions

Like all of the catecholamines, dopamine can be deactivated by alkaline solutions such as sodium bicarbonate. If the patient is taking monoamine oxidase inhibitors (a type of antidepressant), the dose should be reduced. Dopamine may cause hypotension when used concomitantly with phenytoin (Dilantin).

Dosage

The standard method of preparing a dopamine infusion is to place 800 mg in 500 mL of D_5W or by adding 400 mg to 250 mL of D_5W; this gives a

TABLE 7–6

Dopamine Hydrochloride (Intropin) Dosage Phenomena

Physiological effect	2–5 µg/kg/min	5–20 µg/kg/min	More than
Cardiac output	No change	Increase	Increase
Stroke volume	No change	Increase	Increase
Heart rate	No change	Initial increase followed by a decrease toward normal rates as infusion continues	
Myocardial contractility	No change	Increase	Increase
Potential for excessive myocardial oxygen demands	Low[a] Coronary blood flow increased	Low[a] Coronary blood flow increased	Data unavailable
Potential for tachyarrhythmias	Low[a]	Low[a]	Moderate
Total systemic vascular resistance	Slight decrease to no change	No change to slight increase	Increase
Renal blood flow	Increase	Increase	Decrease[b]
Urine output	Increase	Increase	Decrease[b]

[a]Low but needs monitoring.

[b]Relative to peak values achieved at lower dosages.

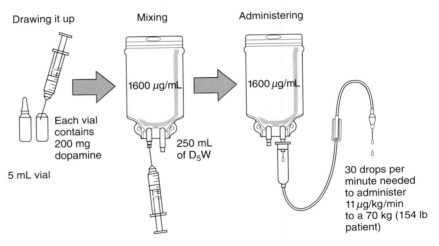

FIGURE 7–2   Preparation of dopamine infusion.

concentration of 1600 µg/mL. The effects of dopamine are dose dependent. Table 7–6 illustrates effects based on common dosages.

The initial infusion rate is from 2 to 5 µg/kg/min. This rate may be increased until blood pressure improves (see Figure 7–2). Dopamine is administered only by IV drip, which should be piggybacked into an already established IV infusion.

How Supplied

Dopamine comes in prefilled syringes, ampules, and premixed bags. The standard preparation is 200 mg in 5 mL of solvent; 400 mg preparations in 5 mL of solvent are also available.

DOBUTAMINE (DOBUTREX)

Class: Sympathetic agonist

Description

Dobutamine is a synthetic catecholamine. It acts primarily on β_1-receptors but is a less potent β-agonist than is isoproterenol.

Mechanism of Action

Dobutamine increases the force of the systolic contraction (positive inotropic effect) with little chronotropic activity. For these reasons, it is useful in the management of congestive heart failure when an increase in heart rate is not desired.

Indication

Dobutamine is used for short-term management of congestive heart failure when an increased cardiac output, without an increased cardiac rate, is desired.

Contraindications

Dobutamine should not be used as the sole agent in hypovolemic shock unless fluid resuscitation is well under way. To increase cardiac output in severe emergencies, such as cardiogenic shock, dopamine is the preferred agent.

Precautions

Tachycardia and an increase in the systolic blood pressure are common following the administration of dobutamine. Increases in heart rate of more than 10 percent may induce or exacerbate myocardial ischemia. Premature ventricular contractions (PVCs) can occur in conjunction with dobutamine administration. Lidocaine should be readily available. As with any sympathomimetic, blood pressure should be monitored.

Side Effects

Dobutamine can cause nervousness, headache, hypertension, dysrhythmias, palpitations, chest pain, dyspnea, nausea, and vomiting. Many of these side effects are dose related.

Interactions

Dobutamine may be ineffective when administered to patients taking beta-blockers because these medications can block the beta-receptors on which dobutamine acts. Patients taking tricyclic antidepressants are at increased risk of hypertension with dobutamine administration.

Dosage

The desired dosage range for dobutamine is between 2 and 20 μg/kg/min. Dobutamine should be administered according to the patient's response (see Figure 7–3).

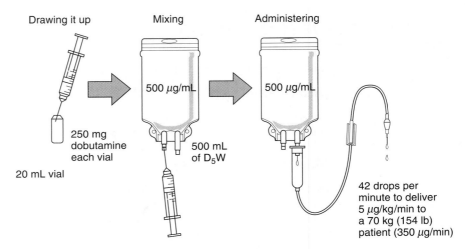

Drawing it up   Mixing   Administering

500 μg/mL

500 μg/mL

250 mg
dobutamine
each vial

20 mL vial

500 mL
of D₅W

42 drops per
minute to deliver
5 μg/kg/min to
a 70 kg (154 lb)
patient (350 μg/min)

FIGURE 7–3   Preparation of dobutamine infusion.

Dobutamine should be diluted in either 500 mL or 1 L of D₅W and administered via IV infusion.

How Supplied

Dobutamine is supplied in 20 mL ampules containing 250 mg of the drug; 250 mg is usually placed in 500 mL of solvent to give a concentration of 0.5 mg/mL (500 μg/mL).

℞ METARAMINOL (ARAMINE)

Class: Sympathetic agonist

Description

Metaraminol is a sympathetic agonist with effects similar to those of norepinephrine. It is much less potent than norepinephrine but has a more prolonged action.

Mechanism of Action

Although metaraminol is not a catecholamine, it is used in the treatment of hypotensive states. It is both an α- and β-agonist. Its vasopressor properties are primarily derived from its action on endogenous catecholamines. It causes the release of norepinephrine from sympathetic nerve endings. In recent years metaraminol has fallen into disuse, with dopamine being the preferred agent.

Indication

Metaraminol is used in hemodynamically significant hypotension not due to hypovolemia.

Contraindications

Metaraminol should not be used in hypovolemia unless fluid resuscitation is well under way.

Precautions

Rapid administration can cause hypertension. Ventricular ectopic activity has been known to occur with the administration of metaraminol. Lidocaine should be readily available.

Side Effects

Metaraminol can cause anxiety, tremulousness, headache, dizziness, nausea, and vomiting. It can also cause bradycardia as a reflex response to increased peripheral vasoconstriction.

Interactions

Metaraminol can be deactivated by alkaline solutions such as sodium bicarbonate. Concomitant administration with beta-blockers can result in markedly elevated blood pressure. Caution should be used when administering metaraminol to patients taking digitalis.

Dosage

The usual dosage of metaraminol is 200 mg in 500 mL of D_5W. This will give a dilution of 0.4 mg/mL. The infusion rate should be titrated according to the blood pressure response. An IV infusion should already be established, into which the metaraminol is piggybacked. Metaraminol can be administered intramuscularly when an IV cannot be established. The initial adult dose should be 5 to 10 mg for intramuscular administration. Many agents, such as dopamine, are far superior to metaraminol and should be used initially.

How Supplied

Metaraminol comes in a concentration of 10 mg/mL. Ampules contain either 1 or 10 mL. Thus, each ampule contains 10 and 100 mg, respectively.

℞ AMRINONE (INOCOR)

Class: Inotrope (phosphodiesterase inhibitor)

Description

Amrinone is a rapidly acting inotropic agent. It is a phosphodiesterase inhibitor and does not act on adrenergic receptors.

Mechanism of Action

Amrinone, like the other medications previously presented, increases cardiac output promptly following intravenous administration. It is a positive inotrope and has some vasodilatory properties. Unlike the other medications, however, it does not stimulate either α- or β-adrenergic receptors. The exact mechanism by which amrinone increases blood pressure is not well understood. It does not increase cardiac output in the same manner as the digitalis preparations. Clinically, amrinone resembles dobutamine in its effects. Because amrinone does not stimulate β-adrenergic receptors, it may be effective in cases of congestive heart failure that do not respond to dobutamine or one of the other inotropic agents.

Indication

Amrinone is used in short-term management of severe congestive heart failure refractory to diuretics, vasodilators, and conventional inotropic agents.

Contraindications

Amrinone should not be administered to patients with a known hypersensitivity to the drug or to the bisulfite class of chemicals.

Precautions

Amrinone should not be used in cases of congestive heart failure occurring immediately after myocardial infarction. Like dobutamine, amrinone may increase myocardial ischemia. As with the other inotropic agents, the blood pressure, pulse, and electrocardiogram (ECG) should be constantly monitored. Amrinone should not be diluted in solutions containing dextrose (i.e., D_5W). Amrinone should be diluted with 0.9 percent sodium chloride (normal saline) or 0.45 percent sodium chloride (one-half normal saline).

Side Effects

Amrinone can cause arrhythmias, hypotension, nausea, vomiting, abdominal pain, and decreased platelets (thrombocytopenia).

Interactions

Furosemide (Lasix) should not be administered into an intravenous line delivering amrinone. A chemical reaction occurs between these two drugs, resulting in the formation of a precipitate in the intravenous line. Amrinone should not be diluted in solutions containing dextrose.

Dosage

Therapy should be initiated with an IV bolus of 0.75 mg/kg given slowly during a 2- to 5-minute interval. This should be followed by a maintenance infusion of 2 to 15 μg/kg/min. This infusion can be prepared by placing one ampule (100 mg) in 500 mL of normal saline solution. This will give a concentration of 0.2 mg/mL (200 μg/mL).

An additional bolus of 0.75 mg/kg given slowly over 2 to 3 minutes can be given 30 minutes later if required.

The overall rate of amrinone administration must be carefully adjusted and based on the patient's clinical response.

Amrinone should only be administered by the IV route, either as a bolus or by infusion, as described earlier.

How Supplied

Amrinone is supplied in 20 mL ampules containing 5 mg/mL.

SYMPATHETIC BLOCKERS

Sympathetic blockers are a unique class of drugs that antagonize adrenergic receptor sites. Certain drugs block only α-receptors, whereas others block only β-receptors. Some of the β-blockers are so selective that they block only β_1- or β_2-receptors. The drugs that block the β-receptors are receiving the most use. They are useful in the treatment of hypertension, cardiac arrhythmias, and angina pectoris. The most popular sympathetic blocker is propranolol (Inderal), a nonselective beta-blocker that is both a β_1- and β_2-antagonist. Although used selectively in emergency medicine, propranolol does play a role in the treatment of certain cardiac arrhythmias.

It is thought that some ventricular arrhythmias, such as ventricular tachycardia and recurrent ventricular fibrillation, can be caused by excessive β-receptor stimulation. Administration of propranolol may inhibit these arrhythmias. Propranolol should not be used in combination with verapamil. The concomitant blocking of slow calcium channels by verapamil, and the β-receptor antagonism caused by propranolol, may result in asystole.

PROPRANOLOL (INDERAL)

Class: Nonselective beta-blocker

Description

Propranolol is a nonselective β-antagonist. It inhibits the effects of circulating catecholamines.

Mechanism of Action

Propranolol nonselectively blocks both β_1- and β_2-adrenergic receptors. It causes a reduction in heart rate (negative chronotropic effect), cardiac contractile force (negative inotropic effect), blood pressure, and myocardial oxygen demand. It is useful in treating recurrent ventricular tachycardia and recurrent ventricular fibrillation that does not respond to lidocaine. It may also be of value in the treatment of tachyarrhythmias resulting from digitalis toxicity and selected supraventricular tachycardias.

Indications

Propranolol is used in ventricular tachycardia refractory to lidocaine and bretylium, recurrent ventricular fibrillation refractory to lidocaine and bretylium, and selected supraventricular tachyarrhythmias.

Contraindications

Propranolol is contraindicated in patients with bradycardia, a history of asthma, COPD, and congestive heart failure.

Precautions

Because propranolol may decrease heart rate, atropine should be readily available. In bradycardia refractory to atropine, transcutaneous pacing should be utilized. Propranolol should be used with caution in diabetics because it may mask the signs and symptoms of hypoglycemia. Glucagon can be used in the management of severe beta-blocker overdose. It helps to maintain the heart rate and blood pressure.

Side Effects

Propranolol may cause bradycardia, hypotension, lethargy, congestive heart failure, dyspnea, wheezing, and weakness.

Interactions

Propranolol should not be administered to patients who have received intravenous verapamil. It should be used with caution in patients taking antihypertensive agents.

Dosage

Propranolol may produce significant, even life-threatening, side effects. When administered intravenously, care must be taken to dilute 1 mg in 10 mL of D_5W. The standard dosage is 1 to 3 mg, diluted in 10 to 30 mL of D_5W. Propranolol should be administered *slowly* (over 2 to 5 minutes). Propranolol should not be administered faster than 1 mg/min. Throughout administration, careful blood pressure monitoring is required. Like all drugs acting on the heart, it should only be administered to patients who are on cardiac monitors. The dosage may be repeated, again under careful monitoring, until a maximum of 3 to 5 mg has been administered. Propranolol should be administered intravenously in the treatment of life-threatening tachyarrhythmias.

How Supplied

The standard preparation of propranolol is 1 mL vials containing 1 mg of the drug.

 ## SOTALOL HCL (SOTACOR, BETAPACE)

Class: Beta-blocker

Description

Sotalol is a nonselective beta-adrenergic blocking agent.

Mechanism of Action

Sotalol blocks stimulation of $beta_1$ (myocardial) and $beta_2$ (pulmonary, vascular, and uterine) adrenergic receptor sites.

Indications

Sotalol is indicated for the treatment of documented life-threatening ventricular arrhythmias such as sustained ventricular tachycardia. It may also be used for the treatment of patients with documented symptomatic ventricular arrhythmias. Sotalol should be reserved for patients in whom the physician believes the benefit of treatment clearly outweighs the risks.

Contraindications

Sotalol is contraindicated in patients with bronchial asthma, allergic rhinitis, severe sinus node dysfunction, sinus bradycardia and second- and third-degree atrioventricular (AV) block (unless a functioning pacemaker is present), cardiogenic shock, severe or uncontrolled heart failure, and known hypersensitivity.

Precautions

Sotalol may cause new or worsen existing arrhythmias. Such proarrhythmic effects range from an increase in frequency of premature ventricular contractions to the development of more severe ventricular tachycardia, ventricular fibrillation, and torsade de pointes.

Side Effects

Central nervous system effects include fatigue, weakness, anxiety, dizziness, drowsiness, insomnia, memory loss, mental status changes, nervousness, and nightmares. Respiratory effects include bronchospasm and wheezing. Cardiovascular effects include arrythmias, bradycardia, congestive heart failure, pulmonary edema, orthostatic hypotension, and peripheral vasoconstriction.

Interactions

General anesthesia, IV phenytoin, and verapamil may cause additive myocardial depression. Additive bradycardia may occur with digitalis glycosides. Additive hypotension may occur with other antihypertensives, acute ingestion of alcohol, or nitrates. Sotalol should be used cautiously within 14 days of monoamine oxidase inhibitor therapy (may result in hypotension). Sotalol may interact with class IA antiarrhythmic drugs such as disopyramide, quinidine, and procainamide and class III drugs such as amiodarone.

Dosage

Oral administration of 80 mg twice daily may be gradually increased (usual maintenance dose is 160 to 320 mg/day in two to three divided doses, up to 480 to 640 mg/day).

How Supplied

Tablets of 80, 120, 160, and 240 mg.

 # METOPROLOL (LOPRESSOR)

Class: Selective beta-blocker

Description

Metoprolol is a β-antagonist that blocks both β_1- and β_2-adrenergic receptors. Unlike propranolol, however, metoprolol is selective for β_1-adrenergic receptors.

Mechanism of Action

Metoprolol causes a reduction in heart rate, systolic blood pressure, and cardiac output following administration because of its selective effects on β_1-adrenergic receptors. In addition, metoprolol appears to inhibit tachycardia, especially in the period following an acute myocardial infarction. Because of these effects, metoprolol is thought to be protective of the heart and is used to reduce potential complications in selected patients who have suffered an acute myocardial infarction. Metoprolol has proved effective in reducing the incidence of ventricular fibrillation and chest pain in these patients, thus reducing overall patient mortality in the post–myocardial infarction period.

Indication

Metoprolol is used in patients with suspected or definite acute myocardial infarction who are hemodynamically stable.

Contraindications

Metoprolol is contraindicated in any patient with a heart rate of less than 45 beats per minute, a systolic blood pressure less than 100 mm Hg, or congestive heart failure. In addition, metoprolol is contraindicated in patients with first-degree heart block with a PR interval greater than 0.24 second, second-degree heart block (either Mobitz I or Mobitz II), or third-degree block. It is also contraindicated in any patient showing either early or late signs of shock. Metoprolol should not be administered to any patient with a history of asthma or bronchospastic disease in the prehospital setting.

Precautions

The blood pressure, pulse rate, ECG, and respiratory status should be continuously monitored during metoprolol therapy. Prehospital personnel should be alert for signs and symptoms of congestive heart failure, bradycardia, shock, heart block, or bronchospasm when administering metoprolol. The presence of any of these signs or symptoms is an indication for discontinuing the medication.

Side Effects

Metoprolol may cause bradycardia, hypotension, lethargy, congestive heart failure, dyspnea, wheezing, and weakness.

Interactions

Metoprolol should not be administered to patients who have received intravenous verapamil. It should be administered with caution to patients taking antihypertensive agents.

Dosage

When administered following an acute myocardial infarction, an initial bolus of 5 mg metoprolol should be given by slow IV injection. If the vital signs remain stable, a second 5 mg bolus should be given 2 minutes after the first. Finally, if the first two boluses are well tolerated, a third 5 mg bolus should be administered 2 minutes after the second bolus. The total dose should not exceed 15 mg. As mentioned previously, the vital signs and ECG should be constantly monitored.

Metoprolol should only be administered by slow IV injection in the manner described earlier.

How Supplied

Metoprolol (Lopressor) is supplied in ampules and prefilled syringes containing 5 mg of the drug in 5 mL of solvent.

LABETALOL (TRANDATE, NORMODYNE)

Class: Nonselective beta-blocker

Description

Labetalol is a nonselective β-blocker and a selective α_1-blocker.

Mechanism of Action

Labetalol differs considerably in its action from the β-blockers previously presented. Like propranolol, labetalol is a nonselective β-adrenergic antagonist showing no preference for either β_1- or β_2-receptors. However, unlike the other β-blockers, labetalol also blocks α_1-adrenergic receptors. Blockage of α_1-receptors inhibits peripheral vasoconstriction, thus causing peripheral vasodilation. Because of these properties, labetalol is a potent agent for lowering blood pressure in cases of hypertensive crisis. It lowers blood pressure by decreasing cardiac output through its β_1-blocking properties and by causing peripheral vasodilation through its α_1-blocking properties.

Indication

Labetalol is indicated for the acute management of hypertensive crisis.

Contraindications

Labetalol is contraindicated in patients with bronchial asthma, congestive heart failure, heart block, bradycardia, or cardiogenic shock.

Precautions

As with all β-blockers the blood pressure, pulse rate, ECG, and respiratory status should be continuously monitored. Prehospital personnel should be alert for signs and symptoms of congestive heart failure, bradycardia, shock, heart block, or bronchospasm when administering labetalol. The appearance of any of these signs or symptoms is an indication for discontinuing the drug. Because of the effects of labetalol on β_1-receptors, postural hypotension might occur and should be anticipated. The patient should be supine at all times during drug administration.

Side Effects

Labetalol may cause bradycardia, hypotension, lethargy, congestive heart failure, dyspnea, wheezing, and weakness.

Interactions

Labetalol should not be administered to patients who have received intravenous verapamil. It should be administered with caution to patients taking antihypertensive agents.

Dosage

The following are two accepted methods of administering labetalol in the treatment of hypertensive crisis:

1. Twenty milligrams of labetalol can be administered by slow IV injection over 2 minutes. Immediately before the injection

and at 5 and 10 minutes after the injection, the supine blood pressure should be recorded. Additional injections of 40 mg can be given every 10 minutes until a desired supine blood pressure is achieved or 300 mg of the drug has been given.

2. Two ampules (200 mg) of labetalol can be added to 250 mL of D_5W. This gives a concentration of 0.8 mg/mL. This solution should be administered at a rate of 2 mg/min (2.5 mL/min). The blood pressure should be continuously monitored.

Labetalol should be administered by slow IV injection or infusion as described earlier.

How Supplied

Labetalol (Trandate, Normodyne) is supplied in ampules containing 100 mg in 20 mL of solvent (5 mg/mL).

ESMOLOL (BREVIBLOC)

Class: Selective beta-blocker

Description

Esmolol is a β_1 selective (cardioselective) β-blocker with a very short half-life.

Mechanism of Action

Esmolol is a selective β_1-blocker. It has a very rapid onset and a short duration of action (9 minutes). Esmolol is used to slow rapid heart rates in patients with supraventricular tachycardia including atrial flutter and atrial fibrillation. Patients with extremely rapid heart rates can develop congestive heart failure or angina because the rapid heart rate may prevent adequate filling of the ventricles. The duration of action of esmolol is so brief that it should be administered by intravenous infusion.

Indication

Esmolol is used in supraventricular tachycardia (including atrial fibrillation and atrial flutter) accompanied by a rapid ventricular rate.

Contraindications

Esmolol should not be used in patients with sinus bradycardia, heart block greater than first degree, cardiogenic shock, or overt congestive heart failure.

Precautions

A significant number of patients receiving esmolol may experience hypotension (systolic less than 90 mm Hg). Hypotension can occur at any dose but primarily is dose related. If hypotension develops, the dosage should be reduced. Patients with congestive heart failure may have worsening of their symptoms with esmolol. Because esmolol may depress cardiac contractility, it should be used with extreme caution in patients prone to congestive heart failure. Patients with bronchospastic disease (e.g., asthma and COPD) should not receive β-blockers, including esmolol, unless the medical control physician deems that the benefits outweigh the risks.

Side Effects

Esmolol may cause bradycardia, dizziness, hypotension, lethargy, congestive heart failure, dyspnea, wheezing, and weakness.

Interactions

Esmolol should not be administered to patients who have received intravenous verapamil. It should be administered with caution to patients taking antihypertensive agents. Morphine can increase the blood levels of esmolol, requiring a reduction in dosage. Esmolol should not be used in cases of supraventricular tachycardia caused by epinephrine, dopamine, and norepinephrine.

Dosage

Esmolol therapy is started by administering a loading dose of 500 μg/kg/min for 1 minute. After 1 minute the dose should be reduced to a maintenance dose of 50 μg/kg/min for 4 minutes. If an adequate therapeutic effect is not seen, the loading dose should be repeated for 1 minute and then the maintenance dose is increased to 100 μg/kg/min. The dose can be titrated at 4-minute intervals by repeating the loading dose for 1 minute and increasing the maintenance dose by 50 μg/kg/min at 4-minute intervals until the desired effect is obtained. The maintenance dose should not exceed 200 μg/kg/min. In the event of an adverse reaction, the dose of esmolol can be reduced or discontinued immediately. The esmolol infusion is prepared by placing two 2.5 g ampules of esmolol in 500 mL of 5 percent dextrose, normal saline, or lactated Ringer's solution. An alternative method is to place one 2.5 g ampule in 250 mL of fluid. Either will provide a 10 mg/mL concentration. Esmolol should be administered intravenously.

How Supplied

Esmolol is supplied in 100 mg vials containing 100 mg in 10 mL (10 mg/mL) for loading-dose administration. It is also supplied in 2.5 g vials for preparation of the infusion.

The 2.5 g vials are for preparation of the infusion only, not for intravenous injection.

ANTIARRHYTHMICS

Many different drugs are useful in the treatment and prevention of cardiac arrhythmias. Some drugs are useful in the treatment of atrial arrhythmias, whereas others are useful in the treatment of ventricular arrhythmias. As a result, it is essential to distinguish between these two types of arrhythmias. The common antiarrhythmic drugs are classified based on their action (see Table 7–7).

The most common antiarrhythmic drugs used in emergency medicine include the following:

Lidocaine (Xylocaine). Lidocaine is the drug of choice in the treatment of ventricular tachycardia and malignant premature ventricular contractions.

TABLE 7–7

Antidysrhythmic Classifications and Examples

General Action	Class	Prototype	ECG Effects
Sodium Channel Blockers	IA	Quinidine, procainamide*, disopyramide	Widened QRS, prolonged QT
	IB	Lidocaine*, phenytoin, tocainide, mexiletine	Widened QRS, prolonged QT
	IC	Flecainide*, propafenone	Prolonged PR, widened QRS
	I (Miscellaneous)	Moricizine*	Prolonged PR, widened QRS
Beta Blockers	II	Propranolol*, acebutolol, esmolol	Prolonged PR, bradycardias
Potassium Channel Blockers	III	Bretylium*, amiodarone	Prolonged QT
Calcium Channel Blockers	IV	Verapamil*, diltiazem	Prolonged PR, bradycardias
Miscellaneous		Adenosine, digoxin	Prolonged PR, bradycardias

*prototype

Procainamide (Pronestyl). Procainamide, like lidocaine, is useful in the suppression of ventricular arrhythmias. It is generally not a first-line drug, and its use is reserved for arrhythmias that do not respond to lidocaine.

Bretylium tosylate (Bretylol). Bretylium is used in the treatment of ventricular fibrillation that is refractory to lidocaine.

Adenosine (Adenocard). Adenosine is a naturally occurring nucleoside useful in the treatment of supraventricular tachycardias and is considered a first-line medication in emergency care of paroxysmal supraventricular tachycardia.

Verapamil (Isoptin). Verapamil is a slow calcium channel blocker. It is used in the treatment of paroxysmal supraventricular tachycardia and other atrial arrhythmias.

Diltiazem (Cardizem). Diltiazem is a calcium channel blocker and is used to slow the rapid ventricular rate that often accompanies atrial flutter and atrial fibrillation.

Amiodarone (Cordarone). Amiodarone is a class III antiarrhythmic agent that decreases sinus automaticity, reduces the speed of conduction, and increases the refractory period of the AV node.

Phenytoin (Dilantin). Phenytoin is infrequently used in the emergency setting as an antiarrhythmic agent. It has proven effectiveness, however, in the management of life-threatening arrhythmias resulting from digitalis toxicity.

Edrophonium chloride (Tensilon). Edrophonium chloride is an anticholinesterase agent that has proven effectiveness in terminating paroxysmal supraventricular tachycardias that do not respond to vagal maneuvers. Its usage is rapidly declining, with verapamil and adenosine being preferred.

Magnesium sulfate. Magnesium is a cofactor in many of the chemical and enzyme reactions that occur in the body. Magnesium deficiency is associated with a high frequency of cardiac arrhythmias and sudden death. Pharmacologically, it functions like a physiological calcium channel blocker.

Propranolol (Inderal). Propranolol, discussed in the previous section, plays a role in the treatment of supraventricular arrhythmias. Students are encouraged to review the section on propranolol and integrate the information with that on the drugs mentioned here.

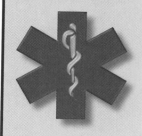

CASE PRESENTATION

EMS is dispatched to a residence for a man with chest pain. The patient is conscious and breathing and has a history of "heart attacks." On arrival paramedics are directed to a 63-year-old male (weight 80 kg) sitting on the couch in the living room. The patient is pale, cool, and diaphoretic.

On Examination

CNS:	The patient is conscious, alert, and oriented × 4
Resp:	Respirations are 24 and of normal depth; lung sounds clear bilaterally; trachea is midline; no signs of trauma
CVS:	Carotid and radial pulses are strong and irregular; skin is pale, cool, and diaphoretic
ABD:	Soft and nontender
Muscl/Skel:	Patient able to move extremities on command; no weaknesses to hand grip

Vital Signs

Pulse:	72/min, irregular, strong
Resp:	24/min, shallow
BP:	122/72 mm Hg
SpO$_2$:	95 percent
ECG:	Regular sinus rhythm with multifocal PVCs at 10/min

Hx:

P	No provoking factors
Q	Crushing pain
R	Radiating to neck
S	10/10, worst pain ever
T	Started suddenly 1/2 hour ago

Past Hx: The patient's wife states that her husband has had several episodes of chest pain brought on by exertion over the past few weeks. He was diagnosed with angina 6 years ago and had a "heart attack" last year. He has nitroglycerin spray, which he has used twice, prior to arrival of the ambulance. The patient takes nitroglycerin spray and ASA.

Treatment

Oxygen was administered by nonrebreather at 15 L/min. An IV was started with an 18-gauge catheter in the left arm and run TKO. The paramedics noticed a change on the ECG monitor to ventricular bigeminy. The patient was given nitroglycerin spray 0.4 mg with no relief; 2.5 mg of morphine was administered and provided slight relief of pain. Lidocaine 120 mg was given IV push, and a lidocaine drip was initiated at 2 mg/min, which converted the patient into a sinus rhythm. ASA was not given because the patient already takes ASA daily. Transport to the hospital was initiated. The pain was rated at 8/10, and another nitroglycerin spray and 2.5 mg of morphine were given. A 12-lead ECG confirmed ST elevation in both the inferior and lateral leads. The destination hospital was informed of a potential candidate for thrombolytic therapy and a second 18-gauge IV was initiated and run TKO. On arrival at the hospital the patient was treated with a thrombolytic medication and then admitted to the CCU to recover.

LIDOCAINE (XYLOCAINE)

Class: Antiarrhythmic

Description

Lidocaine is an amide-type local anesthetic. It is frequently used to treat life-threatening ventricular dysrhythmias.

Mechanism of Action

Lidocaine is probably the most frequently used antiarrhythmic agent in the treatment of life-threatening cardiac emergencies. Moreover, it has been shown to be effective in suppressing premature ventricular contractions, in treating ventricular tachycardia and some cases of ventricular fibrillation, and in increasing the fibrillation threshold in acute myocardial infarction. Lidocaine depresses depolarization and automaticity in the ventricles. It has very little effect on atrial tissues. In therapeutic doses it does not slow AV conduction and does not depress myocardial contractility. The most common cause of ventricular arrhythmias is acute myocardial infarction. Lidocaine suppresses ventricular ectopy in the setting of myocardial infarction and increases the ventricular fibrillation threshold. This prevents PVCs from inducing ventricular fibrillation. After acute myocardial infarction, the ventricular fibrillation threshold is often significantly reduced. Moreover, because electrical defibrillation tends to cause ventricular irritability, patients who have been successfully defibrillated should be treated with lidocaine.

Lidocaine is most apt to suppress ventricular arrhythmias when the level of the drug in the blood is between 1.5 and 6.0 µg/mL of blood. A 75 to 100 mg bolus of lidocaine will maintain adequate blood levels for only 20 minutes (see Figure 7–4). Therefore, once an arrhythmia is suppressed, the lidocaine bolus should be followed by a 2 to 4 mg/min infusion to ensure therapeutic blood levels (see Figure 7–5). It is important to distinguish patterns of premature ventricular contractions that are likely to lead to

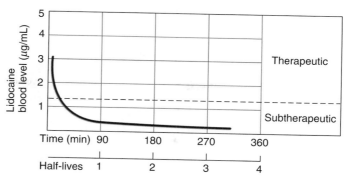

FIGURE 7-4 Blood levels of lidocaine following bolus without drip.

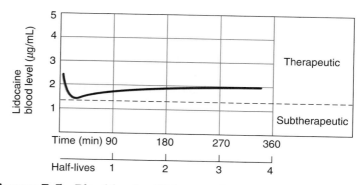

FIGURE 7-5 Blood levels of lidocaine following bolus with drip.

serious arrhythmias. Premature ventricular contractions that may lead to life-threatening arrhythmias are called malignant premature ventricular contractions. These patterns include the following:

- More than six unifocal PVCs per minute
- PVCs that appear to be coming from more than one ectopic focus (i.e., multifocal PVCs)
- PVCs that occur in couplets (two PVCs together without a normal QRS complex in between)
- Runs of more than two PVCs or ventricular tachycardia PVCs falling in the vulnerable period of the preceding normal complex (R on T phenomena)

The aforementioned premature ventricular contractions, as well as ventricular tachycardia and ventricular fibrillation, must be treated vigorously with lidocaine.

Indications

Lidocaine is used in ventricular tachycardia, ventricular fibrillation, and malignant premature ventricular contractions.

Contraindications

Lidocaine is usually contraindicated in second-degree Mobitz II and third-degree blocks. Lidocaine slows conduction of the electrical impulse from the atria to the ventricles. Decreased ventricular rates may accompany high-grade heart block, resulting in escape beats that are premature ventricular contractions. Whenever premature ventricular contractions occur in conjunction with bradycardia (heart rate less than 60 beats per minute), the bradycardia should be treated first. The drug of choice is atropine sulfate, followed by external pacing if atropine is not effective. If PVCs are still present after increasing the rate, lidocaine should be administered.

Precautions

Central nervous system depression may occur when the dosage exceeds 300 mg/hr. Symptoms of central nervous system depression include a decreased level of consciousness, irritability, confusion, muscle twitching, and eventually seizures. Exceedingly high doses can result in coma and death. Routine prophylactic lidocaine therapy in patients with acute myocardial infarction is no longer recommended. However, it may be used in conjunction with thrombolytic therapy to suppress expected reperfusion dysrhythmias.

Side Effects

Lidocaine may cause drowsiness, seizures, confusion, hypotension, bradycardia, heart blocks, nausea, vomiting, and respiratory and cardiac arrest.

Interactions

Lidocaine should be used with caution when administered concomitantly with procainamide, phenytoin, quinidine, and β-blockers because drug toxicity may result.

Dosage

Refractory ventricular fibrillation and pulseless ventricular tachycardia. The initial dose of lidocaine should be 1.0 to 1.5 mg/kg body weight. Lidocaine can be repeated every 3 to 5 minutes at a dose of 0.5 to 0.75 mg/kg to a maximum of 3.0 mg/kg. A single bolus dose of 1.5 mg/kg in cardiac arrest is generally acceptable because plasma lidocaine levels will remain therapeutic as a result of reduced drug elimination during cardiopulmonary resuscitation (CPR). Only bolus therapy should be used during CPR. Once a patient has been resuscitated, IV infusion therapy can be started to maintain therapeutic blood levels of the drug.

Ventricular tachycardia with a pulse and malignant PVCs. The initial dose of lidocaine should be 1.0 to 1.5 mg/kg. Boluses of 0.5 to 0.75 mg/kg can be repeated every 5 to 10 minutes as required to a maximum dose of 3.0 mg/kg. Once the arrhythmia has been suppressed, a lidocaine drip should be initiated at 2 to 4 mg/min.

The dosage of lidocaine should be reduced 50 percent in patients over 70 years of age and in patients with liver disease, heart failure, bradycardias, or conduction disturbances. Lidocaine is generally given in an IV bolus followed by an infusion (see Figure 7–6). It can also be given endotracheally, however, when an IV line cannot be established. The dose should be increased 2 to 2.5 times the intravenous dose when administering it endotra-

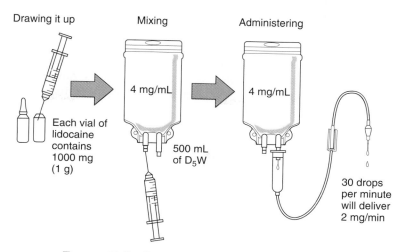

FIGURE 7–6 Preparation of lidocaine infusion.

cheally. A preparation of lidocaine that can be given intramuscularly for ventricular arrhythmias is also available. This usage should be reserved for times when an IV line cannot be established and the patient is not intubated.

How Supplied

Lidocaine is supplied in the following dosages: prefilled syringes, 100 mg in 5 mL of solvent 1 and 2 g additive syringes; ampules, 100 mg in 5 mL of solvent 1 and 2 g vials (in 30 mL of solvent); and premixed bags, 1 to 2 g in 500 mL of 5 percent dextrose.

PROCAINAMIDE (PRONESTYL)

Class: Antiarrhythmic

Description

Procainamide is an ester-type local anesthetic. It is frequently used to treat life-threatening ventricular dysrhythmias refractory to lidocaine.

Mechanism of Action

Procainamide is effective in suppressing ventricular ectopy. It may be effective in cases in which lidocaine has not suppressed life-threatening ventricular arrhythmias. Procainamide reduces the automaticity of the various pacemaker sites in the heart. Procainamide slows intraventricular conduction to a much greater degree than does lidocaine.

Indications

Procainamide is used in persistent cardiac arrest due to ventricular fibrillation and refractory to lidocaine, premature ventricular contractions refractory to lidocaine, and ventricular tachycardia refractory to lidocaine.

Contraindications

Procainamide should not be administered to patients with severe conduction system disturbances, especially second- and third-degree heart blocks.

Precautions

Procainamide must not be administered to patients demonstrating PVCs in conjunction with bradycardia. The heart rate should first be increased with atropine or transcutaneous pacing. Only after increasing the heart rate can the PVCs be treated with lidocaine or procainamide if they persist. Hypotension is common with intravenous infusion. Constant blood pressure monitoring is essential.

Side Effects

Procainamide may cause drowsiness, seizures, confusion, hypotension, bradycardia, heart blocks, nausea, vomiting, and respiratory and cardiac arrest.

Interactions

The hypotensive effects of procainamide may be increased if administered with antihypertensive drugs. The chance of neurological toxicity by both lidocaine and procainamide increases when the medications are administered together.

Dosage

In treating PVCs or ventricular tachycardia, 100 mg should be administered every 5 minutes at a rate of 20 mg/min. This should be discontinued if any of the following occur:

1. Arrhythmia is suppressed
2. Hypotension ensues
3. QRS complex is widened by 50 percent of its original width
4. A total of 17 mg/kg of the medication has been administered

The maintenance infusion of procainamide is 1 to 4 mg/min. The duration of procainamide's effect is shorter than that of lidocaine, requiring a more rigorous approach. Procainamide should be administered by slow IV bolus (20 mg/min) followed by a maintenance infusion. Generally, 1 g of procainamide is placed in 500 mL of D_5W. This gives a final concentration of 2 mg/mL (see Figure 7–7).

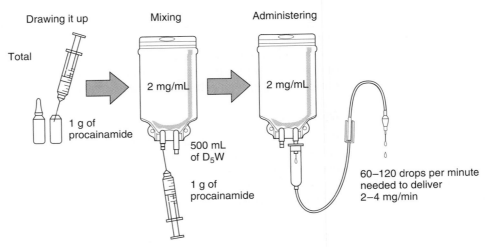

FIGURE 7–7 Preparation of procainamide infusion.

How Supplied

Procainamide is supplied in the following dosages: 10 mL vials containing 1000 mg of the drug and 2 mL vials containing 1000 mg of the drug (for infusion).

℞ BRETYLIUM TOSYLATE (BRETYLOL)

Class: Antiarrhythmic

Description

Bretylium is an antiarrhythmic that exhibits both adrenergic and direct myocardial effects.

Mechanism of Action

Bretylium tosylate causes two effects on adrenergic nerve endings. Once administered, bretylium causes release of norepinephrine from adrenergic nerve endings, which in turn causes a slight increase in heart rate, blood pressure, and cardiac output. These sympathomimetic effects last approximately 20 minutes in the noncardiac arrest setting. Then, norepinephrine reuptake is inhibited, which results in an adrenergic blockade. At this time, hypotension may develop (particularly orthostatic hypotension). Adrenergic blockade usually begins 15 to 20 minutes after drug administration and lasts for several hours (see Figure 7–8). The antiarrhythmic effect of bretylium is

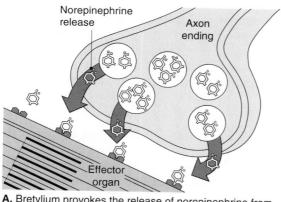

A. Bretylium provokes the release of norepinephrine from the axon ending.

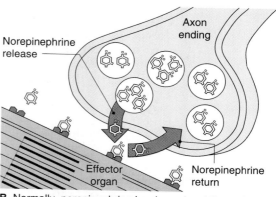

B. Normally, norepinephrine is released and then taken back up to the axon ending.

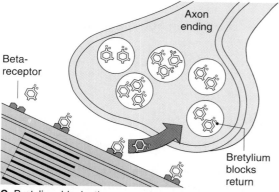

C. Bretylium blocks the return of norepinephrine to the axon ending.

FIGURE 7–8 The pharmacological effects of bretylium.

Antiarrhythmics

poorly understood, but it appears that it elevates the ventricular fibrillation threshold much as lidocaine does. Bretylium sometimes converts ventricular fibrillation or ventricular tachycardia to a supraventricular rhythm. Because of this action, bretylium is sometimes referred to as a chemical defibrillator.

Indications

Bretylium is used in ventricular fibrillation refractory to lidocaine and ventricular tachycardia refractory to lidocaine. At present, bretylium is not considered a first-line antiarrhythmic.

Contraindications

There are no contraindications to bretylium when used in the treatment of life-threatening ventricular arrhythmias.

Precautions

Postural hypotension occurs in approximately 50 percent of patients receiving bretylium. This side effect should be anticipated, and the patient should be kept in a supine position.

Side Effects

Bretylium may cause dizziness, syncope, seizures, hypotension, hypertension, angina, nausea, and vomiting.

Interactions

Arrhythmias caused by digitalis toxicity may be worsened by the initial release of norepinephrine that accompanies bretylium usage. Bretylium can interact with other antiarrhythmic agents, causing antagonistic or additive effects. The hypotensive effects of bretylium may be worsened if administered with class Ia antiarrhythmics such as procainamide, quinidine, or disopyramide.

Dosage

Bretylium should be administered at a dose of 5 mg/kg body weight. If the arrhythmia persists, subsequent doses of 10 mg/kg can be administered at 5-minute intervals. The total dose should not exceed 30 mg/kg. Because bretylium is somewhat slow in its onset, it should be administered by IV bolus.

How Supplied

Bretylium is supplied in ampules containing 500 mg of the drug in 10 mL of solvent.

ADENOSINE (ADENOCARD)

Class: Antiarrhythmic

Description

Adenosine is a naturally occurring nucleoside that slows AV conduction through the AV node. It has an exceptionally short half-life and a relatively good safety profile.

Mechanism of Action

Adenosine is a naturally occurring substance (purine nucleoside) that is present in all body cells. Adenosine decreases conduction of the electrical impulse through the AV node and interrupts AV reentry pathways in paroxysmal supraventricular tachycardia (PSVT). It can effectively terminate rapid supraventricular arrhythmias such as PSVT. The half-life of adenosine is approximately 5 seconds. Because of its rapid onset of action and very short half-life, the administration of adenosine is sometimes referred to as chemical cardioversion. A single bolus of the drug was effective in converting PSVT to a normal sinus rhythm in a significant number (90 percent) of patients in the initial drug studies. Adenosine does not appear to cause hypotension to the same degree as does verapamil.

Indication

Adenosine is used in PSVT (including that associated with Wolff-Parkinson-White syndrome) refractory to common vagal maneuvers.

Contraindications

Adenosine is contraindicated in patients with second- or third-degree heart block, sick sinus syndrome, or those with known hypersensitivity to the drug.

Precautions

Adenosine typically causes arrhythmias at the time of cardioversion. These generally last a few seconds or less and may include PVCs, premature atrial contractions, sinus bradycardia, sinus tachycardia, and various degrees of AV block. In extreme cases, transient asystole may occur. If this occurs, appropriate therapy should be initiated. Adenosine should be used cautiously in patients with asthma.

Side Effects

Adenosine can cause facial flushing, headache, shortness of breath, dizziness, and nausea, among others. Because the half-life of adenosine is so brief, side effects are generally self-limited.

Interactions

Methylxanthines (e.g., aminophylline and theophylline) may decrease the effectiveness of adenosine, thus requiring larger doses. Dipyridamole (Persantine) can potentiate the effects of adenosine. The dosage of adenosine may need to be reduced in patients receiving dipyridamole.

Dosage

The initial dose of adenosine is 6 mg given as a rapid intravenous bolus over a 1- to 2-second period. To be certain that the drug rapidly reaches the central circulation, it should be given directly into a vein or into a proximal medication port of a functioning IV line. It should be followed immediately by a rapid saline flush. If the initial dose does not result in conversion of the PSVT within 1 to 2 minutes, a 12 mg dose may be given as a

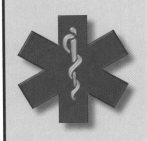

CASE PRESENTATION

At 1900 hours paramedics are dispatched to a residence for a 42-year-old female complaining of shortness of breath and chest pain. The patient is conscious and breathing. On arrival the paramedics are met by the patient's son, who directs the ambulance crew to the kitchen. They find the patient seated in a chair. The patient looks anxious, scared, and pale.

On Examination

CNS: The patient is conscious, alert, and oriented × 4; appears anxious

Resp: Respirations are 24 and shallow, with difficult, labored breathing; lung sounds clear bilaterally; trachea is midline; no signs of trauma

CVS: Carotid and radial pulses are present and rapid, pulse weaker radially; skin is pale and cool

ABD: Soft and nontender

Muscl/Skel: Patient able to move extremities on command; no weaknesses to hand grip

Vital Signs

Pulse: 220/min, regular, weak

Resp: 24/min, shallow, with difficulty breathing normally

BP: 110/60 mm Hg

SpO$_2$: 97 percent

ECG: Supraventricular tachycardia

Hx:
- **P** Was cooking at onset of symptoms
- **Q** Palpitations, squeezing discomfort with a feeling of SOB
- **R** Nonradiating
- **S** 3/10
- **T** Started suddenly about 30 minutes ago

Past Hx: The patient states that this has never happened before. She was cooking dinner when it suddenly "hit" her. She thought it would go away if she sat down, but it seemed to just get worse. She states that her heart feels like it is going to "jump" out of her chest and that she is having a hard time catching her breath. She does not take any medication except vitamins and is not allergic to anything.

Treatment

Oxygen was administered by nonrebreather at 15 L/min and an 18-gauge IV was initiated in her left antecubital vein and run TKO. A 12-lead ECG confirmed the SVT, and paramedics had the patient attempt the Valsalva maneuver without successful conversion of the SVT.

They advised the patient about adenosine, explaining the potential side effects; 6 mg of adenosine was then administered by rapid IV push. Although the patient felt some of the side effects of the adenosine, the first dose did not convert the SVT. The paramedics then administered a second dose of adenosine, this time increasing the dose to 12 mg. After a 4-second interval of a second-degree heart block, the patient's rhythm converted to a regular sinus rhythm. The patient stated that she was free of symptoms. She was transported to the hospital for further assessment, and a 12-lead ECG done en route did not show any acute evidence of a myocardial infarction. The patient was released shortly after with no apparent lasting effects of the SVT.

rapid IV bolus. The 12 mg dose may be repeated a second time if required. Doses greater than 12 mg should not be administered. Adenosine should only be given by rapid IV bolus, directly into the vein, or into the medication administration port closest to the patient.

How Supplied

Adenosine (Adenocard) is supplied in vials containing 6 mg of the drug in 2 mL of saline solvent.

 ## VERAPAMIL (ISOPTIN, CALAN)

Class: Calcium channel blocker

Description

Verapamil is a calcium ion antagonist (calcium channel blocker). Calcium channel blockers cause a relaxation of vascular smooth muscle and slow conduction through the AV node. Verapamil has a greater effect on conduction and a lesser effect on vascular smooth muscle than do other agents in the same class.

Mechanism of Action

Verapamil causes vascular dilation and slows conduction through the AV node. The advantages are twofold. First, verapamil inhibits arrhythmias caused by a reentry mechanism such as with paroxysmal supraventricular tachycardia. Second, it decreases the rapid ventricular response seen with atrial tachyarrhythmias such as atrial flutter and fibrillation. Verapamil also reduces myocardial oxygen demand because of its negative inotropic effects and causes coronary and peripheral vasodilation.

Indication

Verapamil is used in PSVT refractory to adenosine.

Antiarrhythmics

163

Contraindications

Verapamil should not be administered to any patient with severe hypotension or cardiogenic shock. In addition, verapamil should not be administered to patients with ventricular tachycardia in the prehospital setting. Before attempting to treat a patient suffering atrial flutter or atrial fibrillation, it is essential that the paramedic ensure that the patient does not have Wolff-Parkinson-White syndrome.

Precautions

Verapamil can cause systemic hypotension. Thus, it is essential that the blood pressure be constantly monitored following verapamil administration. Calcium chloride can be used to prevent the hypotensive effects of calcium channel blockers and in the management of calcium channel blocker overdosage.

Side Effects

Verapamil can cause nausea, vomiting, dizziness, headache, bradycardia, heart block, hypotension, and asystole.

Interactions

Verapamil should not be administered to patients receiving intravenous β-blockers because of an increased risk of congestive heart failure, bradycardia, and asystole.

Dosage

In the treatment of paroxysmal supraventricular tachycardia, a 2.5 to 5 mg IV dose should be given initially during a 2- to 3-minute interval. A repeat dose of 5 to 10 mg can be given in 15 to 30 minutes if PSVT persists and there have not been any adverse responses to the initial dose. The total dose of verapamil should not exceed 30 mg in 30 minutes.

How Supplied

Verapamil (Isoptin) is supplied in 2 mL ampules containing 5 mg of the drug.

DILTIAZEM (CARDIZEM)

Class: Calcium channel blocker

Description

Diltiazem is a calcium-ion antagonist (calcium channel blocker). Calcium channel blockers cause a relaxation of vascular smooth muscle and slow conduction through the AV node. Diltiazem has a nearly equal effect on vascular smooth muscle and AV conduction.

Mechanism of Action

Diltiazem causes vascular dilation and slows conduction through the AV node. It slows the rapid ventricular rate associated with atrial fibrillation and atrial flutter. It is also used in the treatment of angina because of its negative inotropic effect and because it dilates the coronary arteries.

Indications

Diltiazem is used to control rapid ventricular rates associated with atrial fibrillation and atrial flutter, for angina pectoris, and for PSVT refractory to adenosine.

Contraindications

Diltiazem should not be administered to any patient with severe hypotension or cardiogenic shock. In addition, diltiazem should not be administered to patients with ventricular tachycardia (wide-complex tachycardia) in the prehospital setting. Before attempting to treat a patient suffering atrial flutter or atrial fibrillation, it is essential that the paramedic ensure that the patient does not have Wolff-Parkinson-White syndrome.

Precautions

Diltiazem can cause systemic hypotension. Thus, it is essential that the blood pressure be constantly monitored following diltiazem administration. Calcium chloride can be used to prevent the hypotensive effects of calcium channel blockers and in the management of calcium channel blocker overdosage. Diltiazem should be kept refrigerated; however, it can be kept at room temperature for 1 month but must be discarded if unused.

Side Effects

Diltiazem can cause nausea, vomiting, dizziness, headache, bradycardia, heart block, hypotension, and asystole.

Interactions

Diltiazem should not be administered to patients receiving intravenous β-blockers because of an increased risk of congestive heart failure, bradycardia, and asystole.

Dosage

In the treatment of rapid ventricular rates associated with atrial fibrillation and atrial flutter, a 20 mg intravenous bolus (0.25 mg/kg) of diltiazem should be administered over 2 minutes. The bolus dose should be followed by a maintenance infusion of 5 to 15 mg/hr. For paroxysmal supraventricular tachycardia, a 0.25 mg/kg intravenous bolus should be administered over 2 minutes.

How Supplied

Diltiazem (Cardizem) is supplied in 5 mL vials containing 25 mg of the drug and in 10 mL vials containing 50 mg of the drug.

AMIODARONE HCL (CORDARONE)

Class: Antiarrhythmic agent

Description

Amiodarone is a class III antiarrhythmic agent used to treat ventricular arrhythmias unresponsive to other antiarrythmics.

Mechanism of Action

Amiodarone prolongs the action potential duration in all cardiac tissues.

Indications

Amiodarone is used in life-threatening cardiac arrhythmias such as ventricular tachycardia and ventricular fibrillation.

Contraindications

Amiodarone is contraindicated in breast-feeding patients in cardiogenic shock and those with severe sinus node dysfunction resulting in marked sinus bradycardia, second- or third-degree AV block, symptomatic bradycardia, or known hypersensitivity.

Precautions

Amiodarone should be used with caution in patients with latent or manifest heart failure because failure may be worsened by its administration.

Side Effects

Paramedics should monitor the patient's ECG and be alert for hypotension, bradycardia, increased ventricular beats, prolonged PR interval, QRS complex, and QT interval. The patient should also be monitored for signs of pulmonary toxicity such as dyspnea and cough.

Interactions

Amiodarone may react with warfarin, digoxin, procainamide, quinidine, and phenytoin.

Dosage

Ventricular arrhythmias (adults). Loading dose of 150 mg over 10 minutes (15 mg/min) IV or IO. May be repeated as necessary for recurrent or refractory arrhythmias.

Maintenance dose. 1 mg/min for 6 hours. Then 0.5 mg/min.

How Supplied

Ampule of 150 mg/3 mL.

PHENYTOIN (DILANTIN)

Class: Antiarrhythmic and anticonvulsant

Description

Phenytoin is an anticonvulsant and antiarrhythmic that depresses spontaneous ventricular depolarization.

Mechanism of Action

Phenytoin (Dilantin) is used frequently in the treatment of epilepsy but also has antiarrhythmic properties. It has proved effective in the management of arrhythmias caused by digitalis toxicity or tricyclic antidepressant drug overdoses. It depresses spontaneous depolarization of ventricular tissues and appears to improve atrioventricular conduction. Its use in the management of status epilepticus is discussed in Chapter 10.

Indication

Phenytoin is used in life-threatening arrhythmias resulting from digitalis toxicity or tricyclic antidepressant overdose. Ventricular arrhythmias in the setting of acute myocardial infarction should first be treated with lidocaine.

Contraindications

Phenytoin is contraindicated in cases of bradycardia and high-grade heart block. It should not be administered to patients who take the drug chronically for seizures until the blood level has been determined.

Precautions

Intravenous administration of phenytoin should not exceed 50 mg/min. Signs of central nervous system depression or hypotension may occur. Elderly patients are at increased risk of developing side effects from phenytoin administration. Extravasation should be avoided. Any patient receiving intravenous phenytoin should have continuous cardiac monitoring as well as frequent monitoring of vital signs.

Side Effects

Phenytoin can cause drowsiness, dizziness, headache, hypotension, arrhythmias, itching, rash, nausea, and vomiting.

Interactions

Phenytoin must never be diluted in dextrose-containing solutions such as D_5W. It should be diluted in normal saline or other non-glucose-containing crystalloids.

Dosage

The recommended dose of phenytoin is 100 mg over 5 minutes to a maximum loading dose of 1000 mg, until the arrhythmia is suppressed, or until symptoms of central nervous system depression appear. In the emergency setting, phenytoin should be given by slow IV bolus or IV infusion with constant ECG monitoring.

How Supplied

Phenytoin (Dilantin) is supplied in 2 and 5 mL vials containing 50 mg/mL of the drug. Dilantin is incompatible with solutions containing dextrose. If an infusion of Dilantin is prepared, the drug should be placed in normal saline.

EDROPHONIUM CHLORIDE (TENSILON)

Class: Antiarrhythmic and cholinesterase inhibitor

Description

Edrophonium belongs to a class of drugs referred to as anticholinesterase agents. It is used in the treatment of paroxysmal supraventricular tachycardia refractory to first-line agents.

Mechanism of Action

Edrophonium inhibits the actions of the enzyme *acetylcholinesterase.* This enzyme plays an important role in neurophysiology because it deactivates the neurotransmitter of the parasympathetic nervous system, acetylcholine. Physostigmine, an emergency drug used in the management of atropine-type poisonings and tricyclic antidepressant overdoses, is chemically similar to edrophonium. The neurophysiology of the parasympathetic nervous system is discussed in more detail in the following section on parasympatholytics. Edrophonium has proven effectiveness in the management of paroxysmal supraventricular tachycardias that do not respond to vagal maneuvers. The inhibition of acetylcholinesterase by edrophonium serves to enhance the acetylcholine secreted by the vagus nerve on the heart. This increased parasympathetic effect has been successful in slowing and eventually terminating paroxysmal supraventricular tachycardias. With the introduction of adenosine and the calcium channel blockers (verapamil), edrophonium has fallen into relative disuse.

Indication

Edrophonium is used for PSVT refractory to vagal maneuvers and adenosine.

Contraindications

Edrophonium should not be administered to patients with a history of hypersensitivity to the drug. It should not be used in patients who are hypotensive or bradycardic because it can worsen these conditions.

Precautions

The respiratory pattern should be carefully monitored during and following administration of edrophonium. Also, the patient should be constantly monitored for signs of bradycardia. Atropine sulfate should be readily available in those cases of bradycardia causing hemodynamic problems. Edrophonium should be used with caution in the elderly.

Side Effects

Edrophonium can cause dizziness, weakness, sweating, increased salivation, constricted pupils, hypotension, bradycardia, abdominal cramps, nausea, and vomiting.

Interactions

Edrophonium should not be administered in dextrose solutions because it tends to crystallize in the tubing. The chances of developing a significant bradycardia are enhanced when edrophonium is administered to patients taking digitalis.

Dosage

The standard dosage is 5 mg initially intravenously. If unsuccessful after 10 minutes or so, a second dose of 10 mg may be administered. Physicians frequently order the administration of a test dose of 0.1 to 0.5 mg, particularly to elderly patients, before the administration of the full dose. Edrophonium should be administered intravenously only.

How Supplied

Edrophonium is supplied in ampules containing 10 mg of the drug in 1 mL of solvent.

MAGNESIUM SULFATE

Class: Antiarrhythmic

Description

Magnesium sulfate is a salt that dissociates into the magnesium cation (Mg^{2+}) and the sulfate anion when administered. Magnesium is an essential element in numerous biochemical reactions that occur within the body.

Mechanism of Action

Magnesium is an essential element in many of the biochemical processes that occur in the body. It acts as a physiological calcium channel blocker and blocks neuromuscular transmission. A decreased magnesium level (hypomagnesemia) is associated with cardiac arrhythmias, symptoms of cardiac insufficiency, and sudden death. Hypomagnesemia can cause refractory ventricular fibrillation. Administration of magnesium sulfate in the emergency setting appears to reduce the incidence of ventricular arrhythmias that may follow an acute myocardial infarction. It also appears to decrease the complications associated with acute myocardial infarction. Magnesium sulfate has been used for years in the management of preterm labor and the hypertensive disorders of pregnancy (preeclampsia and eclampsia). Its usage in obstetrics is discussed in Chapter 11.

Indications

Magnesium sulfate is used in severe refractory ventricular fibrillation or pulseless ventricular tachycardia, post–myocardial infarction for prophylaxis of arrhythmias, and torsade de pointes (multiaxial ventricular tachycardia).

Contraindications

Magnesium sulfate should not be administered to patients who are in shock, who have persistent severe hypertension, who have third-degree AV block, who routinely undergo dialysis, or who are known to have a decreased calcium level (hypocalcemia).

Precautions

Magnesium sulfate should be administered slowly to minimize side effects. Any patient receiving intravenous magnesium sulfate should have continuous cardiac monitoring and frequent monitoring of vital signs. If possible, the knee and biceps deep tendon reflexes should be checked prior to beginning magnesium therapy. It should be used with caution in patients with known renal insufficiency. Hypermagnesemia (elevated magnesium level) can occur following magnesium sulfate administration. Calcium salts (calcium chloride or calcium gluconate) should be available as an antidote for magnesium sulfate in case serious side effects occur.

Side Effects

Magnesium sulfate can cause flushing, sweating, bradycardia, decreased deep tendon reflexes, drowsiness, respiratory depression, arrhythmias, hypotension, hypothermia, itching, and rash.

Interactions

Magnesium sulfate can cause cardiac conduction abnormalities if administered in conjunction with digitalis.

Dosage

Ventricular fibrillation or ventricular tachycardia. 1 to 2 g of magnesium sulfate should be diluted in 10 mL of D_5W and administered by slow IV push over 1 to 2 minutes. Alternatively, 1 to 2 grams of magnesium sulfate can be diluted in 100 mL of D_5W and administered IV piggyback over 1 to 2 minutes.

Torsade de pointes. Higher doses are often required in the treatment of torsade de pointes. Typically, 5 to 10 g are diluted in 100 mL of D_5W and administered at a rate of 1 g/min until the arrhythmia is suppressed or the maximum dose has been administered.

Post–myocardial infarction prophylaxis. 1 to 2 g of magnesium sulfate can be diluted in 100 mL of D_5W and administered over 5 to 30 minutes as an IV piggyback.

Magnesium should be administered intravenously in the prehospital setting. However, it can be administered intramuscularly if IV access cannot be obtained. Because of the volume of the drug (5 to 10 mL), the dose should be divided in half and each half administered intramuscularly at a separate site (usually each gluteus).

How Supplied

Magnesium sulfate is supplied in vials and prefilled syringes. The drug is supplied in both 10 percent and 50 percent solutions. The solution should be examined closely prior to preparation to avoid dosing errors.

Drugs that inhibit the actions of the parasympathetic nervous system are referred to as *parasympatholytics*. Sometimes they are referred to as *anticholinergics*. To fully understand the role and actions of the parasympatholytics, we must first review the parasympathetic nervous system.

The parasympathetic, or *cholinergic*, system plays a major role in the maintenance of homeostasis. Parasympathetic stimulation induces peristalsis and causes pupillary constriction and a decrease in the heart rate. The primary nerve of the parasympathetic nervous system is the *vagus nerve*. The vagus nerve descends from the brain along the carotid arteries. It then innervates the heart and the digestive system. Paramedics should be familiar with the manual method of vagal stimulation, carotid sinus massage. Carotid sinus massage is used to slow the heart rate in paroxysmal supraventricular tachycardia.

When the vagus nerve is stimulated, it causes acetylcholine to be released from the presynaptic nerve endings. It then activates acetylcholine receptors on the target organs. These receptors cause the heart rate to slow. Then, after only a fraction of a second, cholinesterase is released, which deactivates acetylcholine. Several drugs act on these junctions. The primary drug of this type is atropine sulfate. Atropine binds to the acetylcholine receptors, thus inhibiting activation. Besides increasing the heart rate, atropine is used frequently as a preoperative medication because it decreases digestive secretions, especially salivation. Certain chemicals, especially the organophosphate insecticides, tend to block, in an irreversible manner, the action of cholinesterase. Excessive levels of acetylcholine can cause serious problems.

Research has shown that some cases of asystole can be caused by an increase in parasympathetic tone. The reason for the increase is not clear. Based on this information, however, the American Heart Association recommends administering 1 mg of atropine sulfate as soon as possible to any patient encountered in asystole.

It is important to remember that abdominal distension with air from CPR can increase parasympathetic tone. This can often go unrecognized and makes it difficult to restore a spontaneous rhythm from asystole. It should be a routine part of advanced life support (ALS) to decompress the stomach if distended. The use of proper CPR, Sellick's maneuver, and endotracheal intubation can help minimize abdominal distension.

ATROPINE SULFATE

Class: Anticholinergic

Description

Atropine is a parasympatholytic (anticholinergic) that is derived from parts of the *Atropa belladonna* plant.

Mechanism of Action

Atropine sulfate is a potent parasympatholytic and is used to increase the heart rate in hemodynamically significant bradycardias. Hemodynamically significant bradycardias are those slow heart rates accompanied by hypotension, shortness of breath, chest pain, altered mental status, congestive heart failure, and shock. Atropine acts by blocking acetylcholine receptors, thus inhibiting parasympathetic stimulation. Although it has positive chronotropic properties, it has little or no inotropic effect. It plays an important role as an antidote in organophosphate poisonings. Atropine has been shown to be of some use in asystole, presumably because some cases of asystole may be caused by a sudden and tremendous increase in parasympathetic tone. The mechanism by which atropine is effective in asystole is not clear. However, despite no definite proof of its value in asystole, there is little evidence that its use is harmful in this setting.

Indications

Atropine is used in hemodynamically significant bradycardia and asystole.

Contraindications

There are no contraindications in emergency situations.

Precautions

Atropine may actually worsen the bradycardia associated with second-degree Mobitz II and third-degree AV blocks. In these cases, the paramedic should go straight to transcutaneous pacing instead of trying atropine. A maximum dose of 0.04 mg/kg body weight of atropine should not be exceeded except in the setting of organophosphate poisoning. If the heart rate fails to increase after a total of 0.04 mg/kg has been given, then transcutaneous pacing is indicated.

Side Effects

Atropine sulfate can cause blurred vision, dilated pupils, dry mouth, tachycardia, drowsiness, and confusion.

Interactions

There are few interactions in the prehospital setting.

Dosage

Hemodynamically significant bradycardia. An initial dose of 0.5 mg should be administered intravenously. This dose can be repeated every 3 to 5 minutes until a maximum dose of 0.04 mg/kg has been administered.

Asystole. In the treatment of asystole, the dose should be increased to 1.0 mg. When an IV cannot be placed, atropine can be administered endotracheally. However, the dose should be increased to 2 to 2.5 times the intravenous dose.

Atropine should be given as an IV bolus in emergency situations or endotracheally when an IV cannot be placed.

How Supplied

Atropine is supplied in prefilled syringes containing 1.0 mg in 10 mL of solution.

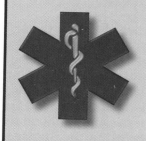

CASE PRESENTATION

Paramedics are called to a local shopping mall for a medical emergency. Reportedly, a patient collapsed and is unconscious and breathing. On arrival the patient is found lying on the floor in the center court with a pillow under her head. The patient appears to be in her early 60s.

On Examination

CNS: The patient is conscious, slow to respond to verbal commands, and disoriented to person, place, and time

Resp: Respirations are 12 and shallow; lung sounds clear bilaterally; trachea is midline; no signs of trauma

CVS: Weak, regular, slow carotid pulse and radial pulses are present; skin is pale, cool, and diaphoretic; no complaint of chest pain

ABD: Soft and nontender

Muscl/Skel: Patient able to move extremities slightly, with delay, on command; weak bilateral hand grip; no obvious injuries

Vital Signs

Pulse: 36/min, regular, weak

Resp: 12/min, shallow

BP: 72/56 mm Hg

SpO$_2$: 86 percent

ECG: Sinus bradycardia

Hx: Unknown; patient was in the mall alone and is unable to give a history or answer questions.

Past Hx: Unknown; no Medic Alert.

Treatment

Oxygen was administered by nonrebreather at 12 L/min and well tolerated by the patient. An IV of normal saline was established. The patient was given 0.5 mg of atropine. Following the atropine the patient's pulse rate increased slightly to 42/min and her blood pressure was 80/62. At this point the pacing pads were placed on the patient as a precautionary measure. A second dose of atropine 0.5 mg was given, and the heart rate improved to 68/min with a blood pressure of 108/82. The patient's level of consciousness improved. The patient was moved to the ambulance and transported to the hospital.

En route to the hospital the patient stated that she was shopping alone when she felt faint. She sat down to let the faintness pass. She does not remember what happened prior to fainting. She remembers waking and seeing the paramedics with her.

CARDIAC GLYCOSIDES

Digitalis, the principal drug in the cardiac glycoside class, is one of the oldest medications known to humans. For hundreds of years it has been used in the treatment of congestive heart failure. Digitalis and the related cardiac glycosides increase the force (inotropic effect) of the myocardial contraction. When given to patients in congestive heart failure, it significantly increases cardiac output, reducing left ventricular diameter; decreases venous pressure; and hastens reduction of peripheral and pulmonary edema. In recent years digitalis has also proved effective in the management of patients with atrial flutter and atrial fibrillation. In these patients rapid atrial rates produce accelerated ventricular rates, which can be reduced by digitalis therapy.

Several digitalis preparations are available:

Digitoxin. Digitoxin is the longest-acting cardiac glycoside. It must not be confused with the shorter-acting digoxin.

Digoxin (Lanoxin). Digoxin is the most commonly prescribed form of digitalis.

Ouabain. Ouabain has a rapid rate of onset and a relatively short duration of effect. Its use is reserved for cases in which rapid digitalization is required.

Deslanoside (Cedilanid-D). Deslanoside is the most rapidly acting digitalis preparation.

Cardiac glycosides have profound effects on cardiac function and rhythm. The therapeutic index (therapeutic dose/toxic dose) is low, which means that the possibility of digitalis toxicity should always be considered in patients with this medication. Signs of digitalis toxicity include cardiac arrhythmias (PVCs, PSVT with 2:1 block, and so on), nausea, vomiting, headache, visual disturbances (yellow vision), and drowsiness. Almost any arrhythmia can be associated with digitalis toxicity.

Digitalis is a potent and potentially toxic drug. Extreme care must be used whenever it is administered. Constant monitoring of vital signs and ECG is essential. In almost all cases digitalization should be deferred until the patient is in the emergency department and under the care of the emergency department physician.

DIGOXIN (LANOXIN)

Class: Cardiac glycoside

Description

Digoxin is a moderately rapid-acting cardiac glycoside used in the management of congestive heart failure and to control the heart rate in atrial fibrillation and atrial flutter.

Mechanism of Action

Digoxin is a cardiac glycoside effective in the treatment of congestive heart failure and rapid atrial arrhythmias. It increases the force of the cardiac contraction through its effects on the sodium-potassium ATPase system.

Digoxin significantly increases the stroke volume, thus increasing the cardiac output. It also decreases AV nodal conduction, thus slowing the heart rate. Therapeutic effects begin in about half an hour and peak at 24 hours.

Indications

Digoxin is used in congestive heart failure and supraventricular tachyarrhythmias, especially atrial flutter and atrial fibrillation.

Contraindications

Digoxin should not be given to any patient showing any of the signs or symptoms of digitalis toxicity. It also should not be administered to patients in ventricular fibrillation.

Precautions

Patients receiving digoxin should be constantly monitored for signs and symptoms of digitalis toxicity. Extreme care should be used when administering digoxin to patients with myocardial infarction, because they are prone to digitalis toxicity. Digitalis toxicity is potentiated in patients with hypokalemia, hypomagnesemia, and hypercalcemia. Digitalis crosses the placenta and thus can affect the fetal heart in much the same manner as the mother's.

Side Effects

Digoxin can cause numerous side effects. Noncardiac side effects include anorexia, nausea, vomiting, abdominal pain, diarrhea, fatigue, depression, drowsiness, yellow vision, headache, dizziness, hallucinations, sweating, itching, and rash. Cardiac side effects include arrhythmias, bradycardias, tachycardias, various degrees of heart block, hypotension, and cardiac arrest.

Interactions

Many drugs have potential interaction problems with digoxin. Quinidine and the calcium channel blockers (verapamil, nifedipine, and diltiazem) can increase serum digoxin levels. The administration of digoxin concomitantly with beta-blockers can cause severe bradycardia. Diuretics can cause potassium depletion, which can lead to digitalis toxicity.

Dosage

The dosage is 0.25 to 0.5 mg given by slow IV push. Digoxin is generally given intravenously in the treatment of supraventricular tachyarrhythmias.

How Supplied

Digoxin (Lanoxin) is supplied in 2 mL ampules containing 0.5 mg of the drug.

THROMBOLYTICS

A myocardial infarction begins with the formation of a blood clot (thrombus) in a coronary artery. This clot results in complete occlusion of the artery and subsequent interruption of blood flow to the area of the myocardium supplied by that artery. Usually, the coronary artery is already partially obstructed by atherosclerosis. These obstructions are often the narrowest (or tightest) portions of the artery and the site of thrombus formation.

Following arterial occlusion, the portion of the myocardium supplied by the obstructed artery becomes ischemic. At this point the ischemia can be reversed with minimal permanent injury to the muscle if the blood supply can be restored. However, if the occlusion continues, the myocardium will become injured and will eventually die. There is a window of 6 hours after the onset of pain to restore perfusion to the injured myocardium. There are several ways perfusion can be restored, including percutaneous transluminal coronary angioplasty (PTCA), coronary artery bypass grafting (CABG), and thrombolytic therapy. PTCA requires access to a cardiac catheterization lab and subsequent coronary arteriogram to identify the occlusion. Then, a special balloon catheter is introduced into the diseased artery. The balloon is placed at the site of the occlusion and filled, resulting in dilation of the occlusion. This process is time-consuming and not available in every hospital. Likewise, CABG requires an initial arteriogram followed by major surgery to bypass the obstruction. Thrombolytic therapy, unlike the other procedures, does not require coronary angiography and can be performed in any community hospital and, in some places, in the prehospital setting.

Thrombolytic therapy is the administration of a drug to dissolve the blood clot in the coronary artery causing an acute myocardial infarction. There are three major types of thrombolytics available in the United States: streptokinase (Streptase), anistreplase (Eminase), and alteplase (tPA, Activase). Aspirin, a platelet aggregation inhibitor, is included in this discussion because it has proved highly effective in reducing mortality following myocardial infarction.

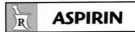 **ASPIRIN**

Class: Platelet aggregator inhibitor and anti-inflammatory agent

Description

Aspirin is an anti-inflammatory agent and an inhibitor of platelet function. This makes it a useful agent in the treatment of various thromboembolic diseases such as acute myocardial infarction.

Mechanism of Action

Aspirin blocks the formation of the substance thromboxane A_2, which causes platelets to aggregate and arteries to constrict. This results in an overall reduction in mortality associated with myocardial infarction. It also appears to reduce the rate of nonfatal reinfarction and nonfatal stroke.

Indications

Aspirin is used for new chest pain suggestive of acute myocardial infarction (AMI) and signs and symptoms suggestive of recent stroke (cerebrovascular accident).

Contraindications

Aspirin is contraindicated in patients with known hypersensitivity to the drug. It is relatively contraindicated in patients with active ulcer disease and asthma.

Precautions

Aspirin can cause gastrointestinal upset and bleeding. Enteric-coated aspirin, if available, should be used in patients who have a tendency for gastric irritation and bleeding with aspirin. Aspirin should be used with caution in patients who report allergies to the nonsteroidal anti-inflammatory (NSAID) class of drugs. Doses higher than recommended can actually interfere with possible benefits.

Side Effects

Aspirin can cause heartburn, gastrointestinal bleeding, nausea, vomiting, wheezing, and prolonged bleeding.

Interactions

When administered together, aspirin and other anti-inflammatory agents may cause an increased incidence of side effects and increased blood levels of both drugs. Administration of aspirin with antacids may reduce the blood levels of the drug by decreasing absorption.

Dosage

The recommended dosage for aspirin is 160 to 325 mg taken as soon as possible after the onset of chest pain. Baby aspirin (160 mg) is often preferred because it can be chewed and swallowed and is often a little more palatable; many myocardial infarction patients are nauseated. Aspirin is often given as part of a thrombolytic therapy protocol.

How Supplied

Aspirin is supplied in tablets (chewable and standard) containing 160 and 325 mg of the drug. Enteric-coated aspirin (Ecotrin) is available for those with a tendency for gastronintestinal upset with aspirin therapy.

STREPTOKINASE (STREPTASE)

Class: Thrombolytic

Description

Streptokinase is a potent thrombolytic. It is derived from the bacteria Group C, β-hemolytic streptococci.

Mechanism of Action

Streptokinase acts with plasminogen (present in the blood) to produce a so-called activator complex. This activator complex converts plasminogen to the enzyme plasmin. Plasmin then digests fibrin and fibrinogen, resulting in the dissolution of clots that cause coronary occlusion.

Indication

Streptokinase is used for acute myocardial infarction.

Contraindications

Streptokinase is absolutely contraindicated in the following cases:

1. Active internal bleeding
2. Suspected aortic dissection
3. Traumatic CPR (rib fractures, pneumothorax)
4. Severe, persistent hypertension
5. Recent head trauma or known intracranial tumor
6. History of stroke in the past 6 months
7. Pregnancy

It is relatively contraindicated (i.e., the risks must be weighed against the potential benefits) in the following cases:

1. History of trauma or major surgery in the past 2 months
2. Initial blood pressure greater than 180 systolic or 110 diastolic that is controlled by medical treatment
3. Active peptic ulcer or blood in stool
4. History of stroke, tumor, brain surgery, or head injury
5. Known bleeding disorder or current use of warfarin (Coumadin)
6. Significant liver dysfunction or kidney failure
7. Exposure to streptokinase or anistreplase during the preceding 12 months
8. Known cancer or illness with possible thoracic, abdominal, or intracranial abnormalities
9. Prolonged CPR

Precautions

Streptokinase may be ineffective if administered within 12 months of prior streptokinase or anistreplase therapy. Anaphylaxis can occur with streptokinase therapy. Emergency resuscitative drugs and equipment should be immediately available. Reperfusion arrhythmias are common once the occluded artery opens. Antiarrhythmic medications should be immediately available.

Side Effects

Streptokinase can cause bleeding, allergic reactions, anaphylaxis, fever, nausea, and vomiting.

Interactions

Streptokinase should be used with caution in patients on anticoagulation therapy.

Dosage

Streptokinase should be administered at 1.5 million units over 1 hour. This is typically part of a streptokinase protocol in which aspirin, an antihistamine, and a corticosteroid are administered before administering streptokinase. The antihistamine and corticosteroid are given to prevent a possible allergic reaction to the drug.

Streptokinase must be reconstituted immediately prior to administration. The manufacturer's recommendations for reconstitution, which accompany the drug, should be followed explicitly. Streptokinase should be administered intravenously, preferably through an IV pump.

How Supplied

Streptokinase is supplied in a box containing a 50-mL infusion bottle and a 6.5-mL vial of the drug.

ANISTREPLASE (EMINASE, APSAC)

Class: Thrombolytic

Description

Anistreplase is a potent thrombolytic. It is a derivative of the plasminogen-streptokinase activator complex and is derived from the bacteria Group C, β-hemolytic streptococci.

Mechanism of Action

Anistreplase is an inactive derivative that is activated when administered. Plasmin is produced from plasminogen (present in the blood). Plasmin then digests fibrin and fibrinogen, resulting in the dissolution of clots that cause coronary occlusion.

Indication

Acute myocardial infarction

Contraindications

Anistreplase is absolutely contraindicated in the following cases:

1. Active internal bleeding
2. Suspected aortic dissection
3. Traumatic CPR (rib fractures, pneumothorax)
4. Severe persistent hypertension
5. Recent head trauma or known intracranial tumor
6. History of stroke in the past 6 months
7. Pregnancy

It is relatively contraindicated (i.e., the risks must be weighed against the potential benefits) in the following cases:

1. History of trauma or major surgery in the past 2 months
2. Initial blood pressure greater than 180 systolic or 110 diastolic that is controlled by medical treatment

3. Active peptic ulcer or blood in stool

4. History of stroke, tumor, brain surgery, or head injury

5. Known bleeding disorder or current use of warfarin (Coumadin)

6. Significant liver dysfunction or kidney failure

7. Exposure to streptokinase or anistreplase during the preceding 12 months

8. Known cancer or illness with possible thoracic, abdominal, or intracranial abnormalities

9. Prolonged CPR

Precautions

Anistreplase may be ineffective if administered within 12 months of prior streptokinase or anistreplase therapy. Anaphylaxis can occur with anistreplase therapy. Emergency resuscitative drugs and equipment should be immediately available. Reperfusion arrhythmias are common once the occluded artery opens. Antiarrhythmic medications should be immediately available.

Side Effects

Anistreplase can cause bleeding, allergic reactions, anaphylaxis, fever, nausea, and vomiting.

Interactions

Anistreplase should be used with caution in patients on anticoagulation therapy.

Dosage

Anistreplase (30 units) should be injected slowly over 4 to 5 minutes in a onetime dose. This is typically part of an Eminase protocol in which aspirin, an antihistamine, and a corticosteroid are administered before administering anistreplase. The antihistamine and corticosteroid are given to prevent a possible allergic reaction to the drug.

Anistreplase must be reconstituted immediately prior to administration and used within 30 minutes of reconstitution. The manufacturer's recommendations for reconstitution, which accompany the drug, should be followed exactly. When mixing the drug, the paramedic must be careful not to shake it. Instead, it should be gently rolled in the vial to mix it.

Anistreplase should be administered by slow intravenous bolus.

How Supplied

Anistreplase is supplied in a 30-unit vial. It is very expensive and should be handled carefully.

ALTEPLASE, TISSUE PLASMINOGEN ACTIVATOR (ACTIVASE)

Class: Thrombolytic

Description

Alteplase (tPA) is a potent thrombolytic. It is a tissue plasminogen activator produced through recombinant DNA technology.

Mechanism of Action

Alteplase is an enzyme that converts plasminogen (present in the blood) to the enzyme plasmin. It also produces a limited amount of fibrinogen in the absence of fibrin. When administered, alteplase binds to the fibrin in a thrombus and converts the plasminogen into plasmin. Plasmin then digests fibrin and fibrinogen, causing the dissolution of clots that cause coronary occlusion.

Indication

Alteplase is used for acute myocardial infarction.

Contraindications

Alteplase is absolutely contraindicated in the following cases:

1. Active internal bleeding
2. Suspected aortic dissection
3. Traumatic CPR (rib fractures, pneumothorax)
4. Severe, persistent hypertension
5. Recent head trauma or known intracranial tumor
6. History of stroke in the past 6 months
7. Pregnancy

It is relatively contraindicated in the following cases:

1. History of trauma or major surgery in the past 2 months
2. Initial blood pressure greater than 180 systolic or 110 diastolic that is controlled by medical treatment
3. Active peptic ulcer or blood in stool
4. History of stroke, tumor, brain surgery, or head injury
5. Known bleeding disorder or current use of warfarin (Coumadin)
6. Significant liver dysfunction or kidney failure
7. Known cancer or illness with possible thoracic, abdominal, or intracranial abnormalities
8. Prolonged CPR

Precautions

Alteplase does not appear to have the problem with readministration associated with streptokinase or anistreplase. Anaphylaxis can occur with alteplase therapy but is very rare. Emergency resuscitative drugs and equipment should be immediately available. Reperfusion arrhythmias are common once the occluded artery opens. Antiarrhythmic medications should be immediately available.

Side Effects

Alteplase can cause bleeding, allergic reactions, anaphylaxis, fever, nausea, and vomiting.

Interactions

Alteplase should be used with caution in patients on anticoagulation therapy.

Dosage

The dosage regimen for alteplase is controversial. The manufacturer recommends a total dose of 100 mg; 10 mg is administered as an IV bolus over 1 to 2 minutes, followed by an infusion of 50 mg over the first hour, 20 mg over the second hour, and 20 mg over the third hour. A more popular dosing regimen is the accelerated or front-loaded regimen. In this case, 15 mg of the drug is administered as an IV bolus over 1 to 2 minutes. This is followed by an IV infusion of 50 mg over the first hour and 35 mg over the second hour. Alteplase must be reconstituted immediately prior to administration. The manufacturer's recommendations for reconstitution, which accompany the drug, should be followed exactly. Alteplase should be administered intravenously. An initial bolus should be administered over 1 to 2 minutes followed by an IV infusion, preferably through an IV pump.

How Supplied

Alteplase is supplied in a box containing vials with 20, 50, or 100 mg of the drug. Alteplase is very expensive and should be handled carefully.

ALKALINIZING AGENTS

Alkalinizing drugs, such as sodium bicarbonate, are used to buffer the acids present in the body during and after cardiac arrest and other serious conditions. Normal body pH is 7.4 (7.35 to 7.45). During hypoxia, the serum pH may fall quickly. Sodium bicarbonate will help correct metabolic (usually lactic acid) acidosis until hypoxia is corrected. The following reaction illustrates the role of sodium bicarbonate in acid-base balance:

$$H^+ \quad + \quad HCO_3^- \quad \leftrightarrow \quad H_2CO_2 \quad \leftrightarrow \quad H_2O \quad + \quad CO_2$$

| Acids (strong) | Bicarbonate | Carbonic acid | Water | Carbon dioxide |

Bicarbonate combines with the strong acids, usually lactic acid, and forms a weak, volatile acid (carbonic acid). This acid then is broken down into carbon dioxide and water. The two end products are then removed via the lungs and the kidneys, respectively.

Excessive administration of sodium bicarbonate may cause metabolic alkalosis, which may be worse than the metabolic acidosis being treated. Primary treatment of metabolic acidosis in the setting of hypoxia or cardiac arrest includes adequate oxygenation and blood pressure support.

SODIUM BICARBONATE

Class: Alkalinizing agent

Description

Sodium bicarbonate is a salt that provides bicarbonate to buffer metabolic acidosis, which can accompany several disease processes.

Mechanism of Action

For many years sodium bicarbonate was the cornerstone of advanced cardiac life support care. Controlled studies have shown that sodium bicarbonate was ineffective in the treatment of cardiac arrest. In many instances it has actually been associated with many adverse reactions. Sodium bicarbonate is occasionally used in the treatment of certain types of drug overdose. The most common example is drugs in the tricyclic class of antidepressants. Overdosage of these drugs has serious effects including life-threatening cardiac arrhythmias. Tricyclic antidepressant excretion from the body is enhanced by making the urine more alkaline (raising the pH). Sodium bicarbonate is sometimes administered to increase the pH of the urine to speed excretion of the drug from the body.

Indications

Sodium bicarbonate is used late in the management of cardiac arrest, if at all. Hyperventilation, prompt defibrillation, and the administration of epinephrine and lidocaine should always precede use of sodium bicarbonate. Because these therapies take at least 10 minutes to carry out, sodium bicarbonate should rarely be administered in the first 10 minutes of a resuscitation. Sodium bicarbonate is also indicated in tricyclic antidepressant overdose, phenobarbital overdose, severe acidosis refractory to hyperventilation, and known hyperkalemia.

Contraindications

When used in the management of the situations described earlier, there are no absolute contraindications.

Precautions

Sodium bicarbonate can cause metabolic alkalosis when administered in large quantities. It is important to calculate the dosage based on patient weight and size.

Side Effects

There are few side effects when sodium bicarbonate is used in the emergency setting.

Interactions

Most catecholamines and vasopressors (e.g., dopamine and epinephrine) can be deactivated by alkaline solutions such as sodium bicarbonate. Sodium bicarbonate should not be administered in conjunction with calcium chloride. A precipitate can form, which may clog the IV line.

Dosage

The usual dose of sodium bicarbonate is 1 mEq/kg body weight initially followed by 0.5 mEq/kg of body weight every 10 minutes. When possible, the dosage of sodium bicarbonate should be based on the results of arterial blood gas studies. Sodium bicarbonate should be administered only as an IV bolus.

How Supplied

Sodium bicarbonate comes in prefilled syringes containing 50 mEq of the drug in 50 mL of solvent.

CARDIAC PAIN MANAGEMENT (ANALGESICS)

Drugs that have proved to be effective in alleviating pain are referred to as analgesics. Although they may be administered in many different types of emergencies, they are used most often for the treatment of emergencies involving the cardiovascular system, especially myocardial infarction. Analgesics are covered in detail in Chapter 15. This section covers morphine and nitrous oxide.

Morphine is derived from the opium plant. It has impressive analgesic and hemodynamic effects. Nitronox, a 50 percent mixture of oxygen and nitrous oxide that can be easily inhaled by the patient, is entirely different from the other analgesic agents discussed. Its analgesic effects are also very potent yet disappear within a few minutes after the cessation of administration. Thus, Nitronox can be given for many types of pain in the field without fear of impairing subsequent physical examination in the emergency department. In addition to its analgesic effects, Nitronox delivers oxygen to the patient, which makes it useful in cardiac emergencies.

℞ MORPHINE SULFATE

Class: Narcotic analgesic

Description

Morphine is a central nervous system depressant and a potent analgesic. Although morphine sulfate is one of the most potent analgesics known to humans, it also has hemodynamic properties that make it extremely useful in emergency medicine.

Mechanism of Action

Morphine sulfate is a central nervous system depressant that acts on opiate receptors in the brain, providing both analgesia and sedation. It increases peripheral venous capacitance and decreases venous return. This effect is sometimes called a chemical phlebotomy. Morphine also decreases myocardial oxygen demand. This action is due to both the decreased systemic vascular resistance and the sedative effects of the drug. Patient apprehension and fear can significantly increase myocardial oxygen demand and in some cases can conceivably increase the size of myocardial infarction. The hemodynamic properties of morphine make it one of the most important drugs used in the treatment of pulmonary edema. Morphine is frequently administered to patients who have signs and symptoms of pulmonary edema but who are not having chest pain.

Indications

Morphine is used for severe pain associated with myocardial infarction, kidney stones, and so forth and pulmonary edema either with or without associated pain.

Contraindications

Morphine should not be used in patients who are volume depleted or severely hypotensive because of the hemodynamic effects described earlier. Morphine should not be administered to any patient with a history of hypersensitivity to the drug or to patients with undiagnosed head injury or abdominal pain.

Precautions

Morphine is a narcotic derivative of opium. It has a high tendency for addiction and abuse and is thus covered under the Controlled Substances Act of 1970. It is classified as a Schedule II drug. Consequently, there are special considerations involved in the handling of the drug. Many emergency medical services (EMS) have opted to use the synthetic analgesics, including nalbuphine and pentazocine, instead of morphine and meperidine because of these problems. Morphine causes severe respiratory depression in high doses. This is especially true in patients who already have some form of respiratory impairment. The narcotic antagonist naloxone (Narcan) should be readily available whenever morphine is administered.

Side Effects

Morphine can cause nausea, vomiting, abdominal cramps, blurred vision, constricted pupils, altered mental status, headache, and respiratory depression.

Interactions

The CNS depression associated with morphine can be enhanced when administered with antihistamines, antiemetics, sedatives, hypnotics, barbiturates, and alcohol.

Dosage

There are many different approaches to the administration of morphine. An initial dose in the range of 2 to 10 mg intravenously is standard. This dose can be augmented with additional doses of 2 mg every few minutes and can be continued until the pain is relieved or until signs of respiratory depression occur.

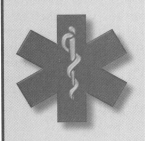

CASE PRESENTATION

At 1300 hours an ALS unit is dispatched to a mobile home park for a 61-year-old male complaining of chest pain. The patient is conscious and breathing.

On arrival paramedics are met at the door by the patient's wife. She states that she and her husband had attended church. During the service, he began to feel short of breath. She noticed that he was sweating heavily and appeared pale. She drove him home. The patient took two nitroglycerin sprays (0.4 mg) with no relief. Initially, he would not let her call the ambulance. Finally, he agreed that she could call the ambulance.

As paramedics approach the patient, they see a man sitting in a reclining chair. The patient appears in obvious distress.

On Examination

CNS: The patient is conscious, alert, and oriented × 4; appears in obvious distress

Resp: Respirations are 24 and shallow; lung sounds clear bilaterally; trachea is midline; no signs of trauma

CVS: Carotid and radial pulses are present and weak; skin is pale, cool, and diaphoretic

ABD: Soft and nontender

Muscl/Skel: Patient able to move extremities on command; no weaknesses to hand grip

Vital Signs

Pulse: 96/min, regular, weak

Resp: 24/min, shallow

BP: 144/94 mm Hg

SpO$_2$: 88 percent

ECG: Regular sinus rhythm with ST elevation

Hx:
P	No provoking factors
Q	Squeezing pain
R	Radiating to left shoulder and jaw
S	8/10, worst pain ever
T	Started suddenly about 2 hours ago

Past Hx: The patient's wife states that her husband has had several episodes of chest pain in the past month but has not seen his doctor during that time. He was diagnosed with angina 2 years ago. He has nitroglycerin spray, which he has used more often this month than ever in the past. Nitroglycerin is the patient's only prescription home medication. The patient has no recent history of operations, ulcers, or hypertension.

Treatment

Oxygen was administered by nonrebreather at 12 L/min and tolerated by the patient. The patient was hooked up to the ECG monitor, and a regular sinus rhythm with ST elevation was noted. The ST elevation was confirmed in MCL leads 1 and 6. An intravenous line with an 18-gauge catheter was established and run TKO. Paramedics administered nitroglycerin spray (0.4 mg) from their drug kit. The patient stated that the pain was not relieved by the oxygen or the nitroglycerin. The base hospital ordered 2.5 mg of morphine IV. The morphine was given, and transport to the hospital was started. En route the patient stated that the chest pain was 6/10 and a second dose of 2.5 mg of morphine was given, with moderate relief. A second 18-gauge IV was started and run TKO. ASA 325 mg was given by mouth. The patient stated the pain was now 2/10. He was pale, cool, and diaphoretic but appeared less anxious. The base hospital was contacted and advised of the patient findings. The base hospital physician agreed with the findings of the paramedics and prepared to follow through with the thrombolytic protocol on the patient's arrival at the hospital pending evaluation of a 12-lead ECG.

To attain desired effects, intramuscular injection usually requires 5 to 15 mg based on the patient's weight. However, morphine is routinely given intravenously in emergency medicine and is often administered with an antiemetic agent such as promethazine (Phenergan) to help prevent the nausea and vomiting that often accompany morphine administration. The antiemetics also tend to potentiate morphine's effects. Morphine can also be given intramuscularly and subcutaneously.

How Supplied

Morphine comes in tamper-proof ampules and Tubex prefilled cartridges. To ease administration, the 10 mg in 1 mL dilution is preferred.

NITROUS OXIDE (NITRONOX AND ENTONOX)

Class: Analgesic and anesthetic gas

Description

Nitronox is a blended mixture of 50 percent nitrous oxide and 50 percent oxygen that has potent analgesic effects. The Entonox unit consists of one tank which contains both nitrous oxide and oxygen. The Entonox tank must be shaken to mix the gases prior to use.

Mechanism of Action

Nitrous oxide is a CNS depressant with analgesic properties. In the prehospital setting it is delivered in a fixed mixture of 50 percent nitrous oxide and 50 percent oxygen. When inhaled, it has potent analgesic effects. These effects quickly dissipate, however, within 2 to 5 minutes after cessation of administration. The Nitronox unit consists of one oxygen and one nitrous oxide cylinder. The gases are fed into a blender that combines them at the appropriate concentration. The mixture is then delivered to a modified demand valve for administration to the patient. Nitronox must be self-administered. It is effective in treating many varieties of pain encountered in the prehospital setting including pain from many types of trauma. The high concentration of oxygen delivered along with the nitrous oxide will increase the oxygen tension in the blood, thus reducing hypoxia.

Indications

Nitrous oxide is used for pain of musculoskeletal origin (particularly fractures), burns, suspected ischemic chest pain, and states of severe anxiety including hyperventilation.

Contraindications

Nitronox should not be used with any patient who cannot comprehend verbal instructions or who is intoxicated with alcohol or other drugs. It should not be administered to any patient with a head injury who exhibits an altered mental status. Nitronox should not be administered to any patient with COPD because the high concentration of oxygen (50 percent) might result in respiratory depression. Nitrous oxide tends to diffuse into closed spaces more readily than either carbon dioxide or oxygen. Many COPD patients have air-containing blebs in their lungs, and nitrous oxide can concentrate in these blebs causing them to swell. Swollen blebs may rupture, causing a pneumothorax.

Nitronox should not be administered to patients with a thoracic injury suspicious of pneumothorax, because the gas may accumulate in the pneumothorax, increasing its size. Also, patients with severe abdominal pain and distention, suggestive of bowel obstruction, should not receive Nitronox. Nitrous oxide can concentrate in pockets of an obstructed bowel, possibly leading to rupture.

Precautions

Nitronox should only be used in areas that are well ventilated. When the gas is used in the patient compartment of an ambulance, it is recommended that a scavenging system be in place. Nitrous oxide exists in a liquid state inside the gas cylinder. Heat present in the air, the cylinder wall, or the various regulators and lines causes the liquid to vaporize. This vaporization process makes the cylinder tank and lines cool to touch. Following prolonged use, frost may develop on the cylinder, regulator, or lines. In very cold environments, generally less than 21 °F (6 °C), the liquid may be slow to vaporize, and administration may be impossible.

Side Effects

The nitrous oxide–oxygen mixture can cause dizziness, light-headedness, altered mental status, hallucinations, nausea, and vomiting.

Interactions

Nitrous oxide can potentiate the effects of other central nervous system depressants such as narcotics, sedatives, hypnotics, and alcohol.

Dosage

Nitronox should only be self-administered. Continuous administration may take place until the pain is significantly relieved or the patient drops the mask. The patient care record should document the duration of drug administration.

How Supplied

The nitrous oxide–oxygen mixture is supplied in a cylinder system in which both gases are fed into a blender that delivers a fixed 50 percent–50 percent mixture to the patient. The blender is designed to shut off if the oxygen cylinder becomes depleted. It will allow continued administration of oxygen if the nitrous oxide cylinder becomes depleted.

In several countries (England, Canada, and Australia) the nitrous oxide–oxygen mixture (Entonox and Dolonox) is premixed and supplied in a single cylinder. This setup is much lighter than the system used in the United States.

DIURETICS

One of the most common cardiovascular emergencies that emergency personnel are called on to treat is congestive heart failure. Congestive heart failure occurs when the heart loses its ability to pump blood effectively. When this occurs, the venous vessels leading to the heart become engorged. Failure of the left side of the heart causes a buildup of blood in the pulmonary circulation. Failure of the right side of the heart results in congestion of the peripheral circulation, which usually manifests as peripheral edema. Common signs of right heart failure include jugular venous distention, ascites, and pedal (ankle or pretibial) edema.

In the treatment of congestive heart failure, the primary objectives are to increase the cardiac output and to reduce pulmonary and peripheral edema. Although the inotropic effects of digitalis preparations will increase cardiac output, the rate of onset is relatively slow, making this drug less than ideal in acute pulmonary edema. In acute heart failure the most effective therapy is to reduce venous filling pressure. Venous filling pressure can be reduced mechanically by applying rotating tourniquets, which are placed on three of the extremities to decrease venous return. Phlebotomy (drawing blood out of the circulatory system) can also be employed. The preferred method, however, is the administration of potent diuretics.

FUROSEMIDE (LASIX)

Class: Diuretic

Description

Furosemide is a potent diuretic that inhibits sodium and chloride reabsorption in the kidneys and causes venous dilation.

Mechanism of Action

Furosemide is a loop diuretic that inhibits the reabsorption of both sodium and chloride in the kidneys. It is extremely useful in the treatment of congestive heart failure and pulmonary edema. The effects of furosemide are twofold.

First, following administration furosemide causes venous dilation. This effect usually occurs within 5 minutes and causes a reduction in preload, thus decreasing cardiac work. The second effect of furosemide is the diuretic effect, which begins 5 to 15 minutes after administration.

Indications

Furosemide is used in congestive heart failure and pulmonary edema.

Contraindications

Usage in pregnancy should be limited to life-threatening situations in which the benefits of furosemide outweigh the risks. Furosemide has been known to cause fetal abnormalities. It should not be administered to patients with a known allergy to the sulfa class of medications.

Precautions

Dehydration, electrolyte depletion, and hypotension can result from excessive doses of potent diuretics. Thus, blood pressure should be frequently monitored when furosemide is administered. Furosemide should be protected from light.

Side Effects

Furosemide can cause headache, dizziness, hypotension, volume depletion, potassium depletion, arrhythmias, diarrhea, nausea, and vomiting.

Interactions

Furosemide should not be administered in the same line as amrinone (Inocor) because a chemical reaction can occur between the two, causing the formation of a precipitate in the intravenous line. Administration of furosemide with other diuretics can lead to severe volume depletion and electrolyte imbalance.

Dosage

The standard dosage of furosemide is 40 mg given by slow IV push in patients already on chronic oral furosemide therapy and 20 mg intravenously in patients who are not taking the drug orally on a regular basis. Dosages as high as 80 to 120 mg intravenously may be indicated in severe cases. Furosemide should be given intravenously in emergency situations.

How Supplied

Furosemide is supplied in ampules and prefilled syringes that contain 10 mg/mL.

BUMETANIDE (BUMEX)

Class: Diuretic

Description

Bumetanide is a potent diuretic with a rapid rate of onset and a short duration of action.

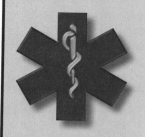

CASE PRESENTATION

Paramedics are called at 0800 hours to a residence for a woman having difficulty breathing. Dispatch states that the woman is conscious and breathing. On arrival paramedics find a 71-year-old female sitting in a recliner in the living room. She is in severe respiratory distress. Paramedics immediately place the chair into the upright position.

On Examination

CNS: The patient is conscious, alert, and oriented × 4; appears in obvious respiratory distress and is very restless

Resp: Respirations are 40 and shallow; lung sounds are diminished bilaterally with loud rales (crackles) audible; two- to three-word dyspnea; trachea is midline; no signs of trauma

CVS: Carotid and radial pulses are weak and regular; skin is pale, lips are blue, and the patient is cool and diaphoretic to touch

ABD: Soft and nontender

Muscl/Skel: Patient able to move extremities on command; no weaknesses to hand grip

Vital Signs

Pulse: 120/min, regular, weak

Resp: 40/min, shallow, bilateral loud rales

BP: 180/108 mm Hg

SpO$_2$: 80 percent

ECG: Sinus tachycardia

Hx: The patient's husband states that his wife has been complaining of mild SOB for the past two days. She has not been able to lie down to sleep because it increases the difficulty of breathing. Therefore she has been sitting in the recliner to sleep. This morning her breathing is worse. She is having difficulty speaking now. He was not sure what to do and finally called the ambulance.

Past Hx: The patient has a history of congestive heart failure and is currently taking Lasix 20 mg twice per day, Slo-K (potassium), and digoxin.

Treatment

Oxygen was administered by nonrebreather at 15 L/min and not well tolerated by the patient. An IV of normal saline was initiated and run TKO. The patient was hooked up to the ECG monitor, and a sinus tachycardia was noted. Nitroglycerin spray was administered, with no relief. Following the nitrospray, paramedics administered 2.5 mg of morphine followed by 80 mg of Lasix (double the patient's home daily dose of Lasix as per their standing orders). Paramedics attempted to assist the patient's respirations with a bag-valve-mask device, but the patient became anxious and combative. The nonrebreather was placed back on the patient. The patient did not experience any improvement from the nitroglycerin spray but seemed more relaxed after administration of morphine. En route the patient was treated with two more doses of nitroglycerin spray, 5 minutes apart, and the patient began to experience some relief of her SOB. She was able to speak short sentences and was no longer cyanotic on arrival at the hospital. At the hospital the patient was started on intravenous nitroglycerin and was given another 80 mg of Lasix, with significant improvement.

Mechanism of Action

Like furosemide, bumetanide is a loop diuretic that inhibits the reabsorption of sodium chloride in the kidneys and thus causes a net diuresis; 1 mg of bumetanide has the diuretic potency of 40 mg of furosemide.

Indications

Bumetanide is used in congestive heart failure and pulmonary edema.

Contraindications

Usage in pregnancy should be limited to life-threatening situations in which the benefits of using bumetanide outweigh the risks.

Precautions

Dehydration and electrolyte depletion can result from excessive doses of potent diuretics. Patients who have experienced allergic reactions to furosemide have not experienced those same reactions when administered bumetanide, which suggests that this drug may be used in patients with furosemide allergy who are in need of rapid diuresis.

Side Effects

Bumetanide can cause muscle cramps, dizziness, hypotension, headache, nausea, and vomiting.

Interactions

Bumetanide can potentiate the effects of the various antihypertensive agents and should be used with caution in patients taking these agents.

Dosage

The usual initial dose of bumetanide is 0.5 to 1.0 mg given during a period of 1 to 2 minutes. A second or third dose can be administered at 2- to 3-hour intervals if required. The total daily dosage should not exceed 10 mg. Bumetanide injection can be given by either the IV or intramuscular route. In the emergency setting, the IV route is preferred.

How Supplied

Bumetanide (Bumex) is supplied in ampules containing 0.5 mg in 2 mL of solvent (0.25 mg/mL). It is also supplied in 2, 4, and 10 mL vials containing 0.25 mg/mL.

ANTIANGINAL AGENTS

A common manifestation of advanced cardiovascular disease is angina pectoris, which results from a narrowing of the coronary arteries due to the buildup of atherosclerotic plaques, or coronary artery vasospasm. In exercise and other stressful situations, the amount of blood that can be carried by the coronary arteries may not be sufficient to meet the oxygen demands of the myocardium. This results in myocardial hypoxia, causing the classic pain syndrome called angina pectoris. Sublingual nitroglycerin usually gives immediate relief by dilating the coronary arteries and decreasing cardiac work. In recent years there have been trials in which nitroglycerin has been administered to patients suffering myocardial infarction in the hope of decreasing the extent of myocardial damage. Nitroglycerin is often administered to patients complaining of chest pain to rule out angina as the cause. When cardiac pain is not relieved by nitroglycerin, morphine and other potent analgesics are administered.

Nitroglycerin is usually administered sublingually. Recently, however, it has been given intravenously in certain cases of unstable angina and acute myocardial infarction.

Calcium-ion antagonists, such as nifedipine (Procardia), have proved effective in the management of angina, especially when there is coronary artery vasospasm.

 ## NITROGLYCERIN (NITROSTAT)

Class: Nitrate

Description

Nitroglycerin is a potent smooth muscle relaxant used in the treatment of angina pectoris.

Mechanism of Action

Nitroglycerin is a rapid smooth muscle relaxant that reduces cardiac work and, to a lesser degree, dilates the coronary arteries. This results in increased coronary blood flow and improved perfusion of the ischemic myocardium. Relief of ischemia causes reduction and alleviation of chest pain. Pain relief following nitroglycerin administration usually occurs within 1 to 2 minutes, and therapeutic effects can be observed up to 30 minutes later. Nitroglycerin also causes vasodilation, which decreases preload; decreased preload leads to decreased cardiac work. This feature, in conjunction with coronary vasodilation, reverses the effects of angina pectoris.

Indications

Nitroglycerin is used for chest pain associated with angina pectoris, chest pain associated with acute myocardial infarction, and acute pulmonary edema (unless accompanied by hypotension).

Contraindications

Nitroglycerin is contraindicated in patients who are hypotensive or who may have increased intracranial pressure. It should not be administered to patients in shock.

Precautions

Patients taking nitroglycerin may develop a tolerance for the drug, which necessitates increasing the dose. Headache is a common side effect of nitroglycerin administration and results from vasodilation of cerebral vessels. Nitroglycerin deteriorates quite rapidly once the bottle is opened. When a bottle of nitroglycerin is opened, it should be dated. Nitroglycerin should also be protected from light. Blood pressure and the other vital signs should always be monitored during nitroglycerin administration.

Side Effects

Nitroglycerin can cause headache, dizziness, weakness, tachycardia, hypotension, orthostasis, skin rash, dry mouth, nausea, and vomiting.

Interactions

Nitroglycerin can cause severe hypotension when administered to patients who have recently ingested alcohol. It can cause orthostatic hypotension when used in conjunction with beta-blockers.

Dosage

One tablet (0.4 mg) is administered sublingually for routine angina pectoris. This dose can be repeated in 3 to 5 minutes as required. Usually, more than three tablets should not be administered in the prehospital setting. Nitroglycerin should be administered sublingually. Care should be taken to ensure that it is not swallowed. IV nitroglycerin is used in the emergency department and intensive care units, but the sublingual route is adequate for most prehospital situations. Nitroglycerin is also available in patches and in ointment form for transdermal administration.

How Supplied

Nitroglycerin is supplied in bottles containing 0.4 mg tablets (1/150 grain). The tablets must be protected from light and air to prevent deterioration.

NITROGLYCERIN PASTE

Class: Nitrate

Description

Nitroglycerin paste contains a 2 percent solution of nitroglycerin in a special absorbent paste. When placed on the skin, nitroglycerin is absorbed into the systemic circulation. In many cases it may be preferred over nitroglycerin tablets because of its longer duration of action.

Mechanism of Action

Nitroglycerin is a rapid smooth muscle relaxant that reduces cardiac work and, to a lesser degree, dilates the coronary arteries. This results in increased coronary blood flow and improved perfusion of the ischemic myocardium. Relief of ischemia causes reduction and alleviation of chest pain. Pain relief following transcutaneous nitroglycerin administration usually occurs within 5 to 10 minutes, and therapeutic effects can be observed up to 30 minutes later. Nitroglycerin also causes vasodilation, which decreases preload; decreased preload leads to decreased cardiac work. This feature, in conjunction with coronary vasodilation, reverses the effects of angina pectoris.

Indications

Nitroglycerin paste is used for chest pain associated with angina pectoris and chest pain associated with acute myocardial infarction.

Contraindications

Nitroglycerin paste is contraindicated in patients with increased intracranial pressure. It should not be administered to patients who are hypotensive or in shock.

Precautions

Patients taking the drug routinely may develop a tolerance and require an increased dose. Headache is a common side effect of nitroglycerin administration and occurs as a result of vasodilation of the cerebral vessels. Postural syncope sometimes occurs following the administration of nitroglycerin; it should be anticipated and the patient kept supine when possible. It is important to monitor blood pressure constantly.

Side Effects

Nitroglycerin can cause headache, dizziness, weakness, tachycardia, hypotension, orthostasis, skin rash, dry mouth, nausea, and vomiting.

Interactions

Nitroglycerin can cause severe hypotension when administered to patients who have recently ingested alcohol. It can cause orthostatic hypotension when used in conjunction with beta-blockers.

Dosage

Generally 1/2 to 1 inch (1.25 to 2.50 cm) of the Nitro-Bid Ointment is applied. Measuring applicators are supplied.

How Supplied

Nitro-Bid Ointment is supplied in 20 and 60 g tubes. Several dose-measuring applicators are also included.

NITROGLYCERIN SPRAY

Class: Nitrate

Description

Nitroglycerin spray is a special preparation of nitroglycerin in an aerosol form that delivers precisely 0.4 mg of nitroglycerin per spray.

Mechanism of Action

Nitroglycerin is a rapid smooth muscle relaxant that reduces cardiac work and, to a lesser degree, dilates the coronary arteries. This results in increased coronary blood flow and improved perfusion of the ischemic myocardium. Relief of ischemia causes reduction and alleviation of chest pain. Pain relief following nitroglycerin administration usually occurs within 1 to 2 minutes, and peak effects occur within 4 minutes. Therapeutic effects can be observed up to 30 minutes later. Nitroglycerin also causes vasodilation, which decreases preload; decreased preload leads to decreased cardiac work. This feature, in conjunction with coronary vasodilation, reverses the effects of angina pectoris.

Indications

Nitroglycerin spray is used for chest pain associated with angina pectoris and chest pain associated with acute myocardial infarction.

Contraindications

Nitroglycerin is contraindicated in patients who are hypotensive, who are in shock, or who may have increased intracranial pressure.

Precautions

Patients taking nitroglycerin routinely may develop a tolerance for the drug. Headache is a common side effect of nitroglycerin administration and results from dilation of cerebral blood vessels. This effect should be anticipated. The blood pressure should be monitored during nitroglycerin therapy.

Side Effects

Nitroglycerin can cause headache, dizziness, weakness, tachycardia, hypotension, orthostasis, skin rash, dry mouth, nausea, and vomiting.

Interactions

Nitroglycerin can cause severe hypotension when administered to patients who have recently ingested alcohol. It can cause orthostatic hypotension when used in conjunction with beta-blockers.

Dosage

One spray (0.4 mg) should be sprayed under the tongue at the onset of an attack of angina. No more than three sprays are recommended in a 25-minute period. (The spray should not be inhaled.) Nitroglycerin spray should be applied to the sublingual mucous membranes in the manner described earlier.

How Supplied

Nitroglycerin spray is supplied in an aerosol container containing 200 doses of nitroglycerin.

ANTIHYPERTENSIVES

A dangerously elevated blood pressure is a hypertensive emergency. A hypertensive crisis is defined as a sudden increase in the systolic and diastolic blood pressure, causing a functional disturbance of the central nervous system, the heart, or the kidneys. Hypertensive emergencies call for prompt and efficient care by prehospital providers.

Hypertensive emergencies are often divided into two categories: hypertensive emergencies and hypertensive urgencies. A hypertensive emergency is a situation in which the blood pressure must be lowered within 1 hour. A hypertensive urgency is a situation in which the blood pressure should be lowered within 24 hours. Hypertensive emergencies develop when the blood pressure exceeds 130 mm Hg diastolic pressure (with or without symptoms) or any elevated blood pressure associated with end-organ symptoms. End-organ symptoms include chest pain, dyspnea, altered mental status, seizures, stroke, nosebleed, or hypertensive encephalopathy. In many cases the emergency develops not from the absolute blood pressure value but from how rapid the value is achieved. Rapid elevations in blood pressure are poorly tolerated by the body and more apt to cause end-organ symptoms.

Hypertensive encephalopathy is the most devastating complication of hypertension. Signs and symptoms include severe headache, nausea and vomiting, and an altered mental state. The altered mental state can range from lethargy or confusion to coma. Neurological symptoms, including blindness, inability to speak, muscle twitches, weakness, or paralysis, may be present as well. The treatment is to lower blood pressure as rapidly and as safely as possible.

Hypertension is a chronic disease. An elevated blood pressure is not uncommon in the emergency setting. Elevated blood pressure should only be treated if there are significant end-organ changes (i.e. altered mental status). In cases where the blood pressure must be lowered, labetalol or sodium nitroprusside should be used. The drug should be initiated at a low dose and increased until the blood pressure is controlled. Nifedipine (Procardia) was used for many years in the acute treatment of hypertensive emergencies. However, complications (i.e. CVA) were reported and the popular press published several articles on the adverse effects of nifedipine. Because of this, it is no longer used in this setting.

 ## NIFEDIPINE (PROCARDIA, ADALAT)

Class: Calcium channel blocker

Description

Nifedipine is a calcium channel blocker that is used in the treatment of hypertension.

Mechanism of Action

Nifedipine causes relaxation of the smooth muscles that encircle the peripheral blood vessels, principally the arterioles. This relaxation results in peripheral vasodilation, a decrease in peripheral vascular resistance, and a decrease in both the systolic and diastolic blood pressure. Nifedipine is also effective in reducing coronary artery spasm in angina. Nifedipine can be used in hypertension associated with pregnancy if hydralazine is not available.

Indications

Nifedipine is used in hypertension and angina pectoris.

Contraindications

Nifedipine is contraindicated in patients with known hypersensitivity to the drug. It should not be administered to patients who are hypotensive.

Precautions

Nifedipine can cause a significant drop in blood pressure. Thus, blood pressure should be frequently monitored. Nifedipine should be used with caution in patients with heart failure. It should not be administered to patients receiving IV β-blockers.

Side Effects

Nifedepine can cause nausea, vomiting, dizziness, headache, bradycardia, heart block, hypotension, and asystole.

Interactions

Nifedepine should not be administered to patients receiving intravenous β-blockers because of an increased risk of congestive heart failure, bradycardia, and asystole.

Dosage

Several small puncture holes should be placed in one 10 mg capsule before placing it under the tongue, where it can be absorbed. Alternatively, the capsule can be bitten by the patient and swallowed with approximately the same rate of onset. In severe hypertension the medical control physician may order an initial dose of 20 mg. Nifedipine should only be administered orally or sublingually, as described earlier.

How Supplied

Nifedipine is supplied in 10 and 20 mg tablets.

SODIUM NITROPRUSSIDE (NITROPRESS, NIPRIDE)

Class: Antihypertensive and vasodilator

Description

Sodium nitroprusside is a potent vasodilating agent used in the management of hypertensive crisis when a prompt reduction in blood pressure is required.

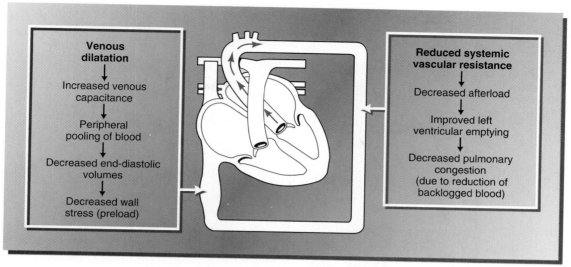

FIGURE 7–9 Actions of sodium nitroprusside.

Mechanism of Action

Sodium nitroprusside acts by dilating both peripheral arteries and peripheral veins. This reduction in peripheral vascular resistance results in an immediate reduction in blood pressure, which is generally proportional to the rate of drug administration. Sodium nitroprusside administration is usually accompanied by an increase in heart rate.

Although not approved for this use, sodium nitroprusside is occasionally used in the management of severe congestive heart failure. The dilation of the peripheral veins results in decreased blood return to the heart (preload). In addition, the dilation of the peripheral arteries reduces the pressure against which the heart has to pump (afterload). This results in a net increase in cardiac output in patients with severe congestive heart failure (see Figure 7–9).

Because sodium nitroprusside is such a potent agent, the blood pressure, pulse rate, respiratory status, and EKG should be constantly monitored during drug administration.

Indication

Hypertensive crisis in which a prompt reduction in blood pressure is essential.

Contraindications

None when used in the management of life-threatening hypertensive crisis.

Precautions

Once the sodium nitroprusside infusion is prepared, it should be immediately wrapped in an opaque material, usually aluminum foil, to protect it from light. Once exposed to light the drug is quickly inactivated. Sodium nitroprusside should not be used in children or pregnant women in the prehospital setting. The dosage should be reduced somewhat in elderly patients. The constant monitoring of blood pressure and pulse is essential throughout sodium nitroprusside administration.

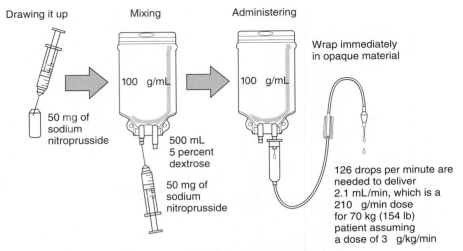

Figure 7–10 Preparation of sodium nitroprusside infusion.

Side Effects

Sodium nitroprusside can cause dizziness, headache, hypotension, chest pain, dyspnea, palpitations, nausea, and vomiting.

Interactions

The effects of sodium nitroprusside can be potentiated when administered with other antihypertensive agents.

Dosage

The standard dose is 50 mg of sodium nitroprusside diluted in 500 mL of D₅W. This will give a concentration of 100 µg/mL. The initial dose should be 0.5 µg/kg/min (see Figure 7–10). The typical dosage range is from 0.5 to 8.0 µg/kg/min. Sodium nitroprusside should only be diluted in D₅W or normal saline and administered by slow IV infusion using a minidrip administration set (preferably through an IV pump). *This medication should never be given by IV bolus.*

How Supplied

Sodium nitroprusside is supplied in 5 mL vials containing 50 mg of the drug.

HYDRALAZINE (APRESOLINE)

Class: Antihypertensive and vasodilator

Description

Hydralazine is a potent vasodilating agent used to lower blood pressure in cases of hypertensive crisis.

Mechanism of Action

Hydralazine, like sodium nitroprusside, relaxes vascular smooth muscle, primarily in the arterial system, thus causing decreased arterial pressure (diastolic greater than systolic), decreased peripheral resistance, and increased cardiac output. Hydralazine causes postural hypotension to a lesser degree than does sodium nitroprusside. The effects of hydralazine are usually seen within 5 to 10 minutes after the initiation of therapy.

Indications

Hydralazine is used in hypertensive crisis in which a prompt reduction in blood pressure is required and hypertension complicating pregnancy (preeclampsia).

Contraindications

Hydralazine should not be administered to patients with a known history of hypersensitivity to the drug, coronary artery disease, or rheumatic heart disease involving the mitral valve.

Precautions

The administration of hydralazine may cause angina pectoris or ECG changes because of the increased cardiac output. This drug should not be used in the prehospital phase of emergency medical care of children because of limited experience with the drug in these cases. The blood pressure, pulse rate, respiratory status, and ECG should be monitored at all times during hydralazine therapy. Headache, nausea, and vomiting have been known to occur following hydralazine therapy and should be expected.

Side Effects

Hydralazine can cause headache, dizziness, altered mental status, tachycardia, arrhythmias, orthostasis, chest pain, nausea, and vomiting.

Interactions

The effects of hydralazine can be potentiated when administered with other antihypertensive agents.

Dosage

The usual dosage of hydralazine in the management of hypertensive crisis is 20 to 40 mg given by slow IV bolus. This dose can be repeated in 4 to 6 hours if required. If an IV line cannot be established, then the same dosage of the drug can be given by intramuscular injection. The blood pressure and ECG should be continuously monitored. Parenteral hydralazine should be administered by slow IV bolus. When necessary, however, the drug can be administered by intramuscular injection.

How Supplied

Hydralazine is supplied in 1 mL ampules containing 20 mg of the drug.

DIAZOXIDE (HYPERSTAT)

Class: Antihypertensive and vasodilator

Description

Diazoxide relaxes vascular smooth muscle and is effective in the treatment of hypertensive crisis.

Mechanism of Action

Diazoxide causes a decrease in both systolic and diastolic pressure by causing vasodilation of the peripheral arterioles. This results in decreased peripheral vascular resistance and a subsequently lowered systolic and diastolic blood pressure.

Indication

Diazoxide is used for severe hypertension in which a prompt decrease in diastolic blood pressure is indicated.

Contraindications

Diazoxide should not be administered to patients with a known hypersensitivity to the drug or to the thiazide class of diuretics. Although there are some additional medical conditions for which diazoxide is contraindicated, the paramedic will most likely be unaware of these in the field.

Precautions

Hypotension may occur and, if severe, should be treated with sympathomimetics. Because of the rapid onset of action of diazoxide, frequent blood pressure monitoring (every minute) to detect possible hypotension is mandatory.

Side Effects

Diazoxide can cause headache, dizziness, altered mental status, tachycardia, arrhythmias, chest pain, congestive heart failure, edema, hyperglycemia, nausea, and vomiting.

Interactions

The effects of diazoxide can be potentiated when administered with other antihypertensive agents. It can also decrease the blood levels of phenytoin and precipitate a seizure.

Dosage

The standard dose of diazoxide is 1 to 3 mg/kg of body weight given intravenously over 30 seconds up to 150 mg/kg. The dose may be repeated at 5- to 15-minute intervals as required. Diazoxide is administered intravenously.

How Supplied

Diazoxide is supplied in ampules containing 300 mg of the drug in 20 mL of solvent.

The following agent does not readily fit into the classes of drugs discussed thus far.

CALCIUM CHLORIDE

Class: Calcium supplement

Description

Calcium chloride provides elemental calcium in the form of the cation (Ca^{2+}). Calcium is required for many physiological activities.

Mechanism of Action

Calcium chloride replaces calcium in cases of hypocalcemia. Calcium chloride causes a significant increase in the myocardial contractile force and appears to increase ventricular automaticity. Although frequently used for many years in the management of cardiac arrest, especially that resulting from asystole and electromechanical dissociation, recent studies have presented data that seriously question the role of calcium chloride, even in these situations. Calcium chloride is an antidote for magnesium sulfate and can minimize some of the side effects of calcium channel blocker usage.

Indications

Calcium chloride is used in acute hyperkalemia (elevated potassium), acute hypocalcemia (decreased calcium), and calcium channel blocker toxicity (nifedipine, verapamil, and diltiazem).

Contraindications

Caution is warranted when calcium chloride is administered to patients receiving digitalis, because it may precipitate digitalis toxicity.

Precautions

It is extremely important to flush the IV line between administrations of calcium chloride and sodium bicarbonate to avoid precipitation. Calcium chloride can cause tissue necrosis at the injection site. It should always be administered through an IV that is patent and running well.

Side Effects

Calcium chloride can cause bradycardia, arrhythmias, syncope, nausea, vomiting, and cardiac arrest.

Interactions

Calcium chloride will interact with sodium bicarbonate and form a precipitate. In addition, calcium chloride can cause elevated digoxin levels, and possibly digitalis toxicity, when administered to patients receiving digitalis preparations.

Dosage

The standard dose for calcium chloride is 2 to 4 mg/kg intravenously. This dose may be repeated every 10 minutes as required. Calcium chloride should only be given intravenously in the emergency setting.

How Supplied

Calcium chloride comes in prefilled syringes containing 1 g of the drug in 10 mL of solvent (10 mL of a 10 percent solution).

SUMMARY

All of the medications discussed in this chapter are only of value when used in conjunction with other treatment modalities. Without appropriate cardiopulmonary resuscitation, the medications used in the management of cardiac arrest are not effective. As mentioned, the dosages presented in this chapter are based on nationally accepted regimens. Paramedics should become familiar with the routine dosages and protocols used in their areas.

KEY WORDS

adrenergic receptors. Receptors specific to norepinephrine- and epinephrine-like substances.

adrenergic system. The part of the nervous system that prepares the body to deal with various stresses, whether real or imagined. Also referred to as the sympathetic nervous system.

aerobic metabolism. The process of generating energy with the aid of oxygen.

agonist. A drug or other substance that causes a physiological response.

anaerobic metabolism. The process of generating energy without the aid of oxygen.

antagonist. A drug or other substance that blocks a physiological response or that blocks the action of another drug or substance.

automaticity. The capacity of self-depolarization. Refers to the pacemaker cells of the heart.

catecholamine. A class of hormones that act on the autonomic nervous system. They include epinephrine, norepinephrine, and similar compounds.

cholinergic system. A division of the autonomic nervous system that is responsible for controlling vegetative functions. Also called the parasympathetic nervous system.

chronotrope. A drug or substance that affects the heart rate.

concomitant. Occurring at the same time.

dopaminergic receptor. Receptor in the renal and splanchnic vessels that maintains vasodilation.

dromotrope. A drug or substance that affects the conduction velocity of the heart.

endogenous. Coming from inside the body.

homeostasis. The natural tendency of the body to maintain the internal environment relatively constant.

hypoxic drive. Respiratory control system commonly present in patients with chronic obstructive pulmonary disease whereby respirations are dependent on changes in the concentration of oxygen concentration as opposed to changes in the concentration of carbon dioxide.

inotrope. A drug or substance that affects the contractile force of the heart.

lactic acid. An organic acid normally present in tissue. One form of lactic acid in muscle and blood is a product of the change of the carbohydrates glucose and glycogen to energy during physical exercise.

neurotransmitter. A substance that is released from the axon terminal of a presynaptic neuron on excitation and that travels across the synaptic cleft to either excite or inhibit the target cell. Examples include acetylcholine, norepinephrine, and dopamine.

pheochromocytoma. A tumor of the adrenal gland that causes too much release of two hormones (epinephrine and norepinephrine). Signs include high blood pressure, headache, sweating, high blood sugar level, nausea, vomiting, and fainting spells.

pulse oximetry. An assessment modality that measures the oxygen saturation level of the blood through a noninvasive sensor placed on a finger or earlobe.

retrolental fibroplasia. A disorder caused by giving excess amounts of oxygen to premature infants. A fiberlike tissue forms behind the lens of the eye.

stroke volume. The amount of blood ejected by the heart in one cardiac contraction.

sympathomimetic. A drug or substance that causes effects such as those of the sympathetic nervous system (also called adrenergic).

Torsade de pointes. A form of ventricular tachycardia in which the morphology of the QRS appears to change (the axis rotates). It is often drug induced but may be the result of low potassium levels in the blood (hypokalemia) or profound slow heart beat (bradycardia).

Wolff-Parkinson-White syndrome. A disorder of the heart characterized by early contraction of the heart muscle.

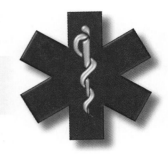

chapter 8

DRUGS USED IN THE TREATMENT OF RESPIRATORY EMERGENCIES

OBJECTIVES

After completing this chapter, the reader should be able to

1. Discuss the devices commonly used to administer oxygen in the field.

2. Discuss pulse oximetry and end-tidal carbon dioxide detection and describe the prehospital use of both.

3. Discuss the pathophysiology and prehospital management of asthma and status asthmaticus.

4. Describe and list the indications, contraindications, and dosages for the following beta agonists used in respiratory emergencies: epinephrine 1:1000, albuterol, racemic epinephrine, terbutaline, isoetharine, metaproterenol, and aminophylline.

5. Describe and list the indications, contraindications, and dosages for the following anticholinergics: atropine and ipratropium.

6. Describe and list the indications, contraindications, and dosages for magnesium sulfate.

7. Describe and list the indications, contraindications, and dosages for the following corticosteroids: methylprednisolone and hydrocortisone.

8. Discuss the indications and considerations in the use of neuromuscular blockers.

9. List the steps in performing rapid-sequence induction (RSI) intubation.

10. List the steps in performing rapid-sequence sedation (RSS) intubation.

11. Describe and list the indications, contraindications, and dosages for the following medications used as neuromuscular-blocking agents: succinylcholine, pancuronium, vecuronium, and rocuronium.

INTRODUCTION

Oxygen is the most important drug for use in the management of respiratory emergencies. In addition to oxygen, however, several pharmacological agents have proved quite effective in relieving respiratory distress. In this chapter medications commonly used in the prehospital treatment of respiratory emergencies are discussed. These medications include the following:

Gases

Oxygen

Beta Agonists

Epinephrine 1:1000

Albuterol/Salbutamol (Proventil, Ventolin)

Racemic epinephrine (Vaponefin)

Terbutaline (Brethine, Bricanyl)

Isoetharine (Bronkosol)

Metaproterenol

Xanthines

Aminophylline

Anticholinergics

Atropine

Ipratropium

Corticosteroids

Methylprednisolone

Hydrocortisone

Neuromuscular Blockers

Succinylcholine

Vecuronium

Pancuronium

Rocuronium

Other

Magnesium sulfate

Sympathomimetics are among the most frequently used agents in the treatment of respiratory emergencies. The principal sympathomimetics include epinephrine, isoetharine, terbutaline, metaproterenol, and albuterol. In treating cardiovascular emergencies it is highly desirable to activate β_1-adrenergic receptors. When treating patients in respiratory distress, however, it is desirable to activate β_2-receptors. Unfortunately, most of the agents that activate β_2-receptors also have some effect on β_1-receptors. When activated, β_1-receptors cause an increase in heart rate and myocardial contractile force, whereas β_2-receptors cause peripheral vasodilation and, most important, bronchodilation. Common side effects of these medications include palpitations, anxiety, and dizziness. Considerable effort has been devoted to isolation of pharmacological agents that act principally on β_2-receptors. Currently, metaproterenol and albuterol are the sympathomimetic agents most frequently used in the prehospital phase of emergency medical care. They are chemically related to epinephrine but tend to be more selective than epinephrine for β_2-receptors.

Another agent used in the management of respiratory emergencies is aminophylline. Aminophylline, chemically unrelated to the catecholamines, belongs to a class of drugs called *xanthines*. A commonly encountered drug within the xanthines class is caffeine. Aminophylline causes relaxation of the bronchiole smooth musculature and bronchodilation.

Although not discussed here, corticosteroids play a major role in the treatment of respiratory diseases. Asthma and many cases of chronic obstructive pulmonary disease (COPD) have inflammation as the underlying cause. Although the β-agonists help reverse bronchospasm, they do little for the underlying inflammation. Corticosteroids have a very long rate of onset (1 to 4 hours), and thus their effects are not usually seen in the prehospital setting.

Some systems have added neuromuscular-blocking agents to their paramedic drug lists. These medications are very effective in providing muscle relaxation for endotracheal intubation. However, because they remove a patient's protective reflexes and cause apnea, they should only be used by personnel with experience in their use.

OXYGEN

Oxygen administration is an important aspect of patient care. It is essential in cases that involve suspected hypoxia of any cause, chest pain due to myocardial ischemia, asthma, and cardiorespiratory arrest.

Oxygen Administration

Administering oxygen to a hypoxic patient raises his or her oxygen level by increasing the

- Inspired percentage of oxygen
- Oxygen concentration at the alveolar level
- Arterial oxygen levels
- Amount of oxygen delivered to the patient's cells

Oxygen administration decreases hypoxia and reduces the volume of respiration necessary to oxygenate the blood. It also reduces the myocardial work demanded to maintain given arterial oxygen tension.

There are no absolute contraindications to oxygen administration. However, it should be used with caution in premature infants and patients who are prone to carbon dioxide retention (hypoxic drive). It should be administered at lower flow rates with COPD patients (1 to 3 L delivered via nasal cannula). If a patient develops respiratory depression, breathing should be assisted with a bag-valve-mask device. When ventilating via a bag-valve-mask device, 100 percent oxygen is used. When providing oxygen to a premature infant, the mask is held over the face, not directly on it.

Oxygen Devices

Devices commonly used to administer oxygen in the field include the nasal cannula, the simple face mask, the nonrebreather mask, and, to a lesser extent, the Venturi mask.

Nasal Cannula

The *nasal cannula* is a frequently used device that is comfortable and is easily tolerated by the patient. It can deliver oxygen concentrations ranging from 24 to 44 percent. The oxygen flow rates for the nasal cannula vary from 1 to 6 L/min.

Simple Face Mask

The *simple face mask* delivers an oxygen concentration of 40 to 60 percent. Flow rates administered through the simple face mask range from 8 to 12 L/min. No fewer than 6 L/min should be administered through this device, because expired carbon dioxide can accumulate in the mask. Flow rates in excess of 8 L/min are needed to "wash out" any expired carbon dioxide.

The simple face mask provides oxygen to patients who are suffering from moderate hypoxia. Disadvantages include that it may feel confining to the patient, it muffles the patient's speech, and it requires a tight face seal. Because the mask covers the patient's face, it should be used with caution in cases that involve nausea or vomiting. With the pediatric patient, a flow rate of 6 to 8 L/min is generally considered acceptable.

Nonrebreather Mask

When the patient inhales, the 100 percent oxygen contained in the reservoir is drawn into the mask and the patient's respiratory passages. Ambient air is prevented from entering the mask by the rubber flap that closes over the inlet-outlet ports during inspiration. When the patient exhales, the flapper valve is open to allow the expired air an exit. A one-way valve situated between the mask and the reservoir prevents the expired air from entering the reservoir bag.

The *nonrebreather mask* delivers the highest concentration of oxygen. When supplied at a flow rate of 10 to 15 L/min, it can deliver an 80 to 100 percent oxygen concentration. No fewer than 8 L/min of oxygen should be administered through this device. Because the nonrebreather mask is a relatively closed system, it restricts the inspiration of ambient air. Therefore, its reservoir bag should not be allowed to deflate totally or be allowed to kink. Otherwise, the patient might suffocate.

The nonrebreather mask is similar to the simple face mask in that it requires a tight seal. A tight seal may be difficult to obtain with some patients because they find the mask confining. This device should be employed with caution in nauseated patients. Its main application lies in the treatment of severely hypoxic patients—those suffering respiratory compromise, shock, acute myocardial infarction, trauma, or carbon monoxide poisoning.

Venturi Mask

With the *Venturi mask*, relatively precise concentrations of oxygen can be provided. This device is not commonly used in prehospital care and is used in the treatment of COPD patients. To control the amount of ambient air taken in by a patient, some Venturi masks are supplied with dial selection, and others come with interchangeable caps. These devices deliver oxygen concentrations of 24 percent, 28 percent, 35 percent, or 40 percent. The liter flow depends on the oxygen concentration desired.

Ventilation

In the field, paramedics are called on in many cases to provide ventilatory support. Situations will range from those that involve apneic patients to less obvious cases in which patients are experiencing depressed respiratory function.

When a patient is unconscious, his or her respiratory center may not function at a satisfactory level. A significant decrease in the patient's rate or depth of breathing will lead to decreased respiratory minute volume, hypercarbia, hypoxia, and a lowered pH. If not corrected, respiratory or cardiac arrest may occur. To achieve effective ventilatory support, an adequate rate and volume of oxygen must be delivered—at least 800 mL of oxygen at a rate of 12 to 20 breaths per minute.

Pulse Oximetry

Pulse oximetry is now widely used in emergency care. The pulse oximeter is a quick and accurate tool that can objectively determine the oxygenation status of the patient. The pulse oximeter provides immediate and continuous evaluation of oxygen delivery to body tissues. It quantifies the effects of interventions including oxygen therapy, medication, suctioning, and ventilatory assistance. In addition, oximetry often detects problems with oxygenation before blood pressure, pulse, and respirations would reveal such a problem. Pulse oximetry, when available, should be used in virtually any patient care situation. In fact, it has been referred to as the fifth vital sign. It should be used during the patient assessment process to determine the patient's baseline value. It should also be used to guide patient care and to monitor the patient's response to paramedic interventions. Normal SpO_2 varies between 95 and 100 percent. Readings between 91 and 94 percent indicate mild hypoxia and warrant further evaluation and supplemental oxygen administration. Readings between 86 and 91 percent indicate moderate hypoxia. These patients should receive 100 percent supplemental oxygen. Readings of 85 percent or lower indicate severe hypoxia and warrant immediate intervention, including the administration of 100 percent oxygen, ventilatory assistance, or both. The goal of therapy is to maintain the SpO_2 in the normal (95 to 99 percent) range.

The incidence of false readings with pulse oximetry is small. When it does occur, the oximeter generates an error signal or a blank screen. Causes of false readings include carbon monoxide poisoning, high-intensity lighting, and certain hemoglobin abnormalities. The absence of a pulse in an extremity will give a false reading. In hypovolemia and in severely anemic patients, the pulse oximetry reading may be misleading. Although the SpO_2 reading may be normal, the total amount of hemoglobin available to carry oxygen may be so markedly decreased that the patient will remain hypoxic at the cellular level.

Pulse oximetry is now an important part of emergency care, including prehospital care. Like the electrocardiogram (ECG) monitor, it provides important information related to the patient. It is important to remember that it is only an additional tool. It does not replace other assessment or monitoring skills. Prehospital care providers cannot depend solely on pulse oximetry reading to guide care; they must always consider and treat the whole patient. The reliability and validity of the pulse oximeter are well documented.

Capnography

Devices that measure the concentration of exhaled carbon dioxide are increasingly used in prehospital care. These devices, called *end-tidal carbon dioxide ($ETCO_2$) detectors*, are most commonly used to assess proper placement of an endotracheal tube. A lack of carbon dioxide in the exhaled air strongly indicates that the tube is placed in the esophagus, whereas the presence of carbon dioxide probably indicates proper tube placement.

End-tidal carbon dioxide detectors are available as either a disposable colorimetric device or an electronic monitor. The device is attached in-line between the endotracheal tube and the ventilation device. Proper tube placement is confirmed by a color change in the colorimetric device or by a light on the electronic monitor.

As with pulse oximetry, an $ETCO_2$ detector should be used only as an adjunct to assessment of endotracheal placement. Paramedics use the device in conjunction with other methods of assessment. It is not a replacement for actually visualizing the endotracheal tube passing through the vocal cords.

ASTHMA

Asthma is a common respiratory illness that affects many persons. Whereas deaths from other respiratory diseases have been steadily declining, deaths from asthma have significantly increased during the past decade. Most of the increased asthma deaths have occurred in patients who are 45 years of age or older. Approximately 50 percent of patients who die from asthma do so before reaching the hospital. Thus, emergency medical service (EMS) personnel are frequently called on to treat patients suffering an asthma attack. Prompt recognition, followed by appropriate treatment, can significantly improve the patient's condition and enhance chances of survival.

Pathophysiology of Asthma

Asthma is a chronic inflammatory disorder of the airways. In susceptible individuals, this inflammation causes symptoms usually associated with widespread but variable airflow obstruction. The major characteristic of asthma is reversible lower airway obstruction. This obstruction is caused by edema, mucus, and smooth muscle spasm; typically, all three factors are involved. Obstruction narrows the diameter of the smaller, smooth muscle–walled bronchioles. The natural dilation of the airways during inhalation allows air to enter these narrowed airways. However, contraction of the airways on exhalation and the obstruction caused by asthma combine to prevent air from escaping.

Air becomes trapped behind the obstruction, preventing continued ventilation of the alveoli, and oxygen–carbon dioxide exchange may be severely impaired. Hypoxemia and hypercarbia result, with the degree of respiratory distress increasing with the severity of obstruction and number of airways involved.

Asthma may be triggered by one of many different factors. These items, commonly referred to as triggers or inducers, vary from one individual to the

Asthma

next. In allergic individuals, environmental allergens are a major cause of inflammation. These allergens may occur both indoors and outdoors. In addition to allergens, asthma may be triggered by cold air, exercise, foods, irritants, and certain medications. Often a specific trigger cannot be identified.

Within minutes of exposure to the offending trigger, a two-phase reaction occurs. The first phase of the reaction is characterized by the release of chemical mediators such as histamine. These mediators cause contraction of the bronchial smooth muscle and leakage of fluid from peribronchial capillaries. This results in both bronchoconstriction and bronchial edema. These two factors can significantly decrease expiratory airflow, causing the typical "asthma attack." Often, the asthma attack resolves spontaneously in 1 to 2 hours or may be aborted by the use of inhaled bronchodilator medications such as albuterol. However, within 6 to 8 hours after exposure to the trigger, a second reaction occurs. This late phase is characterized by inflammation of the bronchioles as cells of the immune system (eosinophils, neutrophils, and lymphocytes) invade the mucosa of the respiratory tract. This leads to additional edema and swelling of the bronchioles and a further decrease of expiratory airflow.

The second phase of the reaction does not typically respond to inhaled beta agonist drugs such as epinephrine or albuterol. Instead, anti-inflammatory agents such as corticosteroids are often required. It is important to point out that the severe inflammatory changes seen in an acute asthma attack do not develop over a few hours or even a few days. The inflammation often begins several days or several weeks before the onset of the actual asthma attack.

Status Asthmaticus

Status asthmaticus is defined as a severe, prolonged asthma attack that cannot be broken by repeated doses of epinephrine or albuterol. It is a serious medical emergency that requires prompt recognition, treatment, and transport. The patient suffering from status asthmaticus frequently has a greatly distended chest from continual air trapping. Breath sounds, and often wheezing, may be absent. The patient is usually exhausted, severely acidotic, and dehydrated. Paramedics should recognize that respiratory arrest is imminent and be prepared for endotracheal intubation. Transport should be immediate, with aggressive treatment continued en route.

Management of Asthma

Treatment of asthma is designed to correct hypoxia, reverse any bronchospasm, and treat inflammatory changes associated with the disease. Oxygen should be administered at a high concentration (100 percent). Intravenous access should be established, and the patient should be placed on an ECG monitor. Initial treatment should be directed at reversing any bronchospasm present. The most commonly used drugs are inhaled beta agonist preparations such as albuterol (Ventolin, Proventil), see Table 8–1. These drugs can be easily administered with a small-volume, oxygen-powered nebulizer. The patient's response to these medications should be monitored and documented.

In addition to beta agonists, early administration of corticosteroids should be considered. Although the inhaled beta agonists will help with bronchoconstriction, they will do little for the underlying inflammation,

TABLE 8-1

Drugs Used in the Treatment of Asthma

Mechanism of Action	Medication
Bronchodilators	
Nonspecific agonists	Epinephrine
	Ephedrine
Beta₂ specific agonists	
Inhaled (short acting)	Albuterol (Ventolin, Proventil)
	Metaproterenol (Alupent)
	Terbutaline (Brethine)
	Bitolterol (Tornalate)
Inhaled (long-acting)	Salmeterol (Serevent)
Methylxanthines	Theophylline (Theo-Dur, Slo-Bid)
	Aminophylline
Anticholinergics	Atropine
	Ipratropium (Atrovent)
Anti-inflammatory agents	
Glucocorticoids	
Inhaled	Beclomethasone (Beclovent)
	Flucticasone (Flovent)
	Triamcinolone (Azmacort)
Oral	Prednisone (Deltasone)
Injected	Methyprednisolone (Solu-Medrol)
	Dexamethasone (Decadron)
Leukotriene Antagonists	Zafirlukast (Accolate)
	Zileuton (Zyflo)
Mast-Cell Membrane Stabilizer	Cromolyn (Intal)

which is the principal problem. If paramedics anticipate a long transport time, medical control may request the administration of methylprednisolone or similar corticosteroid. However, the beneficial effects of corticosteroid administration will probably not be detected until 6 to 8 hours following administration.

If symptoms are severe and do not improve with administration of the inhaled beta agonists, the intravenous administration of aminophylline may be indicated. If the patient is not currently taking a theophylline preparation, paramedics administer a loading dose of 5 to 6 mg/kg of aminophylline over 20 to 30 minutes. This dose should be followed by a maintenance infusion of 0.8 to 1.0 mg/kg/hr. Both the inhaled beta agonists and aminophylline may increase heart rates and/or cause tremors, nausea, and vomiting.

EPINEPHRINE

Class: Sympathetic agonist

Description

Epinephrine is a naturally occurring catecholamine. It is a potent α- and β-adrenergic stimulant; however, its effect on β-receptors is more profound.

Mechanism of Action

Epinephrine acts directly on α- and β-adrenergic receptors. Its effect on β-receptors is much more profound than its effect on α-receptors. The effects of epinephrine include increased heart rate, cardiac contractile force, systemic vascular resistance, and increased blood pressure. It also causes bronchodilation due to its effects on β_2-adrenergic receptors. It is occasionally used to treat the bronchoconstriction accompanying asthma and COPD and is also effective in treating bronchoconstriction associated with anaphylaxis.

Epinephrine's effects usually appear within 90 seconds of administration, and they are usually of short duration. Occasionally the drug must be readministered in 15 to 30 minutes if needed. Epinephrine 1:1000 is given subcutaneously to ensure a steady and prolonged action. Inhaled β-agonists are preferred over epinephrine in the treatment of bronchospasm because they have fewer undesirable side effects.

Indications

Epinephrine is used in bronchial asthma, exacerbation of some forms of COPD, and anaphylaxis.

Contraindications

Because of the cardiac effects seen with the administration of epinephrine, it should not be administered to patients with underlying cardiovascular disease or hypertension. Patients with profound anaphylactic reactions, characterized by hypotension and shock, are usually peripherally vasoconstricted, which will delay absorption of the drug from the subcutaneous site of injection. In these cases, epinephrine 1:10 000 should be administered intravenously.

Precautions

Epinephrine should be protected from light. Also, as with the other catecholamines, it tends to be deactivated by alkaline solutions. Any patient receiving epinephrine 1:1000 should be carefully monitored for changes in blood pressure, pulse, and ECG. Palpitations, anxiety, nausea, and headache are fairly common side effects.

Side Effects

Epinephrine can cause palpitations, anxiety, tremulousness, headache, dizziness, nausea, and vomiting. Because of its strong inotropic and chronotropic properties, epinephrine increases myocardial oxygen demand. Even in low doses it can cause myocardial ischemia. These effects should be kept in mind when administering epinephrine in the emergency setting.

Interactions

The effects of epinephrine can be intensified in patients who are taking antidepressants.

Dosage

The standard dose of epinephrine 1:1000 ranges from 0.3 to 0.5 mg administered subcutaneously, depending on the patient's weight and overall medical condition; 0.3 mg is the usual starting dose for adults. The dose for pediatric patients is 0.01 mg/kg administered subcutaneously. In the pre-hospital phase of emergency medical care, epinephrine 1:1000 should only be administered subcutaneously (except in the case of pediatric cardiac arrest).

How Supplied

Epinephrine is supplied in ampules and prefilled syringes containing 1 mg of the drug in 1 mL of solvent.

ALBUTEROL (UNITED STATES) (PROVENTIL)
SALBUTAMOL (CANADA) (VENTOLIN)

Class: Sympathetic agonist

Description

Albuterol is a sympathomimetic that is selective for β_2-adrenergic receptors.

Mechanism of Action

Albuterol is a selective β_2-agonist with a minimal number of side effects. It causes prompt bronchodilation and has a duration of action of approximately 5 hours.

Indications

Albuterol is used in bronchial asthma and reversible bronchospasm associated with chronic bronchitis and emphysema.

Contraindications

Albuterol should not be administered to any patient with a known history of hypersensitivity to the drug.

Precautions

As with any sympathomimetic, the patient's vital signs must be monitored. Caution should be used when administering albuterol to elderly patients and those with cardiovascular disease or hypertension. Lung sounds should be auscultated before and after each treatment. Ideally, the patient's peak flow rate should be measured both before and after drug administration.

Side Effects

Albuterol can cause palpitations, anxiety, dizziness, headache, nervousness, tremor, hypertension, arrhythmias, chest pain, nausea, and vomiting.

Interactions

The possibility of developing unpleasant side effects increases when albuterol is administered with other sympathetic agonists. β-blockers may blunt the pharmacological effects of albuterol.

Dosage

Albuterol can be administered by metered-dose inhaler or small-volume nebulizer. A common initial dose is two sprays when using a metered-dose inhaler. Each spray delivers 90 μg of albuterol. When using a small-volume nebulizer, the standard adult dose is 2.5 mg (0.5 mL of a 0.5 percent solution diluted in 2.5 mL of normal saline). This amount is typically delivered over 5 to 15 minutes. Albuterol (Ventolin) is also available in the Rotohaler form. A special 200 μg Rotocap is placed in the device and inhaled by the patient. Albuterol should only be administered by inhalation.

How Supplied

Albuterol is supplied in metered-dose inhalers that contain approximately 300 90 μg sprays. The solution for inhalation is supplied in single-patient vials containing 0.5 mL of the drug in 2.5 mL of normal saline. Rotocaps for inhalation are supplied in special 200 μg capsules.

RACEMIC EPINEPHRINE (microNEFRIN, VAPONEFRIN)

Class: Sympathetic agonist

Description

Racemic epinephrine is slightly different chemically from the epinephrine compounds that have been discussed previously. Compounds that differ only in their chemical arrangement are called *isomers*. This particular form is frequently used in children to treat croup.

Mechanism of Action

Racemic epinephrine stimulates both α and β-adrenergic receptors. However, racemic epinephrine has a slight preference for β_2-adrenergic receptors and causes bronchodilation. It also has some effect in relieving the subglottic edema associated with croup. Racemic epinephrine should only be administered by inhalation.

Indication

Racemic epinephrine is used to treat croup (laryngotracheobronchitis).

Contraindications

Racemic epinephrine should not be used in the management of epiglottitis.

Precautions

Racemic epinephrine can result in tachycardia and possibly arrhythmias. Vital signs should be monitored. Many patients develop "rebound worsening" 30 to 60 minutes after the initial treatment and after the effects of racemic epinephrine have worn off. Thus, all children who receive racemic epinephrine should be transported to the hospital. Most hospitals have an institutional policy that requires all children who have received racemic epinephrine to be admitted for at least 24 hours in case rebound worsening occurs.

Dosage

A standard dose is 0.25 to 0.75 mL racemic epinephrine diluted with 2 mL normal saline (2.25 percent) and administered via a standard aerosol nebulizer. It should only be used initially and not repeated. Racemic epinephrine should be given only by inhalation, generally by small-volume nebulizer, diluted with 2 to 3 mL of normal saline.

How Supplied

Racemic epinephrine is supplied in inhaler or nebulizer bottles containing either 7.5, 15, or 30 mL.

℞ TERBUTALINE (BRETHINE, BRICANYL)

Class: Sympathetic agonist

Description

Terbutaline is a synthetic sympathomimetic that is selective for β_2-adrenergic receptors.

Mechanism of Action

Terbutaline, because of its effects on β_2-adrenergic receptors, causes immediate bronchodilation with minimal cardiac effects. Its onset of action is similar to that of epinephrine. Terbutaline is also used to suppress preterm labor.

Indications

Terbutaline is used in bronchial asthma and reversible bronchospasm associated with chronic bronchitis and emphysema.

Contraindications

Terbutaline should not be administered to any patient with a history of hypersensitivity to the drug.

Precautions

As with any sympathomimetic, the patient's vital signs must be monitored. Caution should be used when administering terbutaline to elderly patients and those with cardiovascular disease or hypertension. Lung sounds should be auscultated before and after each treatment. Ideally, the patient's peak flow rate should be measured both before and after drug administration.

Side Effects

Terbutaline can cause palpitations, anxiety, dizziness, headache, nervousness, tremor, hypertension, arrhythmias, chest pain, nausea, and vomiting.

Interactions

The possibility of developing unpleasant side effects increases when terbutaline is used with other sympathetic agonists. β-blockers may blunt the pharmacological effects of terbutaline.

Dosage

The standard dose is two inhalations, 1 minute apart, from a metered-dose inhaler. Terbutaline can also be administered by subcutaneous injection. The usual dose is 0.25 mg. This dose can be repeated in 15 to 30 minutes if needed. Terbutaline should only be administered by inhalation or by subcutaneous injection as described herein.

How Supplied

Terbutaline is supplied in aerosol canisters. Each spray delivers approximately 0.20 mg of the drug. Terbutaline for subcutaneous injection is supplied in vials containing 1 mg of the drug in 1 mL of solvent.

 ## ISOETHARINE (BRONKOSOL)

Class: Sympathetic agonist

Description

Isoetharine is a sympathomimetic similar in chemical structure to epinephrine. It exhibits a slight specificity for β_2-adrenergic receptors, thus reducing the potential for cardiac toxicity.

Mechanism of Action

Isoetharine is a β-agonist with slight selectivity for β_2-adrenergic receptors, causing pulmonary bronchodilation. Its onset of action is similar to that of epinephrine. However, it has a longer duration of effect.

Indications

Isoetharine is used in bronchial asthma and reversible bronchospasm associated with chronic bronchitis and emphysema.

Contraindications

Isoetharine should not be administered to any patient with a history of hypersensitivity to any of the ingredients.

Precautions

As with any sympathomimetic, the patient's vital signs must be monitored. Caution should be used when administering isoetharine to elderly patients and those with cardiovascular disease or hypertension. Lung sounds should be auscultated before and after each treatment. Ideally, the patient's peak flow rate should be measured both before and after drug administration.

Side Effects

Isoetharine can cause palpitations, anxiety, dizziness, headache, nervousness, tremor, hypertension, arrhythmias, chest pain, nausea, and vomiting.

Interactions

The possibility of developing unpleasant side effects increases when isoetharine is administered with other sympathetic agonists. β-blockers may blunt the pharmacological effects of isoetharine.

Dosage

There are three major ways to administer isoetharine, each with different dosages. They are as follows:

Method of Administration	Usual Dose	Dilution
Metered Dose Inhaler	2 inhalations	Undiluted
Oxygen Aerosolization	0.5 milliliters	1:3 with saline
Intermittent positive-pressure breathing	0.5 milliliters	1:3 with saline

Isoetharine should be administered only by one of the methods listed.

How Supplied

Isoetharine is supplied in a 2 mL unit dose containing a 1 percent solution.

 ## METAPROTERENOL (ALUPENT)

Class: Sympathetic agonist

Description

Metaproterenol is a sympathomimetic that is selective for β_2-adrenergic receptors.

Mechanism of Action

Metaproterenol is a selective β_2-agonist and is an effective bronchodilator. Its duration of effect is up to 4 hours.

Indications

Metaproterenol is used in bronchial asthma and reversible bronchospasm associated with chronic bronchitis and emphysema.

Contraindications

Metaproterenol should not be used in patients with cardiac arrhythmias or significant tachycardia.

Precautions

As with any sympathomimetic, the patient's vital signs must be monitored. Caution should be used when administering metaproterenol to elderly patients and those with cardiovascular disease or hypertension. Lung sounds should be auscultated before and after each treatment. Ideally, the patient's peak flow rate should be measured both before and after drug administration.

Side Effects

Metaproterenol can cause palpitations, anxiety, dizziness, headache, nervousness, tremor, hypertension, arrhythmias, chest pain, nausea, and vomiting.

Interactions

The possibility of developing unpleasant side effects increases when metaproterenol is administered with other sympathetic agonists. β-blockers may blunt the pharmacological effects of metaproterenol.

Dosage

Metaproterenol may be administered by metered-dose inhaler. Each spray contains 0.65 mg of metaproterenol. The usual single dose is two to three inhalations, a minute apart, as needed. Metaproterenol may also be administered by small-volume nebulizer. The typical adult dose is 0.2 to 0.3 mL of metaproterenol diluted in 2.5 mL of normal saline. This dose is usually administered over 5 to 15 minutes. Metaproterenol should be administered by inhalation only in the emergency setting.

How Supplied

Metaproterenol is supplied in metered-dose inhalers, with each spray delivering 0.65 mg of the drug. The solution for nebulization is supplied in single-dose units of 0.4 percent (0.2 mL of Alupent in 2.5 mL of saline) and 0.6 percent (0.3 mL of Alupent in 2.5 mL of saline).

℞ AMINOPHYLLINE (SOMOPHYLLIN)

Class: Xanthine

Description

Aminophylline is a xanthine bronchodilator that sometimes proves effective in cases in which sympathomimetics have not been effective.

Mechanism of Action

Aminophylline achieves its bronchodilation effects via a different mechanism than the sympathomimetics. It relaxes bronchial smooth muscle but does not act on adrenergic receptors. Aminophylline also stimulates the respiratory center in the brain. This effect is particularly useful in the treatment of infants with apnea. In addition to bronchodilation, aminophylline has mild diuretic properties, increases the heart rate and cardiac output, and may precipitate arrhythmias. Because of its mild diuretic and inotropic effects, aminophylline is also used in the management of congestive heart failure and pulmonary edema. In prehospital emergency care, aminophylline is usually given by slow IV infusion. Some systems also carry aminophylline suppositories for use in special situations.

Indications

Aminophylline is used in bronchial asthma, reversible bronchospasm associated with chronic bronchitis and emphysema, congestive heart failure, and pulmonary edema.

Contraindications

Aminophylline should not be administered to any patient with a history of hypersensitivity to the drug. It should not be used in patients who have uncontrolled cardiac dysrhythmias.

Precautions

Extreme caution should be used when administering aminophylline to any patient with a history of cardiovascular disease or hypertension. Any patient receiving aminophylline should have a cardiac monitor. One should be alert for any signs of cardiac irritability, especially premature ventricular contractions (PVCs) and tachycardia. Hypotension can occur following rapid administration.

Side Effects

Aminophylline can cause tachycardia, arrhythmias, palpitations, chest pain, nervousness, headache, seizures, nausea, and vomiting.

Interactions

Aminophylline should not be administered to patients who are on chronic theophylline therapy (Slo-Bid, Theo-Dur, and so on) until the amount of drug in the blood has been obtained (theophylline level). Concomitant use with β-blockers and drugs of the erythromycin class of antibiotics may lead to theophylline toxicity.

Dosage

Two major regimens are used in administering aminophylline. The first is for use in patients in whom fluid overload or edema does not appear to be present (i.e., acute bronchial asthma): Place 250 or 500 mg in 90 or 80 mL of 5 percent dextrose, respectively. This can be done with a 100 mL IV bag or with a Buretrol- or Volutrol-type administration set. This solution is then infused over 20 to 30 minutes. This mechanism of slow infusion tends to reduce the chances of arrhythmias. In patients with congestive heart failure, or for whom any additional fluid might be dangerous, a more concentrated infusion is prepared: Place 250 or 500 mg (2 to 5 mg/kg) in 20 mL of 5 percent dextrose in water. This solution is then infused over 20 to 30 minutes using a Buretrol- or Volutrol-type administration set. Parenteral aminophylline should only be given by slow intravenous (IV) infusion by one of the regimens discussed earlier.

How Supplied

Aminophylline is supplied in ampules containing 250 mg in 10 mL of solvent or containing 500 mg in 20 mL of solvent.

ATROPINE SULFATE

Class: Anticholinergic

Description

Atropine is a parasympatholytic (anticholinergic) that is derived from parts of the *Atropa belladonna* plant.

Mechanism of Action

Atropine sulfate is a potent parasympatholytic. It is used in the treatment of respiratory emergencies, because it causes bronchodilation and drying of respiratory tract secretions. Atropine acts by blocking acetylcholine receptors, thus inhibiting parasympathetic stimulation. With the release of ipratropium, atropine has fallen into relative disuse in the treatment of reactive airway disease.

Indications

Atropine is used in bronchial asthma and reversible bronchospasm associated with chronic bronchitis and emphysema.

Contraindications

Atropine sulfate should not be used in patients hypersensitive to the drug. It is not indicated for the acute treatment of bronchospasm, for which rapid response is required.

Precautions

The patient's vital signs must be monitored during therapy with atropine. Caution should be used when administering atropine to elderly patients and those with cardiovascular disease or hypertension. Lung sounds should be auscultated before and after each treatment. Ideally, the patient's peak flow rate should be measured both before and after drug administration.

Side Effects

Atropine can cause palpitations, anxiety, dizziness, headache, nervousness, rash, nausea, and vomiting.

Interactions

There are few interactions in the prehospital setting.

Dosage

Atropine is usually administered with a β-agonist. Typically, 0.5 to 1.0 mg of atropine is placed in 2 to 3 mL of normal saline. This dose is administered by small-volume nebulizer with or without a β-agonist.

How Supplied

Atropine is supplied in ampules and vials containing 1.0 mg in 1 mL of solution.

IPRATROPIUM (ATROVENT)

Class: Anticholinergic

Description

Ipratropium is an anticholinergic (parasympatholytic) bronchodilator that is chemically related to atropine.

Mechanism of Action

Ipratropium is a parasympatholytic used in the treatment of respiratory emergencies. It causes bronchodilation and dries respiratory tract secretions. Ipratropium acts by blocking acetylcholine receptors, thus inhibiting parasympathetic stimulation.

Indications

Ipratropium is used in bronchial asthma and reversible bronchospasm associated with chronic bronchitis and emphysema.

Contraindications

Ipratropium should not be used in patients hypersensitive to the drug. It is not indicated for the acute treatment of bronchospasm, for which rapid response is required.

Precautions

The patient's vital signs must be monitored during therapy with ipratropium. Caution should be used when administering it to elderly patients and those with cardiovascular disease or hypertension. Lung sounds should be auscultated before and after each treatment. Ideally, the patient's peak flow rate should be measured both before and after drug administration.

Side Effects

Ipratropium can cause palpitations, anxiety, dizziness, headache, nervousness, rash, nausea, and vomiting.

Interactions

There are few interactions in the prehospital setting.

Dosage

Ipratropium is usually administered with a β-agonist. Typically, 500 μg of Atrovent is placed in a small-volume nebulizer. A β-agonist can be added if desired. This solution is then administered by small-volume nebulizer with or without a β-agonist. Atrovent is also available in a metered-dose inhaler.

How Supplied

Atrovent is supplied in unit dose vials containing 500 μg (0.02 percent inhalation solution) of the drug already diluted in 2.5 mL saline.

MAGNESIUM SULFATE

Class: Mineral

Description

Magnesium sulfate is a salt that dissociates into the magnesium cation (Mg^{2+}) and the sulfate anion when administered. Magnesium is an essential element in numerous biochemical reactions that occur within the body.

Mechanism of Action

Magnesium acts as a physiological calcium channel blocker and blocks neuromuscular transmission. Magnesium sulfate has been used for years in the management of preterm labor and the hypertensive disorders of pregnancy (preeclampsia and eclampsia). Its usage in obstetrics is discussed in Chapter 11.

Indications

Magnesium sulfate is used in severe bronchospasm, in severe refractory ventricular fibrillation or pulseless ventricular tachycardia, after myocardial infarction for prophylaxis of arrhythmias, and in torsade de pointes (multiaxial ventricular tachycardia).

Contraindications

Magnesium sulfate should not be administered to patients who are in shock, who have persistent, severe hypertension, who have a third-degree atrioventricular (AV) block, who routinely undergo dialysis, or who are known to have a decreased calcium level (hypocalcemia).

Precautions

Magnesium sulfate should be administered slowly to minimize side effects. Any patient receiving intravenous magnesium sulfate should have continuous cardiac monitoring as well as frequent monitoring of vital signs. If possible, the knee and biceps deep tendon reflexes should be checked prior to magnesium therapy. It should be used with caution in patients with known renal insufficiency. Hypermagnesemia (elevated magnesium) can occur following magnesium sulfate administration. Calcium salts (calcium chloride or calcium gluconate) should be available as an antidote for magnesium sulfate in case serious side effects occur.

Side Effects

Magnesium sulfate can cause flushing, sweating, bradycardia, decreased deep tendon reflexes, drowsiness, respiratory depression, arrhythmias, hypotension, hypothermia, itching, and rash.

Interactions

Magnesium sulfate can cause cardiac conduction abnormalities if administered in conjunction with digitalis.

Dosage

The standard dosage is 2 g over 2 to 5 minutes.

How Supplied

Magnesium sulfate is supplied in vials and prefilled syringes. The drug is supplied in both 10 percent and 50 percent solutions. Paramedics should closely examine the solution prior to preparation to avoid dosing errors.

℞ METHYLPREDNISOLONE (SOLU–MEDROL)

Class: Corticosteroid and anti-inflammatory

Description

Methylprednisolone is a synthetic steroid with potent anti-inflammatory properties.

Mechanism of Action

The pharmacological actions of the steroids are vast and complex. In general medical practice, steroids have a wide range of uses. Effective as anti-inflammatory agents, they are used in the management of allergic reactions, asthma, and anaphylaxis. Methylprednisolone is considered an intermediate-acting steroid with a plasma half-life of about 3 to 4 hours.

Indications

Methylprednisolone is used in severe anaphylaxis, asthma or COPD, and urticaria.

Contraindications

There are no major contraindications to the use of methylprednisolone in the acute management of severe anaphylaxis.

Precautions

A single dose of methylprednisolone is all that should be given in the prehospital phase of care. Long-term steroid therapy can cause gastrointestinal bleeding, prolonged wound healing, and suppression of adrenocortical steroids.

Side Effects

Methylprednisolone can cause fluid retention, congestive heart failure, hypertension, abdominal distention, vertigo, headache, nausea, malaise, and hiccups.

Interactions

There are few interactions in the prehospital setting.

Dosage

The standard dosage of methylprednisolone in the management of severe anaphylaxis is 125 to 250 mg administered intravenously. Methylprednisolone may be administered intravenously or intramuscularly, but the intravenous route is preferred in emergency medicine.

How Supplied

Methylprednisolone is supplied in Mix-O-Vials containing 125 mg of the drug. It is supplied in powder form that must be reconstituted in the supplied Mix-O-Vial system. Once reconstituted, it should be used within 48 hours.

Asthma

HYDROCORTISONE (SOLU-CORTEF)

Class: Corticosteroid and anti-inflammatory

Description

Hydrocortisone is a potent corticosteroid with anti-inflammatory properties.

Mechanism of Action

The pharmacological actions of the steroids are vast and complex. Hydrocortisone is considered a short-acting steroid with a plasma half-life of 90 minutes. Like the other adrenocorticosteroids, it is effective as an adjunct in the management of severe anaphylaxis.

Indications

Hydrocortisone is used in severe anaphylaxis, asthma or COPD, and urticaria (hives).

Contraindications

There are no major contraindications to the use of hydrocortisone in the acute management of anaphylaxis.

Precautions

A single dose of hydrocortisone is all that should be given in the prehospital phase of care. Long-term steroid therapy can cause gastrointestinal bleeding, prolonged wound healing, and suppression of adrenocortical steroids.

Side Effects

Hydrocortisone can cause fluid retention, congestive heart failure, hypertension, abdominal distention, vertigo, headache, nausea, malaise, and hiccups.

Interactions

There are few interactions in the prehospital setting.

Dosage

The standard dosage of hydrocortisone in the management of severe anaphylaxis is 40 to 250 mg administered intravenously.

Route

The IV route is preferred in emergency medicine. However, hydrocortisone can be administered intramuscularly when an IV cannot be started.

How Supplied

Hydrocortisone is supplied in Mix-O-Vials containing 100 and 250 mg of the drug.

NEUROMUSCULAR BLOCKERS

Establishment and protection of the airway has the highest priority in emergency care. On certain occasions patients who are still responsive may have trouble maintaining their airway and may require endotracheal intubation. This situation most commonly occurs in patients with drug overdoses, in patients with status epilepticus, and in trauma patients with closed-head injuries. Often, however, intubation is difficult because of the presence of gag reflexes, clenched teeth, or general combativeness. In these cases endotracheal intubation can be carried out after administration of a neuromuscular-blocking agent.

Neuromuscular-blocking agents are drugs that cause muscle relaxation, thus facilitating endotracheal intubation. All skeletal muscles, including the muscles of respiration, respond to these drugs. Following administration, the patient will become apneic and require mechanical ventilation. Neuromuscular-blocking agents have no effect on the patient's level of consciousness or pain sensation. Neuromuscular-blocking drugs are classified as *depolarizing* and *nondepolarizing* based on their mechanism of action. The most commonly used depolarizing drug is succinylcholine, and vecuronium and pancuronium are the most frequently used nondepolarizing agents.

1. *Succinylcholine (Anectine).* Succinylcholine is a depolarizing neuromuscular blocker commonly used in emergency medicine. It acts in approximately 60 to 90 seconds and lasts approximately 3 to 5 minutes. Succinylcholine causes muscle fasciculations progressing to total paralysis, including paralysis of the diaphragm.

2. *Pancuronium (Pavulon).* Pancuronium is a long-acting, nondepolarizing neuromuscular-blocking agent. It acts in 2 to 5 minutes and lasts 40 to 60 minutes.

3. *Vecuronium (Norcuron).* Vecuronium is a nondepolarizing neuromuscular-blocking agent with a rapid onset and short duration of action. It has fewer cardiovascular side effects than succinylcholine and does not cause fasciculations.

4. *Rocuronium (Zemuron).* Rocuronium is a nondepolarizing neuromuscular-blocking agent with a rapid to intermediate onset, depending on dose, and an intermediate duration of action. At equivalent doses, rocuronium has approximately the same clinically effective duration of action as vecuronium. However, the onset of action is approximately 40 percent shorter for rocuronium than for vecuronium.

Depolarizing Blocking Agents

Succinylcholine is the only therapeutic depolarizing blocking agent. Although it is similar to nondepolarizing blockers in its therapeutic effect, its mechanism of action differs. Because succinylcholine is absorbed poorly from the gastrointestinal tract, the preferred administration route is IV. Succincylcholine is metabolized in the liver and excreted via the kidneys.

Pharmacodynamics

Succinylcholine has a biphasic effect. In phase I blockade, it acts like acetylcholine and depolarizes the synaptic membrane of the muscle. However, succinylcholine is not inactivated by cholinesterase, so the depolarization persists, resulting in brief periods of excitation, manifested by muscle fasciculations (uncoordinated contractions of muscle fibers), followed by muscle paralysis and flaccidity. Phase II is normally not seen except in high drug concentrations. Succinylcholine is the drug of choice for short-term muscle relaxation, such as during intubation. The primary adverse drug reactions to succinylcholine are the same as those to nondepolarizing blockers: prolonged apnea and cardiovascular alterations. Patients commonly experience muscle pain from the fasciculations that occur in phase I.

SUCCINYLCHOLINE (ANECTINE)

Class: Depolarizing neuromuscular blocker

Description

Succinylcholine is a short-acting, depolarizing skeletal muscle relaxant used to facilitate endotracheal intubation.

Mechanism of Action

Succinylcholine is a short-acting, depolarizing skeletal muscle relaxant. Like acetylcholine, it combines with cholinergic receptors in the motor nerves to cause depolarization. Neuromuscular transmission is thus inhibited, which renders the muscles unable to be stimulated by acetylcholine. Following IV injection, complete paralysis is obtained within 60 to 90 seconds and persists for approximately 4 to 5 minutes. Effects then start to fade, and a return to normal is seen within 6 minutes. Muscle relaxation begins in the eyelids and jaw. It then progresses to the limbs, the abdomen, and finally the diaphragm and intercostals. It has no effect on consciousness.

Indication

Succinylcholine is used to achieve temporary paralysis when endotracheal intubation is indicated and muscle tone or seizure activity prevents it.

Contraindications

Succinylcholine is contraindicated in patients with a history of hypersensitivity to the drug. It should not be used with penetrating eye injuries or in patients with a history of narrow-angle glaucoma. Succinylcholine should not be administered by persons inexperienced with its use.

Precautions

Succinylcholine should not be administered unless personnel skilled in endotracheal intubation are present and ready to perform the procedure. Oxygen therapy equipment should be readily available, as should all emergency resuscitative drugs and equipment. Fractures have been reported in children following the use of depolarizing neuromuscular blockers due to strong and sustained muscle fasciculations. Cardiac arrest and ventricular arrhythmias have been reported when succinylcholine was administered to patients with severe burns and severe crush injuries.

Side Effects

Succinylcholine can cause wheezing, respiratory depression, apnea, aspiration, arrhythmias, bradycardia, sinus arrest, hypertension, hypotension, increased intraocular pressure, and increased intracranial pressure.

Interactions

Certain drugs can enhance the neuromuscular-blocking action of succinylcholine: lidocaine, procainamide, β-blockers, magnesium sulfate, and other neuromuscular blockers.

Dosage

The dosage for succinylcholine is 1 to 1.5 mg/kg administered intravenously. The preferred route for succinylcholine administration is intravenously. It can be administered intramuscularly if required, however.

How Supplied

Succinylcholine is supplied in vials containing 10 mL of a 20 mg/mL concentration (200 mg total).

Nondepolarizing Blocking Agents

The nondepolarizing blocking agents, also called competitive or stabilizing agents, are derived curare alkaloids and their synthetic analogues. We discuss three such agents: pancuronium bromide, vecuronium bromide, and rocuronium bromide. These drugs produce intermediate to prolonged muscle relaxation, such as that required for intubation and ventilation during surgery. Because nondepolarizing blockers are poorly absorbed from the gastrointestinal tract, they are administered parenterally, with the IV route preferred. A variable but large proportion of the nondepolarizing agents is excreted unchanged in the urine. Some of the newer drugs, such as pancuronium and vecuronium, are metabolized partially in the liver.

Pharmacodynamics

The nondepolarizing blockers compete with acetylcholine at the cholinergic sites of the skeletal muscle membrane. This action blocks acetylcholine's neurotransmitter action, preventing the muscle membrane from depolarizing. The effect can be counteracted clinically by anticholinesterase drugs, such as neostigmine or pyridostigmine, which inhibit the action of acetylcholinesterase, the enzyme that destroys acetylcholine.

The initial muscle weakness produced by the drugs quickly changes to flaccid paralysis that affects the muscles in a specific sequence. The first muscles to exhibit flaccid paralysis are those innervated by the motor portions of the cranial nerves and small, rapidly moving muscles in the eyes, face, and neck. Next, the limb, abdomen, and trunk muscles become flaccid. Finally, the intercostal muscles and diaphragm are paralyzed. Recovery from the paralysis usually occurs in the reverse order.

Because these drugs do not cross the blood-brain barrier, no alterations in consciousness or pain perception occur. Thus patients are aware of what is happening to them and may experience extreme anxiety and pain, but they cannot communicate their feelings.

Nondepolarizing blockers are used for intermediate or prolonged muscle relaxation. They facilitate endotracheal intubation and are used during surgery to decrease the amount of anesthetic required and to facilitate manipulations. They are also used to paralyze patients who need ventilatory support but who fight the endotracheal tube and ventilator.

Pancuronium selectively blocks the vagus nerve and may result in tachycardia, cardiac arrhythmias, and hypertension.

℞ PANCURONIUM BROMIDE (PAVULON)

Class: Nondepolarizing neuromuscular blocker

Description

Pancuronium bromide is a derivative of curare and is used to provide muscle relaxation to facilitate endotracheal intubation.

Mechanism of Action

Pancuronium competes with acetylcholine for cholinergic receptor sites on the postjunctional membrane. This results in paralysis of muscle fibers served by the occupied neuromuscular junction. It does not cause an initial depolarization wave, as does succinylcholine. The onset of action of pancuronium is 30 to 40 seconds, and the effect may persist for up to 60 minutes. Effects may begin to subside after 35 to 45 minutes.

Indication

Pancuronium is used to achieve temporary paralysis when endotracheal intubation is indicated and muscle tone, seizures, or laryngospasm prevents it.

Contraindications

Pancuronium is contraindicated in patients with a history of hypersensitivity to the drug. It should not be administered by persons inexperienced with its use.

Precautions

Pancuronium should not be administered unless personnel skilled in endotracheal intubation are present and ready to perform the procedure. Oxygen therapy equipment should be readily available, as should all emergency resuscitative drugs and equipment. Hypotension can occur. Thus, the vital signs must be constantly monitored. Pancuronium can increase intracranial pressure. In patients with head injuries, vecuronium is often preferred.

Side Effects

Pancuronium can cause wheezing, respiratory depression, apnea, aspiration, arrhythmias, bradycardia, sinus arrest, hypertension, hypotension, increased intraocular pressure, and increased intracranial pressure.

Interactions

Certain drugs can enhance the neuromuscular-blocking action of pancuronium: lidocaine, procainamide, β-blockers, magnesium sulfate, certain antibiotics (aminoglycosides), and other neuromuscular blockers.

Dosage

The adult and pediatric dosage for pancuronium is 0.04 to 0.1 mg/kg administered intravenously. Repeat doses of 0.01 to 0.02 mg/kg administered intravenously may be required every 20 to 40 minutes.

How Supplied

Pancuronium is supplied in 2 and 5 mL vials containing 2 mg/mL of the drug.

VECURONIUM (NORCURON)

Class: Nondepolarizing neuromuscular blocker

Description

Vecuronium is a derivative of pancuronium and is used to provide muscle relaxation to facilitate endotracheal intubation.

Mechanism of Action

Vecuronium has a similar mechanism of action as pancuronium. However, it is approximately one-third more potent, with a shorter duration of effect. Vecuronium competes with acetylcholine for cholinergic receptor sites on the postjunctional membrane. This competition results in paralysis of muscle fibers served by the occupied neuromuscular junction. It does not cause an initial depolarization wave, as does succinylcholine. The onset of action of vecuronium is 1 minute, with good to excellent intubation conditions within 2.5 to 3 minutes.

Indication

Vecuronium is used to achieve temporary paralysis when endotracheal intubation is indicated and muscle tone or seizure activity prevents it.

Contraindications

Vecuronium is contraindicated in patients with a history of hypersensitivity to the drug.

Precautions

Vecuronium should not be administered unless personnel skilled in endotracheal intubation are present and ready to perform the procedure. Oxygen therapy equipment should be readily available, as should all emergency resuscitative drugs and equipment.

Side Effects

Vecuronium can cause wheezing, respiratory depression, apnea, aspiration, arrhythmias, bradycardia, sinus arrest, hypertension, hypotension, increased intraocular pressure, and increased intracranial pressure.

Interactions

Certain drugs can enhance the neuromuscular-blocking action of vecuronium: lidocaine, procainamide, β-blockers, magnesium sulfate, and other neuromuscular blockers.

Dosage

The adult dosage for vecuronium is 0.08 to 0.10 mg/kg administered intravenously. Neuromuscular blockade should last 25 to 30 minutes.

How Supplied

Vecuronium is supplied in 10 mL vials containing 10 mg of the drug. It must be reconstituted with the diluent provided.

℞ ROCURONIUM BROMIDE (ZEMURON)

Class: Nondepolarizing neuromuscular blocker

Description

Rocuronium is a nondepolarizing neuromuscular-blocking agent with a rapid to intermediate onset, depending on dose, and intermediate duration of action.

Mechanism of Action

Rocuronium acts by binding competitively to cholinergic receptors at the motor end plate to antagonize the action of acetylcholine, an effect that is reversible in the presence of acetylcholinesterase inhibitors, such as neostigmine and edrophonium.

Indications

Rocuronium is indicated as an adjunct to general anesthesia to facilitate both rapid-sequence (initiated at 60 to 90 seconds postadministration) and routine endotracheal intubation and to provide skeletal muscle relaxation during surgery or mechanical ventilation.

Contraindications

Rocuronium is contraindicated in patients with a history of hypersensitivity to the drug.

Precautions

Rocuronium should be administered in carefully adjusted dosages by or under the supervision of experienced clinicians who are familiar with its actions and the possible complications of its use. Rocuronium is associated with a slight elevation of heart rate and blood pressure; tachycardia may occur in children.

Side Effects

Bronchospasm is a side effect of rocuronium.

Interactions

Intensity and duration of paralysis may be prolonged by pretreatment with succinylcholine, general anesthesia (inhalation), lidocaine, quinidine, procainamide, beta-adrenergic-blocking agents, potassium-losing diuretics, or magnesium.

Dosage

Rapid-sequence tracheal intubation dosage is 600 μg (0.6 mg)/kg. Maintenance dose is 100 to 200 μg (0.1 to 0.2 mg)/kg continuous infusion.

How Supplied

Rocuronium is supplied in 10 mg/mL in 5 mL vials.

Before administering any neuromuscular-blocking agent, it is essential that paramedics have equipment ready for airway management as soon as the patient becomes apneic. In addition, because a neuromuscular-blocking agent has no effect on pain sensation and mental status, it should not be administered to alert patients without first administering a sedative or analgesic. Most emergency patients have eaten or drunk something in the hours prior to the onset of the emergency. Thus, virtually every emergency patient is considered to have a full stomach.

Neuromuscular blockade and endotracheal intubation may cause vomiting, which increases the risk of aspiration. Consequently, special precautions must be taken to gain rapid control of the airway as soon as the drug is administered. As a result, this procedure is often referred to as *rapid-sequence induction*.

RAPID-SEQUENCE INDUCTION

The procedure for rapid-sequence induction (RSI) is as follows: Place the patient in a supine position. Preoxygenate with 100 percent oxygen for 5 minutes (spontaneous respirations) or ventilate with a bag-valve-mask device and 100 percent oxygen for at least five tidal volumes prior to intubation to facilitate nitrogen washout (allows 3 to 5 minutes of apnea without serious hypoxemia).

1. Establish IV normal saline with large-bore catheter (two IVs if time and personnel permit).
2. Monitor ECG, Sao_2, and vital signs as closely as possible throughout procedure.
3. Perform a thorough neurological exam.
4. Prepare for rapid administration of fentanyl, midazolam, lidocaine, atropine, and succinylcholine.
5. Assemble and prepare equipment (suction, endotracheal tube, endotracheal tube stylet, syringe, lubricant, and cricothyrotomy and PTTV kits).
6. Administer lidocaine 1.5 mg/kg IV push if head is injured or increased intracranial pressure is suspected.

7. Administer atropine 1.0 mg IV push if
   - Bradycardia is present (fentanyl may induce bradydys-rhythmias)
   - Cervical-spine injury
   - Patients under age 16 (pediatric dose 0.02 mg/kg IV push)
8. Prepare paralytic agents.
9. Administer fentanyl 1.0 to 3.0 µg/kg slow IV push.
10. Administer midazolam 0.05 to 0.1 mg/kg slow IV push or for the adult patient, 2.5 to 5.0 mg if the blood pressure is over 100 systolic.
11. As patient becomes relaxed approximately 1 to 2 minutes after administration of midazolam, apply cricoid pressure (Sellick's maneuver) to occlude the esophagus and maintain pressure until the endotracheal tube is in place and the cuff is inflated.
12. Check adequacy of sedation and administer 1.5 mg/kg succinylcholine or 0.01 mg/kg vecuronium IV push and stop ventilating if doing so.
13. Apnea and jaw relaxation are indications that the patient is sufficiently relaxed to proceed with endotracheal intubation. If patient is not adequately relaxed, then administer atropine and a second dose of succinylcholine 1.5 mg/kg.
14. Position head, visualize larynx, and intubate.
15. Observe lung inflations, check endotracheal tube for fogging, and auscultate the chest for adequate ventilation. Ventilate with 100 percent oxygen at 16 to 20 per minute. (Use $ETCO_2$ to determine effective ventilatory rate.)
16. Inflate cuff on endotracheal tube.
17. Release cricoid pressure.
18. Reassess patient's vital signs.
19. The effects of the succinylcholine will wear off in 3 to 5 minutes (vecuronium will wear off in 25 to 30 minutes).
20. Medical control or standing orders may request the administration of pancuronium or vecuronium if continued paralysis is warranted.
21. The maintenance dose of pancuronium is 0.01 mg/kg; the maintenance dose of vecuronium is 0.01 mg/kg.
22. Assess patient for adequacy of sedation. It may be necessary to administer more fentanyl or midazolam for long transports; the effects of both generally last approximately 30 minutes.

RAPID-SEQUENCE SEDATION

An alternative to rapid-sequence induction is the use of many of the same medications, without the use of paralytics. This procedure is referred to as rapid-sequence sedation (RSS). The advantage to this procedure is that paralytics are not used, and a reversal of some of the respiratory depressant effects (from the narcotic fentanyl) is possible with the administration of Narcan. A disadvantage to this procedure occurs in the patient with trismus or a clenched jaw. In spite of the administration of the RSS medications, it may be impossible to pass the endotracheal tube. In this case a surgical airway may be warranted.

The procedure for rapid-sequence sedation is as follows: Place the patient in a supine position. Preoxygenate with 100 percent oxygen for 5 minutes (spontaneous respirations) or ventilate with a bag-valve-mask device and 100 percent oxygen for at least five tidal volumes prior to intubation to facilitate nitrogen washout (allows 3 to 5 minutes of apnea without serious hypoxemia).

1. Establish IV normal saline with large-bore catheter. Monitor ECG SaO_2, and vital signs as closely as possible throughout procedure.

2. Prepare for rapid administration of fentanyl, midazolam, lidocaine, and atropine. Assemble and prepare equipment (suction, endotracheal tube, endotracheal tube stylet, syringe, lubricant, and cricothyrotomy and PTTV kits).

3. Administer lidocaine 1.5 mg/kg IV push.

4. Administer atropine 1.0 mg IV push if

   • Bradycardia is present (fentanyl may induce bradydysrhythmias)

   • Cervical-spine injury

   • Patients under age 16 (pediatric dose 0.02 mg/kg IV push)

5. Administer fentanyl 1.0 μg/kg IV push or for the adult patient 100 μg initially, redosing with 50 μg or 0.5 μg/kg increments as necessary to a maximum of 4 μg/kg.

6. Administer midazolam 0.09 to 0.3 mg/kg slow IV push or for the adult patient 2.5 to 5.0 mg if the patient is responsive to voice or pain and blood pressure is over 100 systolic. Redose with up to three 1 mg boluses if necessary, the blood pressure is over 100 systolic, and the patient becomes responsive to voice or pain.

7. As patient becomes relaxed, approximately 1 to 2 minutes after administration of midazolam, apply cricoid pressure.

8. Check adequacy of sedation and administer additional fentanyl and midazolam if required.

9. Position head, visualize larynx, apply lidocaine spray, and intubate. Observe lung inflations, check endotracheal tube for fogging, and auscultate the chest for adequate ventilation. Ventilate with 100 percent oxygen at 16 to 20 per minute. Monitor ECG, vital signs, and SaO_2 every 3 to 5 minutes.

Maintenance of Sedation

Fentanyl may be repeated 0.5 μg/kg or 50 μg for the adult patient every 20 to 30 minutes, as needed. Midazolam may be repeated 0.05 mg/kg or 2.5 mg for the adult patient every 20 to 30 minutes, as needed. Lorazepam

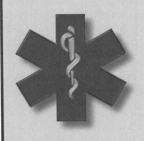

CASE PRESENTATION

EMS is called to a residence for a female patient complaining of shortness of breath. The patient is conscious and breathing. En route dispatch informs the paramedics that the patient has a history of COPD and uses an inhaler. On arrival paramedics are met by the patient's son, who takes them to the bedroom where the patient is sitting up in bed. The patient, an 88-year-old woman, is in obvious respiratory distress. She is leaning forward and struggling to breathe.

On Examination

CNS:	The patient is conscious, alert, and oriented × 4; she is able to answer questions with short answers only (less than 4 words); patient is clearly frightened
Resp:	Respirations are 42 and shallow; patient is wheezing; wheezes are heard throughout all lung fields on expiration; trachea is midline; no signs of trauma
CVS:	Carotid and radial pulses are present and weak; skin is warm and dry
ABD:	Soft and nontender
Muscl/Skel:	Patient able to move extremities on command; no weaknesses to hand grip

Vital Signs:

Pulse:	120/min, irregular, weak
Resp:	42/min, shallow
BP:	152/110 mm Hg
SpO$_2$:	88 percent
ECG:	Sinus rhythm with unifocal PVCs at four to six per minute
Hx:	Patient has emphysema and was recently hospitalized for it and then discharged 2 days ago. She has had a cold for the past 2 weeks and states that changes in weather cause her "lungs to act up." She has been getting progressively worse, and her son states that the inhaler that she uses ran out this afternoon. She has no chest pain and denies any recent trauma.
PHx:	She has had emphysema, which seems to get worse during the winter months, for 20 years. She has been hospitalized numerous times for "breathing problems." The patient had a "heart attack" 2 years ago. Medications include Ventolin and Becloforte inhalers, synthroid, and verapamil; she has no allergies.

Treatment

Oxygen was administered by nasal cannula at 6 1/min, and 5 mg of salbutamol (Ventolin) was administered by an oxygen-powered nebulizer. With coaching, the patient relaxed and her breathing improved slightly. The patient was hooked up to the ECG monitor and a sinus tachycardia was noted. En route to the hospital a second dose of 5 mg of salbutamol and 500 mg of ipratropium bromide (Atrovent) were administered via a nebulizer. On arrival at the hospital, the patient was able to speak normally and the wheezing had diminished significantly. The SpO_2 had increased to 96 percent. Her prescription for the inhalers was refilled, and after an overnight stay in the hospital she was released.

0.05 to 0.1 mg/kg (<2 mg/min) or 2.0 to 4.0 mg, may be given for the adult patient every 4 to 8 hours to a maximum of 8 mg.

Notes

A Glasgow Coma Scale score of 9 or less indicates the need for intubation unless the decreased loss of consciousness can be readily reversed (e.g., hypoglycemia or narcotic overdose).

The sedative effect of midazolam diminishes after approximately 2 hours. The duration of action of fentanyl may be as short as 30 minutes (and reversible with naloxone).

Lorazepam may be used for patients with seizure disorder.

The dosage of benzodiazepines should be reduced in patients over 50 years of age or if hypotension is present.

SUMMARY

Respiratory emergencies are a serious and potentially fatal condition if not treated immediately. Prompt recognition of the signs and symptoms of respiratory distress is essential. Oxygen is the primary drug for treating any respiratory problem. Many types of medical problems, especially asthma and anaphylaxis, respond only to the medications discussed in this chapter.

KEY WORDS

allergens.   A foreign substance that can cause an allergic response in the body but is only harmful to some people.

bronchospasm.   An abnormal contraction of the bronchi, resulting in narrowing and blockage of the airway. A cough with wheezing is the usual symptom. Bronchospasm is the main feature of asthma and bronchitis.

capnography.   A system for measuring the concentration of exhaled carbon dioxide.

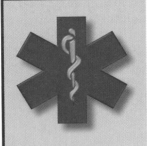

CASE PRESENTATION

At 1830 hours paramedics are called to a rural residence 45 minutes from the hospital for a 45-year-old woman complaining of shortness of breath. She is conscious and breathing. On arrival paramedics are met by the patient's husband, who leads them to the living room. There, paramedics find a patient leaning forward in a chair. The patient is using home oxygen by nasal cannula and an oxygen-powered nebulizer. The patient appears very anxious and in severe respiratory distress.

On Examination

CNS: The patient is conscious, alert, and oriented × 4; in extreme respiratory distress

Resp: Respirations are 36 and shallow; wheezes are heard unaided by stethoscope; there are tight, barely audible wheezes in the apices bilaterally and no sounds heard in the bases; trachea is midline; no signs of trauma

CVS: Carotid and radial pulses are present and weak; skin is pale and cool

ABD: Soft and nontender

Muscl/Skel: Patient able to move extremities on command; no weaknesses to hand grip

Vital Signs

Pulse: 140/min, regular, weak

Resp: 36/min, shallow

BP: 144/94 mm Hg

SpO$_2$: 82 percent

ECG: Sinus tachycardia

Hx: Patient has a 20-year history of asthma and was taking Ventolin by inhaler twice a day, Becloforte twice a day, and home oxygen by nasal cannula at 4 L/min as needed and during sleep. The patient was talking to her granddaughter on the phone. She became very upset during the telephone call and then became short of breath. The patient put on her oxygen (which provided no relief) and also took one dose (2.5 mg) of albuterol with an oxygen-powered nebulizer (which also provided no relief).

Treatment

Paramedics administered 5 mg of Ventolin and 500 μg of Atrovent by nebulizer mask as per standing orders, and the patient was coached to take a breath and hold it. The patient was very agitated, and the coaching had little effect. An IV was initiated and run TKO. The patient was hooked up to the ECG monitor and a sinus tachycardia was noted. The base hospital was contacted, and the paramedics were directed to administer 125 mg of Solu-Medrol IV push and to continue administering Ventolin. The patient's condition deteriorated en route to the hospital. Although the patient was conscious, she was fatigued and unable to follow verbal commands. The base hospital was contacted, and the paramedics were directed to sedate and intubate the patient. The procedure was explained to the patient; 100 µg of fentanyl (Sublimaze) and 2.5 mg of midazolam (Versed) were administered IV. Sellick's maneuver was applied to occlude the esophagus, at which point 1.5 mg/kg of succinylcholine (Anectine) was given IV. Once the jaw relaxed, the patient was intubated and bilateral breath sounds were confirmed. The patient was admitted to the intensive care unit on arrival at the hospital.

chronic obstructive pulmonary disease (COPD). A pulmonary disease characterized by a decreased ability of the lungs to perform the function of ventilation.

edema. An abnormal pooling of fluid in the tissues.

hypercapnia. An increased level of carbon dioxide in the body.

hypoxia. A state in which insufficient oxygen is available to meet the oxygen requirements of the cells.

pH. A scientific method of expressing the acidity or alkalinity of a solution. It is the logarithm of the hydrogen ion concentration divided by 1. The higher the pH, the more alkaline the solution. The lower the pH, the more acidic the solution.

pulse oximetry. An assessment modality that measures the oxygen saturation level of the blood through a noninvasive sensor placed on a finger or earlobe.

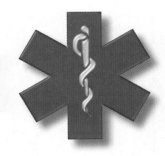

Drugs Used in the Treatment of Metabolic-Endocrine Emergencies

After completing this chapter, the reader should be able to

1. Define the term *hormone.*
2. Discuss the function and location of the pancreas.
3. List two functions of the islets of Langerhans.
4. Discuss the function of glucagon.
5. Define *diabetes mellitus.*
6. Discuss the function of insulin and its relation to glucose metabolism.
7. Compare and contrast type I (insulin-dependent) and type II (non-insulin-dependent) diabetes mellitus.
8. Compare and contrast diabetic ketoacidosis and hypoglycemia.
9. Describe and list the indications, contraindications, and dosages for insulin, glucagon, $D_{50}W$, and thiamine.

240

INTRODUCTION

Glands that secrete hormones directly into the blood, without the aid of ducts, are called *endocrine glands.* With the exception of the pancreas, they rarely cause emergency disorders. Occasionally the thyroid, the endocrine gland that controls metabolic rate, begins secreting excess thyroid hormones. This disorder, called hyperthyroidism, is characterized by increased heart rate, loss of body weight, insomnia, dry skin, hair loss, and nervousness. A rare but severe form of thyroid dysfunction is called *thyroid storm.* Thyroid storm causes fever, tachycardia, dehydration, and a change in mental status. Although this chapter is devoted to metabolic-endocrine emergencies, we primarily discuss the pancreatic disorder *diabetes mellitus.*

DIABETES MELLITUS

The pancreas is located in the retroperitoneal space, within the folds of the small intestine. Within the pancreas is an area called the *islets of Langerhans.* The islets of Langerhans have three types of cells that secrete three different hormones. The α cells secrete the hormone *glucagon.* The β cells secrete *insulin.* A third hormone, called *somatostatin*, is secreted from the delta cells. Insulin is required for the passage of glucose into the cells. Without insulin the blood glucose level rises. Glucagon causes stored carbohydrates, especially glycogen, to be broken down to glucose. When the blood sugar level falls, glucagon is released, which then causes a release of stored carbohydrates. Somatostatin inhibits the secretion of both insulin and glucagon. Functionally, it is similar to growth hormone.

Diabetes mellitus is caused when β cells of the pancreas reduce the amount of insulin secreted. In addition, the relative number of insulin receptors decreases. These two factors contribute to an increasing level of glucose in the blood, which results in increased thirst (polydipsia), increased hunger (polyphagia), and increased urination (polyuria). The hunger results because the various body cells are glucose depleted. The thirst is due to a relative dehydration that occurs when glucose spills over into the urine. Glucose spillage into the urine takes water with it, which results in the polyuria and polydipsia characteristic of hyperglycemia. If allowed to progress untreated, the patient will eventually lapse into diabetic coma. Patients in diabetic coma have warm, dry skin. Clinically they are dehydrated. They may exhibit rapid, deep respirations (Kussmaul respirations), which are part of the body's attempt to rid itself of accumulated acids. Because the signs and symptoms occur early, most patients seek medical care before coma ensues. Once diagnosed, the patient will most likely be placed on hypoglycemic agents. If an excessive amount of insulin is taken, or if the patient fails to eat properly, then *hypoglycemia* can develop (see Table 9–1).

TYPES OF DIABETES

Generally, diabetes mellitus can be divided into two different categories. Type I diabetes, or insulin-dependent diabetes, usually begins in the early years. Patients who have type I diabetes must take insulin. Type II, or non-insulin-dependent diabetes, usually begins later in life and tends to be associated with obesity. Type II diabetes can often be controlled without using insulin. It is important for paramedics to understand the difference between these two forms of diabetes.

TABLE 9-1

Typical findings in Diabetic-Induced Altered Mental Status

Hypoglycemia

Scene Size-up	Initial Assessment	Signs and Symptoms	Vitals/Physical	History	Causes	Management
Presence of syringes, insulin, glucometers, lower extremity prosthetic devices	Chief complaint may reveal patient or family awareness of diabetic condition; may complain of confusion, restlessness, weakness Acute onset Airway compromise (vomitus, tongue)	Weakness/ uncoordination Lethargy/confusion Headache Irritable, nervous behavior Hunger, thirst, polyuria Chest pain Shortness of breath Nausea, vomiting, diarrhea Malaise Abdominal pain May appear intoxicated Coma (severe cases)	**Vitals** Weak or full, rapid pulses Cold clammy skin Diaphoresis Pupils normal to dilated	History of diabetes, cardiac, renal, or vascular disease Obesity, endocrine problems; exertion, infection Slow healing wounds, poor peripheral perfusion, scarring of fingers; provisional amputations	Patient has taken too much insulin Patient has overexerted, thus reducing glucose levels	Check blood sugar level Administer dextrose as per protocol/ standing order

Diabetic Ketoacidosis (DKA/Hyperglycemia)

Scene Size-up	Initial Assessment	Signs and Symptoms	Vitals/Physical	History	Causes	Management
Presence of syringes, insulin, glucometers, lower extremity prosthetic devices	Chief complaint may reveal patient or family awareness of diabetic condition; may complain of confusion, restlessness, weakness Gradual onset "Fruity" smell of ketones on patient's breath Airway compromise	Polyuria, polydypsia, polyphagia Nausea, vomiting Tachycardia Deep, rapid respirations Warm, dry skin Fruity odor on breath Abdominal pain Falling blood pressure Fever (occasionally) Decreased level of consciousness	**Vitals** Weak, rapid pulses Kussmaul's respirations Low blood pressure in later stages Poor skin turgor, pallor, delayed capillary refill related to dehydration **Physical** Injection sites; medical alert jewelry Slow healing wounds, poor peripheral perfusion; Scarring of fingers; Provisional amputations	History of diabetes, cardiac disease, renal disease, vascular disease, obesity, endocrine problems Family history of diabetes	Patient has not taken insulin Patient has overeaten, flooding the body with carbohydrates Patient has infection that disrupts glucose/insulin balance	Check blood sugar level Fluids Insulin

Type I Diabetes Mellitus

Type I diabetes mellitus is a serious disease characterized by inadequate production of insulin by the endocrine pancreas. The cause of type I diabetes is not well understood. One theory is that a viral infection attacks the pancreatic β cells, thus slowing or stopping insulin production. Another theory proposes that the body's immune system mistakenly targets the pancreatic β cells as foreign and attacks them. In either case, heredity appears to be a factor in increasing a person's chances of contracting the disease.

With type I diabetes mellitus, the patient must take daily doses of insulin. In the normal state, the intake of glucose, such as in a meal, results in the release of insulin. Insulin promotes the uptake of glucose by the cells. Type I diabetes generally begins with decreased insulin secretion, subsequently leading to elevated blood glucose levels. However, because insulin is required for glucose to enter into the various body cells, they become glucose depleted despite increased blood glucose levels.

In diabetes, a drop in insulin levels is accompanied by a steady accumulation of glucose in the blood. As the cells become glucose depleted, they begin to use other sources of energy. Therefore, various harmful by-products, such as *ketones* and *organic acids,* are produced. When these by-products start to accumulate, several of the classic findings of diabetic ketoacidosis appear. If the various acids and ketones continue to collect in the blood, severe metabolic acidosis occurs and coma ensues. Severe acidosis can result in serious brain damage or death.

As the concentration of glucose in the blood continues to rise, the kidneys begin excreting glucose in the urine. When glucose is spilled into the urine, it takes water with it, resulting in osmotic diuresis, which dehydrates the patient.

Type II Diabetes Mellitus

Type II diabetes mellitus occurs more commonly than type I does. Like type I, it is characterized by decreased insulin production by the endocrine pancreas. As mentioned previously, type II diabetes usually begins later in life. It is often associated with obesity but can occur in nonobese patients. Increased body weight causes a relative decrease in the number of available insulin receptors. In addition, the insulin receptors become defective and less responsive to insulin. The pancreas also becomes less responsive to stimulation from increased blood glucose levels. Thus, insulin is not secreted as needed, increasing blood glucose levels even further.

The first approach in treating type II diabetes is to encourage the patient to lose weight by reducing the intake of carbohydrates. Physicians may also prescribe oral hypoglycemic agents. These medications tend to stimulate increased insulin secretion from the pancreas and to promote an increase in the number of insulin receptors on the cells. Both actions tend to lower blood glucose levels. If diet and oral agents fail, insulin may be required.

Type II diabetes does not usually result in diabetic ketoacidosis. In type II diabetes, the patient makes enough insulin to maintain pH homeostasis but not enough to supply all of the body's needs. It can, however, develop into a life-threatening emergency termed *nonketotic hyperosmolar coma.* In type II diabetes, when blood glucose levels exceed 600 mg/dL, the high osmolality of the blood causes an osmotic diuresis and dehydration of body cells. It is difficult to distinguish diabetic ketoacidosis from nonketotic hyperosmolar coma in the field. Therefore, the prehospital treatment of both emergencies is identical.

DIABETIC KETOACIDOSIS (DIABETIC COMA)

Diabetic ketoacidosis is a serious complication of diabetes mellitus. It occurs when insulin levels become inadequate to meet the metabolic demands of the body.

Pathophysiology

Diabetic ketoacidosis develops as blood glucose levels increase and individual cells become glucose depleted. The body begins spilling sugar into the urine, which causes a significant osmotic diuresis and serious dehydration, evidenced by dry, warm skin and mucous membranes. As cellular glucose depletion continues, ketones and acids are produced. Subsequently, the blood becomes acidotic. Deep respiration begins as the body tries to compensate for the metabolic acidosis. If ketoacidosis is uncorrected, coma will follow.

Clinical Presentation

The onset of diabetic ketoacidosis is slow, lasting from 12 to 24 hours. In its early stages, the signs and symptoms include increased thirst, excessive hunger, excessive urination, and malaise. Increased urination results from osmotic diuresis accompanying glucose spillage into the urine. Intensified thirst is caused by the body's attempt to replace fluids lost by increased urination. Diabetic ketoacidosis is characterized by nausea, vomiting, marked dehydration, tachycardia, and weakness. The skin is usually warm and dry. Coma is not uncommon. The breath may have a sweet or acetone-like character because of the increased ketones in the blood. Very deep, rapid respirations, called *Kussmaul respirations,* also occur. Kussmaul respirations represent the body's attempt to compensate for the metabolic acidosis produced by ketones and organic acids present in the blood.

Diabetic ketoacidosis is often associated with infection or decreased insulin intake. It may be complicated by several electrolyte imbalances. The most significant is decreased potassium. Decreased potassium (hypokalemia) can lead to serious dysrhythmias or even death.

Ketoacidosis can occur in patients who fail to take their insulin or who take an inadequate amount over an extended period. Persons not previously diagnosed as diabetic occasionally present in ketoacidosis.

HYPOGLYCEMIA (INSULIN SHOCK)

Hypoglycemia occurs when insulin levels are excessive. Hypoglycemia is an urgent medical emergency because a prolonged hypoglycemic episode can result in serious brain injury.

Pathophysiology

Hypoglycemia, sometimes called insulin shock, lies at the other end of the spectrum from diabetic ketoacidosis. Hypoglycemia can occur if a patient accidentally or intentionally takes too much insulin or eats an inadequate

TABLE 9–2			
Route	Onset	Peak	Duration
SC (rapid acting)	30 min to 1 hr	2 to 10 hr	5 to 16 hr
SC (intermediate acting)	1 to 2 hr	4 to 15 hr	22 to 28 hr
SC (long acting)	4 to 8 hr	10 to 30 hr	36 hr

amount of food after taking insulin. If the patient is untreated, the insulin will cause the blood glucose level to drop to a very low level. *Hypoglycemia is a true medical emergency.* If the patient is not treated quickly, he or she can sustain serious injury to the brain because it receives most of its energy from glucose metabolism.

Clinical Presentation

The clinical signs and symptoms of hypoglycemia are many and varied. An abnormal mental status is the most important. In the earliest stages of hypoglycemia, the patient may appear restless or impatient or complain of hunger. As the blood sugar level falls lower, he or she may display inappropriate anger (even rage) or a variety of bizarre behaviors. Sometimes the patient may be placed in police custody for such behaviors or be involved in an automobile accident.

Physical signs may include diaphoresis and tachycardia. If the blood sugar level falls to a critically low level, the patient may sustain a *hypoglycemic seizure* or become comatose.

In contrast to diabetic ketoacidosis, hypoglycemia can develop quickly. A change in mental status can occur without warning. When encountering a patient behaving bizarrely, paramedics should always consider the possibility of hypoglycemia.

In this chapter we discuss *insulin, glucagon, 50 percent dextrose in water ($D_{50}W$),* and *thiamine.* All of these agents, except thiamine, are primarily used in the management of the diabetic patient. Thiamine may be administered before $D_{50}W$ to patients with coma of an unknown origin and in whom alcoholism is suspected.

There are three major classifications of injectable insulin. *Regular insulin* is classified as rapid acting. *Lente* or *NPH insulin* is classified as intermediate acting. Long-lasting insulin is called *ultralente.* Table 9–2 helps illustrate the relationship among the three classes.

INSULIN

Patients with type I diabetes mellitus require insulin to control their blood glucose level. Insulin may also be given to type II diabetics. Four sources of insulin are available:

- Beef insulin: from bovine pancreas
- Pork insulin: from porcine pancreas
- Human insulin: from recombinant deoxyribonucleic acid (DNA)
- Human insulin: from an enzymatic conversion of pork insulin through which the pork insulin molecule becomes identical to the insulin produced by the human pancreas

Insulin is available in three concentrations:

- U 40, or 40 units of insulin per milliliter
- U 100, or 100 units of insulin per milliliter
- U 500, or 500 units of insulin per milliliter

Insulin is not effective when taken orally because the gastrointestinal (GI) tract breaks down the protein molecule before it reaches the bloodstream. All insulin, however, may be given by subcutaneous (SC) injection. Absorption of SC insulin varies according to the injection site and the vascular supply and degree of tissue hypertrophy at the injection site. Regular (unmodified) insulin may be given intravenously (IV) or intramuscularly (IM) as well.

After absorption into the bloodstream, insulin is distributed throughout the body. Insulin-response tissues are located in the liver, adipose tissue, and muscle. Insulin is metabolized primarily in the liver and to a lesser extent in the muscle tissue; it is excreted in the feces and urine.

The exact times for onset, peak, and duration are not absolute. They may vary not only from patient to patient but from injection to injection in the same patient. If insulin absorption is altered, the onset of action, peak concentration level, and duration of action are also altered. If insulin absorption occurs more rapidly, the onset of action and peak concentration times occur more rapidly. Conversely, if insulin absorption is prolonged, onset of action and peak concentration is delayed, and duration of action is prolonged.

Insulin is an anabolic, or building, hormone. It promotes the storage of glucose as glycogen, increases protein and fat synthesis, and inhibits the breakdown of glycogen, protein, and fat.

Insulin is indicated for type I diabetes mellitus. It may also be required for patients with type II diabetes mellitus when other methods of maintaining normal blood glucose level are ineffective. Patients with type II diabetes mellitus may find the usual methods of maintaining a normal blood glucose level ineffective during times of emotional or physical stress (such as surgery and infection) or contraindicated because of pregnancy or hypersensitivity. These patients may need insulin to control blood glucose levels more stringently. Insulin is also indicated for two of the comas that are complications of diabetes: diabetic ketoacidosis (more common with type I diabetes mellitus) and hyperosmolar hyperglycemic nonketotic syndrome (more common with type II diabetes mellitus).

Sometimes insulin is prescribed for patients who do not have diabetes mellitus. Because insulin stimulates cellular uptake of potassium, it may be administered with hypertonic glucose to patients with severe hyperkalemia. This insulin and glucose mixture produces a shift of serum potassium into cells and lowers the serum potassium level for a short time.

All insulin has the same effect in the body. The advantages or disadvantages of a particular kind of insulin reflect the differences in onset of action, peak concentration, and duration of action, as well as concentration, source, and purity. Many different insulin preparations are available; several are available in more than one concentration.

INSULIN (HUMULIN, NOVOLIN, ILETIN)

Class: Hormone and antihyperglycemic

Description

Insulin is a protein secreted by the β cells of the islets of Langerhans. It is responsible for promoting the uptake of glucose by the cells. In diabetics, in whom insulin secretion has diminished, supplemental insulin must be obtained by injection. Older forms of insulin are derived from animals (bovine and porcine). However, animal insulin is not identical to human insulin. Consequently, many patients develop antibodies to animal insulin, rendering it less effective. Human insulin can be manufactured through genetic engineering (recombinant DNA technology). Genetically engineered insulin (Humulin, Novolin) is chemically identical to the insulin hormone secreted by the pancreas. Patients do not develop antibodies to human insulin as they do to animal insulin.

Mechanism of Action

Insulin, when administered, is distributed throughout the body. It combines with insulin receptors present on the cell membranes, which promotes glucose entry into the cell and lowers the blood glucose level.

Indications

Insulin is used in diabetic ketoacidosis, hyperglycemia, and hyperkalemia.

Contraindications

Insulin should be administered only when hyperglycemia or ketoacidosis has been confirmed. A blood glucose approximation should be obtained in all diabetic emergencies. Every emergency medical service (EMS) unit carrying insulin and 50 percent dextrose should also carry Dextrostix reagent strips or an electronic glucose determination device for approximating blood glucose levels. Based on the results of the blood glucose test, and in conjunction with the physical examination, the differential diagnosis between hypoglycemia and ketoacidosis can usually be made. If there is any doubt about the etiology of diabetic coma, glucose should be administered. Insulin is almost always administered in the emergency department and not during the prehospital phase of emergency medical care.

Precautions

Repeated measurements of the blood glucose level, including possible administration of glucose, are necessary.

Side Effects

Insulin may cause hypoglycemia. Itching, swelling, redness, and frank allergic reactions may occur following administration of animal-derived insulins.

Interactions

Certain drugs, such as the corticosteroids, can increase the blood glucose level. Patients receiving these drugs may require a higher dose of insulin. The signs and symptoms of hypoglycemia may be masked in patients receiving β-blockers. Paramedics must always determine the blood glucose level.

Dosage

A standard dose for diabetic coma is 5 to 10 units of regular insulin IV followed by an infusion at 0.1 unit per kilogram per hour; 5 to 20 units of regular insulin can be administered subcutaneously or intramuscularly if there is not an immediate need for intravenous insulin. In an emergency setting insulin should be given intravenously, intramuscularly, or subcutaneously.

How Supplied

Insulin injection is supplied in 10 mL vials containing 100 units per milliliter.

GLUCAGON

Unlike insulin and the oral antidiabetic agents, which decrease the blood glucose level, glucagon increases it. This hyperglycemic agent is a hormone normally produced by the α cells of the islets of Langerhans in the pancreas. After SC, IM, or IV injection, glucagon is absorbed rapidly (Table 9–3). It cannot be taken orally because it is a protein, and it would be destroyed in the GI tract. Glucagon is distributed throughout the body, although its effect occurs primarily in the liver. The exact metabolic fate of glucagon is unknown, although it is degraded extensively in the liver. Glucagon is removed from the body by the liver and the kidneys.

Glucagon regulates the rate of glucose production through glycogenolysis, gluconeogenesis, and lipolysis. A glucagon deficiency results in hypoglycemia. Although glucagon stimulates insulin secretion, insulin antagonizes glucagon's action through a negative feedback system.

Glucagon is used for emergency treatment of severe hypoglycemia. It is also used as an antidote for β-blocker overdose. Glucagon is ineffective in poorly nourished or starving patients.

TABLE 9–3			
Absorption Rate of Glucagon			
Route	*Onset*	*Peak*	*Duration*
SC, IM, IV	5 to 20 min	30 min	1 to 2 hr

GLUCAGON

Class: Hormone and antihypoglycemic

Description

Glucagon is a protein secreted by the α cells of the pancreas. Glucagon for parenteral administration is extracted from beef and pork pancreas. It is used to increase the blood glucose level in cases of hypoglycemia in which an IV cannot be immediately placed.

Mechanism of Action

Glucagon is a hormone secreted by the pancreas. When released it causes a breakdown of stored glycogen to glucose. It also inhibits the synthesis of glycogen from glucose. Both actions tend to cause an increase in circulating blood glucose. In hypoglycemia the administration of glucagon increases blood glucose levels. The drug of choice in the management of insulin-induced hypoglycemia is still $D_{50}W$. A return to consciousness is seen almost immediately following the administration of glucose. A return to consciousness following the administration of glucagon usually takes from 5 to 20 minutes. Glucagon is only effective if there are sufficient stores of glycogen in the liver. Glucagon exerts a positive inotropic action on the heart and decreases renal vascular resistance.

Indications

Glucagon is used in hypoglycemia and β-blocker overdose.

Contraindications

Because glucagon is a protein, hypersensitivity may occur. Glucagon should not be administered to patients with a known hypersensitivity to the drug.

Precautions

Glucagon is only effective if there are sufficient stores of glycogen within the liver. In an emergency situation intravenous glucose is the agent of choice. Glucagon should be administered with caution to patients with a history of cardiovascular or renal disease.

Side Effects

Although side effects are rare, glucagon can cause hypotension, dizziness, headache, nausea, and vomiting.

Interactions

Few interactions with glucagon are reported in the emergency setting.

Dosage

A standard initial dose is 0.25 to 0.5 units administered intravenously. If an IV cannot be obtained, 1 mg of glucagon can be administered intramuscularly.

Route

Glucagon can be administered intravenously, intramuscularly, or subcutaneously.

How Supplied

Glucagon must be reconstituted before administration. It is supplied in rubber-stoppered vials containing 1 unit of powder and 1 mL of diluting solution. It must be used or refrigerated after reconstitution.

50 PERCENT DEXTROSE IN WATER ($D_{50}W$)

Class: Carbohydrate

Description

Dextrose is used to describe the six-carbon sugar *d-glucose*, which is the principal form of carbohydrate used by the body.

Mechanism of Action

Dextrose supplies supplemental glucose in cases of hypoglycemia. Serious brain injury can occur if hypoglycemia is prolonged. Thus, in hypoglycemia the rapid administration of glucose is essential. When the hypoglycemic patient is comatose, glucose cannot be given by mouth and should be given as an IV $D_{50}W$ solution.

Indications

Dextrose is used in hypoglycemia and coma of unknown origin.

Contraindications

There are no major contraindications to the IV administration of $D_{50}W$ to a patient with suspected hypoglycemia. Even if a patient were suffering from ketoacidosis, the amount of glucose present in 50 mL of 50 percent dextrose would not adversely affect the clinical outcome; 50 percent dextrose should be used with caution in patients with increased intracranial pressure because the dextrose load may worsen cerebral edema.

Precautions

It is important to perform a Dextrostix or obtain a Glucometer reading and draw a sample of blood before initiating an IV infusion and giving 50 percent dextrose. Localized venous irritation may occur when smaller veins are used. Infiltration of 50 percent dextrose may result in tissue necrosis.

Side Effects

Side effects can include tissue necrosis and phlebitis at the injection site.

Interactions

There are no interactions in the emergency setting.

Dosage

The standard dosage of 50 percent dextrose in hypoglycemia is 25 g (50 mL of a 50 percent solution) administered intravenously. If an initial dose is ineffective, a second dose of 25 g may also be given; 50 percent dextrose should be diluted 1:1 with sterile water for pediatric administration (thus forming $D_{25}W$). The pediatric dose is 0.5 to 1.0 g/kg of body weight by slow, intravenous bolus.

Route

Dextrose is only given intravenously. Concentrated glucose solutions can cause venous irritation if administered for an extended period.

How Supplied

Dextrose is supplied in prefilled syringes containing 25 g of *d-glucose* in 50 mL of water.

THIAMINE

Thiamine is used primarily to prevent and treat thiamine deficiency syndromes such as beriberi, Wernicke's encephalopathy, and peripheral neuritis associated with pellagra. Thiamine malabsorption may occur in patients with alcoholism, cirrhosis, or GI disease, requiring supplements. In most cases thiamine administration does not result in adverse reactions or toxicity. Various nonspecific reactions that have been reported include nausea, anxiety, sweating, and sensations of warmth. Allergic reactions, ranging from itching and uticaria to cardiovascular failure and death, have occurred with parenteral administration.

℞ THIAMINE

Class: Vitamin

Description

Thiamine is an important vitamin commonly referred to as vitamin B_1. It is required for the conversion of pyruvic acid to acetyl coenzyme A.

Mechanism of Action

A vitamin is a substance that the body cannot manufacture but that is required for metabolism. Most of the vitamins required by the body are obtained through the diet. Thiamine is required for the conversion of pyruvic acid to acetyl coenzyme A. Without this step, a significant amount of the energy available in glucose cannot be obtained. The brain is extremely sensitive to thiamine deficiency. Chronic alcohol intake interferes with the absorption, intake, and use of thiamine. A significant percentage of alcoholics have thiamine deficiency. During extended periods of fasting, neurological symptoms owing to thiamine deficiency may occur. These symptoms include Wernicke's encephalopathy and Korsakoff's psychosis. Wernicke's encephalopathy is an acute and reversible encephalopathy characterized by an unsteady gait, eye muscle weakness, and mental derangement. Korsakoff's psychosis is a significant memory disorder and may be irreversible. Any comatose patients,

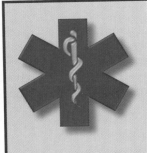

CASE PRESENTATION

At 1630 hours on a Thursday afternoon, paramedics are called to respond to a suburban residence for a patient who is unresponsive. The emergency medical dispatcher reports that the caller is a 9-year-old girl who just came home from school and cannot wake up her mother.

Paramedics are met by the young girl as they arrive at the small frame residence. Tearfully she tells them that her mother is a diabetic and that the ambulance has been called several times before. As paramedics enter the residence, they notice that someone had been preparing a meal. They find the mother lying on the floor in the living room. The girl tells them that her mother's name is Tanya. Paramedics call to Tanya and gently shake her shoulder, but there is no response. There is no evidence of trauma or of a fall. The patient is a 30-year-old woman who is unconscious and unresponsive. She is breathing adequately and has both a radial and a carotid pulse. Both, however, are weak.

On Examination

CNS:	The patient is unconscious and unresponsive
Resp:	Respirations are 30 per minute and shallow; lungs are clear bilaterally, with equal air entry; trachea is midline; no signs of trauma
CVS:	Radial and carotid pulses present but weak; skin is pale and quite diaphoretic
ABD:	Soft and nontender in all four quadrants; no sign of vomiting
Musc/Skel:	No apparent injuries; no pitting edema

Vital Signs

Pulse:	112/min
Resp:	30/min, shallow
BP:	118/78 mm Hg
SpO$_2$:	92 percent
ECG:	Sinus tachycardia
Past Hx:	Her daughter states that the patient has been a diabetic for as long as she can remember. She also shows you insulin vials in the refrigerator (Humulin N and Humulin R). The daughter does not know when her mother last ate. However, they usually eat at 5 P.M.

Treatment

Based on physical findings, the patient history obtained from the daughter, and the presence of insulin in the refrigerator, paramedics suspect that the patient is hypoglycemic. To confirm, they decide to determine the blood glucose level. While one paramedic prepares to do this, another administers oxygen by nonrebreather mask at 12 L/min. By medical control protocol, they are able to begin definitive advanced life support procedures. Paramedics perform venipuncture with an 18-gauge catheter and, prior to connecting the IV tubing, draw a red-top blood tube for analysis. They also use the hub of the needle to obtain a blood sample for glucose testing. An IV of D_5W (normal saline is also acceptable) is initiated and run at a TKO rate. The blood glucose reading is 40 mg/dL (2.2 mmol/L). At this time 50 mL (25 g) of $D_{50}W$ is administered. Following administration of the $D_{50}W$, a fluid bolus of 25 mL of D_5W is administered to flush the IV line.

Almost immediately following the $D_{50}W$ administration, the patient begins to make sounds and move about. The patient awakens and is surprised to see the paramedics. She is very apologetic and somewhat embarrassed. She insists that she is fine now and refuses transport to the hospital. After paramedics are sure that the patient is conscious, alert, and in no further danger, they inform her of the risks of refusing transport. She acknowledges the risks and signs the release form. Paramedics aseptically discontinue the IV, apply an adhesive strip, and leave the scene.

especially those who are suspected to be alcoholic, should receive IV thiamine in addition to the administration of 50 percent dextrose or naloxone.

Indications

Thiamine is used for coma of unknown origin, especially if alcohol may be involved, and delirium tremens.

Contraindications

There are no contraindications to the administration of thiamine in the emergency setting.

Precautions

A few cases of hypersensitivity to thiamine have been reported.

Side Effects

Few side effects are reported with thiamine usage. However, hypotension, dyspnea, and respiratory failure have been reported with its use.

Interactions

There are no interactions in the emergency setting.

Dosage

The emergency dose of thiamine is 100 mg administered intravenously or intramuscularly.

Route

Thiamine can be given either intravenously or intramuscularly. The intravenous route is preferred in emergency medicine.

How Supplied

Thiamine is supplied in 1 mL ampules containing 100 mg of the vitamin.

Thiamine

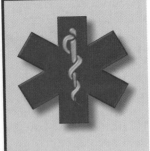

CASE PRESENTATION

Late in the afternoon on a warm September day, paramedics are dispatched to a residence for a patient "not feeling well." The emergency medical dispatcher reports that the patient is a 60-year-old man who is reportedly conscious and alert. On arrival paramedics are directed into the patient's bedroom by his wife. The patient is lying in bed, propped up by two pillows. The patient says he has been feeling ill for over 48 hours. He also reports that he has had rather severe abdominal pain accompanied by nausea and vomiting. However, he has been able to tolerate some clear liquids. He has not been able to keep down any food. He denies any diarrhea or any other problems and is sure that this is the flu.

On Examination

CNS: The patient is conscious, alert, and oriented × 4

Resp: Respirations are 32/minute, deep and labored; lungs are clear bilaterally, with equal air entry; trachea is midline; no signs of trauma

CVS: Both radial and carotid pulses are present but weak; skin is slightly pale and dry

ABD: Soft and nontender in all four quadrants.

Musc/Skel: No apparent injuries; no pitting edema

Vital Signs

Pulse: 140/min

Resp: 32/min, shallow, labored

BP: 92/54 mm Hg

SpO$_2$: 94 percent

ECG: Sinus tachycardia

Past Hx: Past medical history includes insulin-dependent diabetes mellitus (type I). His wife states that the patient has not taken insulin since he has been sick.

Treatment

Oxygen is administered by nonrebreather mask at 12 L/min. The rapid, deep respirations are consistent with Kussmaul respirations. One paramedic prepares an IV of normal saline while another performs venipuncture with a 16-gauge catheter. Blood is drawn for a red-top tube and the hub of the needle is used to obtain a blood sample for glucose testing. The IV of normal saline is connected to the catheter and run at 150 mL/hr. The blood glucose reading exceeds 400 mg/dL (approx 20 mmol/L). Paramedics suspect the patient is in early diabetic ketoacidosis. Care provided during transport to the hospital is primarily supportive and includes monitoring of vital signs and fluid replacement.

At the emergency department the patient's blood glucose reading is 880 mg/dL. His serum ketones are positive at 1:16 dilution. An arterial blood gas reveals a pH of 7.16, pCO_2 of 30 Torr, and pO_2 of 190 Torr (on 40 percent mask), which is generally consistent with a partially compensated metabolic acidosis. He is started on an insulin drip and admitted to the hospital. A chest X ray reveals a right lower lobe pneumonia, which the emergency department physician feels contributed to the development of diabetic ketoacidosis. Following a three-day course of antibiotics and aggressive fluid therapy, the patient is discharged.

SUMMARY

Diabetes mellitus is probably the most common metabolic-endocrine emergency seen in the prehospital phase of emergency medical care. Hypoglycemia, if not immediately treated, can result in serious and permanent brain damage. It is important to remember that acute metabolic-endocrine disorders can cause a wide range of signs and symptoms, from bizarre behavior to coma.

Prehospital drug administration should be guided by available data. Paramedics should always determine the blood glucose level. If it is low, 50 percent dextrose is administered. If alcoholism is suspected, administration of thiamine should be considered. If narcotic abuse is possible, administration of naloxone is considered. The "coma cocktail" is a thing of the past. Prehospital care should be based on physical exam findings and the patient's medical history.

KEY WORDS

diabetes mellitus. An endocrine disorder characterized by inadequate insulin production by the β cells of the islets of Langerhans in the pancreas.

endocrine glands. Glands that secrete hormones directly into the blood.

hormones. Chemical substances released by a gland that control or affect other glands or body systems.

hyperglycemia. A complication of diabetes characterized by excessive levels of blood glucose.

hypoglycemia. A complication of diabetes characterized by low levels of blood glucose. It often occurs from too high a dose of insulin or from inadequate food intake following a normal insulin dose. Sometimes called *insulin shock*, hypoglycemia is a true medical emergency.

ketoacidosis. A complication of diabetes due to decreased insulin secretion or intake. It is characterized by high levels of glucose in the blood, metabolic acidosis, and, in advanced stages, coma. Ketoacidosis is often called *diabetic coma*.

Kussmaul respirations. A very deep, gasping respiratory pattern found in diabetic coma.

chapter 10

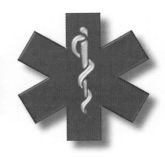

Drugs Used in the Treatment of Neurological Emergencies

OBJECTIVES

After completing this chapter, the reader should be able to

1. Describe the treatment for a patient with a blunt or penetrating head injury.

2. Describe and list the indications, contraindications, and dosages for dexamethasone, mannitol, and methylprednisolone.

3. List three acute, nontraumatic neurological disorders.

4. Describe and list the indications, contraindications, and dosages for the following drugs used in the treatment of seizures: diazepam, lorazepam, midazolam, phenytoin, and phenobarbital.

INTRODUCTION

Emergencies involving the nervous system can be devastating. In addition, they are also notoriously difficult to manage. Signs and symptoms of neurological disorders can range from slight headache to coma. They may be temporary or permanent. Prompt recognition and treatment are essential.

Head injuries are an all-too-common result of automobile and motorcycle accidents. Although encased within the protective skull, the brain is quite susceptible to injury. Following craniocerebral trauma, cerebral edema occurs within 24 hours.

The primary treatment of patients with blunt or penetrating head injury is supportive. Airway management is of paramount importance, and continuous monitoring of blood pressure to detect occult blood loss in major trauma is mandatory. Pharmacological agents that have proved effective in the management of neurological emergencies include *dexamethasone*, which is thought to be of use in reducing brain edema, and *mannitol*, an osmotic diuretic that is also useful in reducing brain edema and is faster acting than dexamethasone.

The management of spinal cord injuries is principally supportive. Recently, a protocol has been established whereby methylprednisolone (Solu-Medrol) is promptly administered to patients with spinal cord injuries. The initial results are favorable: Many patients regain spinal cord function. The severity of the injury depends on the anatomical location of the spinal cord damage. Sometimes, following injury to the spinal cord, shock occurs (neurogenic shock). In these cases the body loses control over peripheral vascular tone. Vasopressor agents, such as norepinephrine, are indicated to ensure maintenance of blood pressure.

The drugs described in this chapter are frequently used in the prehospital phase of emergency medical care in the management of traumatic neurological emergencies.

 # DEXAMETHASONE (DECADRON, HEXADROL)

Class: Corticosteroid

Description

Dexamethasone is a synthetic steroid chemically related to the natural hormones secreted by the adrenal cortex.

Mechanism of Action

Dexamethasone is a long-acting steroid with a plasma half-life of about 5 hours. In general medical practice, steroids have a wide range of uses. Effective as anti-inflammatory agents, they are used in the management of allergic reactions and occasionally as an adjunctive agent in the management of shock. The role of steroids in the management of cerebral edema remains controversial. The mechanism by which and extent to which dexamethasone decreases cerebral edema, if indeed it does, are unclear. It is generally agreed that a large single dose of steroids has little harmful effect. Consequently, it is used frequently in patients with cerebral edema, both in the emergency department and in the prehospital setting.

Indications

Dexamethasone is used in cerebral edema, anaphylaxis, asthma, and exacerbation of chronic obstructive pulmonary disease (COPD).

Contraindications

There are no major contraindications to the use of dexamethasone in the emergency setting.

Precautions

A single dose of dexamethasone is all that should be given in the prehospital phase of care. Long-term steroid therapy can cause gastrointestinal bleeding, prolonged wound healing, and suppression of adrenocortical steroids.

Side Effects

Dexamethasone can cause fluid retention, congestive heart failure, hypertension, abdominal distention, vertigo, headache, nausea, malaise, and hiccups.

Interactions

There are few interactions in the prehospital setting.

Dosage

The dose of dexamethasone varies considerably from physician to physician. The usual range is 4 to 24 mg; 12 mg administered intravenously (IV) is a commonly used dose. High-dose dexamethasone therapy, however, with up to 100 mg of the drug, is sometimes given.

Route

Dexamethasone is administered intravenously or intramuscularly; the intravenous route is preferred in the emergency setting.

How Supplied

Decadron is supplied in two concentrations. The most common is 4 mg/mL. It is supplied in prefilled syringes containing 1 mL of the drug and in vials containing 5 mg.

A second concentration, containing 24 mg/mL, is also available. It is supplied in 5 and 10 mL ampules. This concentration should only be used intravenously.

MANNITOL (OSMOTROL)

Class: Osmotic diuretic

Description

Mannitol is a six-carbon sugar compound that has osmotic diuretic properties.

Mechanism of Action

Mannitol is an osmotic diuretic that inhibits sodium and water absorption in the kidneys. It promotes movement of fluid from the intracellular into the extracellular space. Because it dehydrates brain tissue, mannitol has proved effective in the management of cerebral edema and reduces intracranial pressure.

Indications

Mannitol is used for acute cerebral edema and blood transfusion reactions.

Contraindications

Mannitol should not be used in any patient with acute pulmonary edema or severe pulmonary congestion. It should not be used in any patient who is profoundly hypovolemic.

Precautions

Rapid administration of mannitol can cause a transitory increase in intravascular volume and can result in congestive heart failure. The diuresis that accompanies mannitol therapy can cause sodium depletion.

One problem in the use of mannitol in the prehospital phase of emergency medical care is crystallization of the drug. The more concentrated the solution, the more tendency it has to crystallize at low temperatures. Crystallization begins as temperatures approach 45 °F. Anytime a concentrated solution of mannitol is used, usually 15 percent or greater, an in-line filter should be present. It is important to remember that microscopic crystals appear long before those that can be seen by the naked eye. If mannitol solution crystallizes, it should be warmed slowly in boiling water until the crystals disappear. It should be removed from emergency medical service (EMS) vehicles that are not parked in heated areas during colder weather.

Side Effects

Mannitol can cause chills, headache, dizziness, lethargy, mental status change, chest pain, nausea, and vomiting.

Interactions

Mannitol should not be administered with whole blood or packed red blood cells because it can damage the red blood cells.

Dosage

The typical adult dose of mannitol is 1.5 to 2.0 g/kg of body weight administered intravenously. This dose can be given as a slow IV bolus or IV infusion. The slower rate of infusion helps eliminate the chances of inducing circulatory overload and congestive heart failure.

Route

Mannitol should be given intravenously.

How Supplied

Mannitol is supplied in 250 and 500 mL of a 20 percent solution for IV infusion. A 25 percent solution in 50 mL is available for slow IV bolus.

METHYLPREDNISOLONE (SOLU-MEDROL)

Class: Corticosteroid and anti-inflammatory

Description

Methylprednisolone is an intermediate-acting corticosteroid related to the natural hormones secreted by the adrenal cortex.

Mechanism of Action

Methylprednisolone is an intermediate-acting synthetic steroid. In general medical practice, steroids have a wide range of uses. Effective as anti-inflammatory agents, they are used in the management of allergic reactions and occasionally as an adjunctive agent in the management of shock. The role of steroids in the management of neurological emergencies remains controversial. It is generally agreed that a large single dose of steroids has little harmful effect. Consequently, it is used in patients with spinal cord injury both in the emergency department and in the pre-hospital setting.

Indications

Methylprednisolone is used in spinal cord injury, anaphylaxis, asthma, and exacerbation of COPD.

Contraindications

There are no major contraindications to the use of methylprednisolone in the emergency setting.

Precautions

A single dose of methylprednisolone is all that should be given in the pre-hospital phase of care. Long-term steroid therapy can cause gastrointestinal bleeding, prolonged wound healing, and suppression of adrenocortical steroids.

Side Effects

Methylprednisolone can cause fluid retention, congestive heart failure, hypertension, abdominal distention, vertigo, headache, nausea, malaise, and hiccups.

Interactions

There are few interactions in the prehospital setting.

Dosage

Spinal cord injury. High-dose methylprednisolone is used in treating spinal cord injuries. An initial bolus of 30 mg/kg is administered intravenously over a 15-minute period. This dose is followed 45 minutes later by a maintenance infusion of 5.4 mgs/kg/hr.

Asthma, COPD, or allergic reactions. For other emergencies, 80 to 125 mg is usually administered intravenously or intramuscularly.

How Supplied

Methylprednisolone is supplied in vials containing 125 and 250 mg of the drug. The drug must be reconstituted prior to administration.

NONTRAUMATIC NEUROLOGICAL EMERGENCIES

There are many acute nontraumatic neurological disorders. Drugs, poisonings, and metabolic derangements can precipitate neurological emergencies. Little can be done for stroke and brain tumors in the prehospital phase of emergency medical care. Seizures attributable to epilepsy and other disorders can be managed in the field, however.

Seizures are one of the most frequently encountered neurological emergencies. One seizure followed by another seizure, without an intervening period of consciousness, is called *status epilepticus* and constitutes a serious threat to life. Status epilepticus should be terminated as quickly as possible.

The most common drug used to terminate seizure activity is IV diazepam (Valium). Phenytoin (Dilantin) and phenobarbital are also effective, however. In the following section of this chapter, we discuss these three drugs and their roles in prehospital care.

Benzodiazepines

Benzodiazepines produce many effects, including daytime and preanesthetic sedation, sleep inducement, relief of anxiety and tension, skeletal muscle relaxation, and anticonvulsant activity. In the prehospital setting, benzodiazepines are primarily used as skeletal muscle relaxants, for preprocedure sedation (such as cardioversion), and for anticonvulsant activity.

Benzodiazepines are absorbed well from the gastrointestinal (GI) tract and distributed widely in the body. In the prehospital setting, benzodiazepines are almost always given parenterally. All benzodiazepines are metabolized in the liver and excreted primarily in the urine. Onset of action when administered IV is 1 to 5 minutes, with peak immediate and duration of 15 minutes to 1 hour.

The principle sites of action for benzodiazepines are the cerebral cortex and the limbic, thalamic, and hypothalamic levels of the central nervous system (CNS).

In most cases benzodiazepines are preferred over barbiturates because of their effectiveness and safety. Benzodiazepines offer many advantages, including fewer adverse reactions, decreased potential for abuse, fewer drug interactions, a wide margin of safety between therapeutic and toxic dosages that makes overdoses less likely, and a reduced risk of physical and psychological dependence with therapeutic dosages.

DIAZEPAM (VALIUM)

Class: Anticonvulsant and sedative

Description

Diazepam is a benzodiazepine that is frequently used as an anticonvulsant, sedative, and hypnotic.

Mechanism of Action

In emergency medicine, diazepam is principally used for its anticonvulsant properties. It suppresses the spread of seizure activity through the motor cortex of the brain. It does not appear to abolish the abnormal discharge focus, however. Diazepam, one of the most frequently prescribed medications in the United States, is used in the management of anxiety and stress. It is effective in treating the tremors and anxiety associated with alcohol withdrawal. It is also an effective skeletal muscle relaxant, which makes it an effective adjunct in orthopedic injuries. It is a good premedication for minor operative procedures and cardioversion because it induces amnesia, which diminishes the patient's recall of such procedures.

Indications

Diazepam is used in major motor seizures, status epilepticus, premedication before cardioversion, skeletal muscle relaxant, and acute anxiety states.

Contraindications

Diazepam should not be administered to any patient with a history of hypersensitivity to the drug.

Precautions

Because diazepam is a relatively short-acting drug, seizure activity may recur. In such cases, an additional dose may be required. Flumazenil (Romazicon), a benzodiazepine antagonist, should be available to use as antidote if required. Injectable diazepam can cause local venous irritation. To minimize irritation, it should only be injected into relatively large veins and should not be given faster than 1 mL/min.

Side Effects

Diazepam can cause hypotension, drowsiness, headache, amnesia, respiratory depression, blurred vision, nausea, and vomiting.

Interactions

Diazepam is incompatible with many medications. Whenever diazepam is given intravenously in conjunction with other drugs, the IV line should be adequately flushed. The effects of diazepam can be additive when used in conjunction with other CNS depressants and alcohol.

Dosage

In the management of seizures, the usual dose of diazepam is 5 to 10 mg IV. In many instances it may be necessary to give diazepam directly into the vein, because the seizure activity will prevent the insertion of an indwelling catheter. When given directly into a vein, it is essential that a large vein, preferably in the antecubital fossa, be used. In acute anxiety reactions, the standard dosage is 2 to 5 mg administered intramuscularly.

To induce amnesia prior to cardioversion, a dosage of 5 to 15 mg of diazepam is given intravenously. Peak effects are seen in 5 to 10 minutes. Diazepam should be given intravenously by slow IV push. It can be injected intramuscularly, but absorption via this route is variable. When an IV line cannot be started, parenteral diazepam can be administered rectally with a similar onset of action.

How Supplied

Diazepam is supplied in ampules and prefilled syringes containing 10 mg in 2 mL of solvent.

LORAZEPAM (ATIVAN)

Class: Anticonvulsant and sedative

Description

Lorazepam is a benzodiazepine that is used as an anticonvulsant, sedative, and hypnotic.

Mechanism of Action

Lorazepam is a benzodiazepine with a shorter half-life than that of diazepam. Its onset of action is approximately the same. It is used in the management of anxiety and stress. It is a good premedication for minor operative procedures and cardioversion because it induces amnesia, which diminishes the patient's recall of such procedures. Lorazepam is often used in pediatrics as an anticonvulsant because of its shorter half-life. Like diazepam, lorazepam suppresses the spread of seizure activity through the motor cortex of the brain. It does not appear to abolish the abnormal discharge focus.

Indications

Lorazepam is used in major motor seizures, in status epilepticus, as premedication before cardioversion, and for acute anxiety states.

Contraindications

Lorazepam should not be administered to any patient with a history of hypersensitivity to the drug.

Precautions

Lorazepam should be diluted with normal saline or D_5W prior to intravenous administration. Because lorazepam is a relatively short-acting drug, seizure activity may recur. In such cases, an additional dose may be required. Flumazenil (Romazicon), a benzodiazepine antagonist, should be available to use as antidote if required.

Side Effects

Lorazepam can cause hypotension, drowsiness, headache, amnesia, respiratory depression, blurred vision, nausea, and vomiting.

Interactions

The effects of lorazepam can be additive when used in conjunction with other CNS depressants and alcohol.

Dosage

The usual dose of lorazepam is 0.5 to 2.0 mg when given intravenously. The dose can be increased to 1.0 to 4.0 mg when given intramuscularly. It can be given rectally when an IV cannot be placed. The medication should be drawn up into a syringe. A small, red, rubber pediatric feeding tube can be attached to the syringe. The feeding tube should be inserted 2 to 4 cm into the rectum and the drug administered. Often it is necessary to hold the buttocks together to help the patient retain the drug.

How Supplied

Lorazepam is supplied in ampules and Tubex syringes containing 1, 2, and 4 mg in 2 mL of solvent.

MIDAZOLAM (VERSED)

Class: Sedative and hypnotic

Description

Midazolam is a benzodiazepine with strong hypnotic and amnestic properties.

Mechanism of Action

Midazolam is a potent but short-acting benzodiazepine used widely in medicine as a sedative and hypnotic. It is three to four times more potent than diazepam. Its onset of action is approximately 1.5 minutes when administered intravenously and 15 minutes when administered intramuscularly. Midazolam has impressive amnestic properties. Like the other benzodiazepines, it has no effect on pain.

Indication

Midazolam is used as a premedication before cardioversion and other painful procedures.

Contraindications

Midazolam should not be administered to any patient with a history of hypersensitivity to the drug. It should not be used in patients who have narrow-angle glaucoma. Midazolam should not be administered to patients in shock, with depressed vital signs, or who are in alcoholic coma.

Precautions

Emergency resuscitative equipment must be available prior to the administration of midazolam. Vital signs must be continuously monitored during and after drug administration. Midazolam has more potential than the other benzodiazepines to cause respiratory depression and respiratory arrest. Flumazenil (Romazicon), a benzodiazepine antagonist, should be available to use as antidote if required.

Side Effects

Midazolam can cause laryngospasm, bronchospasm, dyspnea, respiratory depression and arrest, drowsiness, amnesia, altered mental status, bradycardia, tachycardia, premature ventricular contractions, and retching.

Interactions

The effects of midazolam can be accentuated by CNS depressants such as narcotics and alcohol.

Dosage

When used for sedation, midazolam must be administered cautiously, because the amount of medication required to achieve sedation varies from individual to individual. Typically, 1 to 2.5 mg are administered by slow IV injection. Usually, it is best to dilute midazolam with normal saline or D_5W prior to IV administration. Midazolam can be administered intramuscularly at a dose of 0.07 to 0.08 mg/kg (average adult dose of 5 mg). Recently, many centers have been administering midazolam intranasally or by mouth to sedate children prior to suturing of lacerations.

How Supplied

Midazolam is supplied in ampules and vials containing 5 mg/mL of the drug.

Hydantoins

Phenytoin and phenytoin sodium are the most commonly prescribed anticonvulsant agents. In the prehospital setting, phenytoin may be used as a second-line drug for the treatment of seizures and as a second-line antiarrhythmic.

Hydantoin anticonvulsants are usually absorbed slowly, rapidly distributed, and extensively protein bound. They are metabolized in the liver and excreted in the urine.

In most cases, the hydantoin anticonvulsants can stabilize nerve cells against hyperexcitability. Phenytoin's primary site of action appears to be the motor cortex, where the drug inhibits the spread of seizure activity. Phenytoin also exhibits antiarrhythmic properties similar to those of quinidine or procainamide. Because of its clinical efficacy and relatively low toxicity, phenytoin is the most commonly prescribed anticonvulsant.

PHENYTOIN (DILANTIN)

Class: Anticonvulsant and antiarrhythmic

Description

Phenytoin is a long-acting anticonvulsant. It is also used as an antiarrhythmic because it depresses spontaneous ventricular depolarization.

Mechanism of Action

Phenytoin is an effective anticonvulsant. Its onset of action, however, is considerably longer than that of diazepam. In most emergency situations the seizure should first be controlled with Valium. If seizure activity recurs, phenytoin can be administered. Phenytoin also is used to treat arrhythmias caused by digitalis toxicity. This use of the drug is discussed in Chapter 7.

Indications

Phenytoin is used in major motor seizures, status epilepticus, and arrhythmias caused by digitalis toxicity.

Contraindications

Phenytoin should not be given to any patient with a history of hypersensitivity to the drug. It is contraindicated in cases of bradycardia and high-grade heart block. It should not be administered to patients who take the drug chronically for seizures until the blood level has been determined.

Precautions

Intravenous administration of phenytoin should not exceed 50 mg/min. Signs of central nervous system depression or hypotension may occur. Elderly patients are at increased risk of developing side effects from phenytoin administration. Extravasation should be avoided. Any patient receiving intravenous phenytoin should have continuous cardiac monitoring as well as frequent monitoring of vital signs.

Side Effects

Phenytoin can cause drowsiness, dizziness, headache, hypotension, arrhythmias, itching, rash, nausea, and vomiting.

Interactions

Phenytoin must never be diluted in dextrose-containing solutions such as D_5W. It should be diluted in normal saline or other non-glucose-containing crystalloids.

Dosage

The loading dose of phenytoin is typically 10 to 15 mg/kg. This dose should be administered no faster than 50 mg/min. Phenytoin should be diluted with normal saline, because dilution with 5 percent dextrose may result in precipitation of the drug. In emergency medicine phenytoin should be administered intravenously only.

How Supplied

Phenytoin is supplied in 2 and 5 mL ampules containing 50 mg/mL. A 2-mL prefilled syringe is also available. Dilantin is incompatible with solutions containing dextrose. If an infusion of Dilantin is prepared, the drug should be placed in normal saline.

Barbiturates

The long-acting barbiturate phenobarbital is also one of the most widely employed anticonvulsants. Phenobarbitol is used in the long-term treatment of epilepsy and is prescribed selectively for acute treatment of status epilepticus.

The barbiturate anticonvulsants are metabolized in the liver, and metabolites and unchanged drug are excreted in the urine. Phenobarbitol provides an onset of action within 30 minutes after oral administration. Peak anticonvulsant effect occurs in 8 to 12 hours. The onset after IV administration occurs within 5 minutes, with peak anticonvulsant effect within 30 minutes. Phenobarbitol has an extremely long half-life of 50 to 170 hours.

PHENOBARBITAL (LUMINAL)

Class: Anticonvulsant and barbiturate

Description

Phenobarbital belongs to a class of drugs called *barbiturates*. It is used as a sedative and an anticonvulsant.

Mechanism of Action

Barbiturates have many uses in medicine. They are central nervous system depressants and are used as anticonvulsants and in the management of insomnia and anxiety. Phenobarbital is an effective anticonvulsant of relatively low toxicity. It depresses the sensory cortex, decreases motor activity, alters cerebellar function, and causes drowsiness, sedation, and hypnosis.

Indications

Phenobarbital is used in major motor seizures, status epilepticus, and acute anxiety states.

Contraindications

Phenobarbital should not be administered to any patient with a history of hypersensitivity to barbiturates.

Precautions

Respiratory depression and hypotension can occur following IV administration of phenobarbital. Constant monitoring of respiratory pattern and blood pressure is essential. Administration of phenobarbital to children may result in hyperactive behavior.

Side Effects

Phenobarbital can cause drowsiness, altered mental status, agitation, hypoventilation, apnea, bradycardia, hypotension, syncope, headache, nausea, and vomiting.

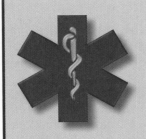

CASE PRESENTATION

At 2130 hours on a Saturday evening, paramedics are called to respond to a residence for a patient who is unconscious and unresponsive. Dispatch reports that the caller is unable to "wake up" his wife. The husband meets the paramedics as they arrive. He says that his wife is a diabetic and that the ambulance has been called several times before. Paramedics find the patient lying in bed in the master bedroom. The man says that his wife has been sick for a couple of days now and has been in bed for most of that time. Paramedics try to awaken the patient by gently shaking her, but there is no response. There is no evidence of trauma or of a fall. The patient is a 40-year-old woman who is unconscious and unresponsive. She is breathing adequately and has both a radial and a carotid pulse. Both, however, are weak.

On Examination

CNS: The patient is unconscious and unresponsive

Resp: Respirations are 24 per minute and shallow; lungs are clear bilaterally, with equal air entry; trachea is midline; no signs of trauma

CVS: The radial and carotid pulses are present but weak; skin is pale and quite diaphoretic

ABD: Soft and nontender in all four quadrants; no sign of vomiting

Musc/Skel: No apparent injuries; no pitting edema

Vital Signs

Pulse: 112/minute

Resp: 24/minute, shallow

BP: 118/78 mm Hg

SpO$_2$: 92 percent

ECG: Sinus tachycardia

Past Hx: The patient's husband states that the patient has been a diabetic for most of her life. He also shows paramedics the insulin vials in the refrigerator (Humulin N and Humulin R). The patient has had a low-grade fever for two days and has not been eating because of nausea. She is also alcoholic.

Treatment

To confirm your diagnosis of hypoglycemia, paramedics decide to take a blood glucose reading. While one paramedic prepares to check the level, another administers oxygen by nonrebreather mask at 15 L/min. An IV is initiated with an 18-gauge catheter and, prior to connecting the IV tubing, paramedics draw a red-top blood tube for analysis. They also use the hub of the needle to obtain a blood sample for glucose testing. An IV of normal saline is initiated and run at a TKO rate. The blood glucose reading is 40 mg/dL (2.2 mmol/L). At this time paramedics administer 100 mg of thiamine IV because of the history of alcoholism and 50 mL (25 g) of $D_{50}W$. Following administration of the $D_{50}W$, a fluid bolus of 20 mL of normal saline is administered to flush the IV line. Almost immediately following the $D_{50}W$ administration, the patient begins to make sounds and move about. The patient awakens and is surprised to see the paramedics. After a few minutes she is alert and oriented, although still a little lethargic. Paramedics decide to transport her to the hospital for assessment and monitor both vital signs and blood glucose levels en route. During the transport she tells paramedics that although she has not been eating normally, she was taking her regular amount of insulin.

Interactions

Phenobarbital may enhance the sedative effects of other sedatives including alcohol, narcotics, antihistamines, and antidepressants.

Dosage

The standard dosage of phenobarbital in the management of status epilepticus is 100 to 250 mg given slowly by IV.

How Supplied

Phenobarbital is supplied in 1 mL ampules containing either 15, 30, 60, or 100 mg of the drug.

SUMMARY

In the management of acute head injury, mannitol has proved effective in reducing cerebral edema. Hyperventilation is even more important in minimizing cerebral edema. It is important to remember that stabilization of the cervical spine, maintenance of the airway, and supplemental delivery of oxygen are of primary importance.

In a general motor seizure, as occasionally occurs, the primary treatment is that of protecting the patient from injury. It is important to remember that most epileptic patients are already taking orally one or two anticonvulsant medications. The judicious use of the parenteral agents discussed in this chapter is therefore indicated. It is helpful to the emergency physician to obtain blood samples from seizure patients prior to the administration of an anticonvulsant. Some authorities believe that a significant percentage of patients who have general motor seizures do so because they fail to follow instructions on ordered medications. Blood studies taken before the administration of anticonvulsants will aid the physician in making a diagnosis.

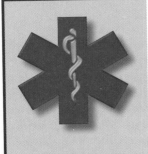

CASE PRESENTATION

At 2:30 P.M. paramedics are called with fire department first responders to a motorcycle collision. On arrival they find an 18-year-old male, unhelmeted rider. Bystanders state that he lost control of the motorcycle on a corner and slid headfirst into the cement retaining wall.

The patient is unconscious and unresponsive to deep pain. He is lying on his left side. His head is being supported by a bystander, who states that the patient has been unconscious and unresponsive since he arrived.

On Examination

CNS: The patient is unconscious and unresponsive; pupils are bilaterally constricted; abnormal flexion (decorticate posture) bilaterally

Resp: Respirations are 30 per minute and deep; lungs are clear bilaterally with equal air entry; trachea is midline; no signs of trauma to the neck or chest

CVS: Both radial and carotid pulses are present and weak; skin is pale and diaphoretic

ABD: Soft and nontender in all four quadrants

Muscl/Skel: No other injuries noted

Vital Signs

Pulse: 50/min

Resp: 30/min, deep

BP: 160 by palpation

SpO$_2$: 87 percent

ECG: Sinus bradycardia

Past Hx: The patient's history is unknown.

Treatment

Fire department first responders assist with spinal immobilization while a paramedic inserts an oropharyngeal airway and begins to ventilate the patient with a bag-valve-mask device and 100 percent oxygen. The patient is moved to an ALS ambulance following rapid immobilization and stabilization on a long spine board. During transport the patient's condition remains largely unchanged except as follows: (1) respiration rate increases to 36 per minute, (2) blood pressure increases to 210/120 mm Hg, (3) oxygen saturation (as measured by pulse oximetry) increases to 91 percent, and (4) pupils become uneven (right > left). Because of the critical nature of this patient's injuries, the following procedures were completed: endotracheal intubation with in-line c-spine stabilization, IV line × 2, 14-gauge catheter (per trauma protocol), normal saline TKO, and mannitol 1.5 g/kg. Total scene time was 10 minutes, and transport time to the hospital was 8 minutes. There were no changes in patient condition en route. On arrival at the hospital the patient was immediately taken to CT, where an epidural hematoma was visualized. The patient was taken emergently to surgery, where the epidural hematoma was decompressed. The patient was transferred to the neurology ICU, where he remains.

KEY WORDS

amnesia. A loss of memory.

benzodiazepine. A class of drugs frequently used to relieve anxiety and insomnia and to induce sedation.

central nervous system. The central portion of the nervous system, namely the brain and spinal cord.

epilepsy. A group of nervous system disorders characterized by the presence of seizures.

intracranial pressure. The pressure in the intracranial space (skull). Increased intracranial pressure can have a deleterious effect on the brain tissue.

neurogenic shock. A state of inadequate tissue perfusion caused by peripheral vasodilation due to loss or interruption of nervous system control.

seizures. A sudden change in nervous function. The symptoms can range from a slight alteration in mental status to violent, generalized, uncontrollable contraction of muscles.

status epilepticus. A state of repeated seizures without an intervening period of consciousness.

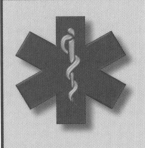

CASE PRESENTATION

At 0900 hours paramedics are called to the local high school for a 16-year-old boy with reported seizures. Dispatch reports that the boy has had one seizure in the last 10 minutes and is now into his second seizure. The boy has a history of epilepsy and takes medication for it. He is unconscious and unresponsive. Three minutes later paramedics arrive at the school and are met by a very frantic teacher, who leads them to a classroom. There they find the patient lying on the floor. The desks have been moved away from the patient, and the patient has been placed in the recovery position. The patient appears to be postictal now.

On Examination

CNS:	The patient is unconscious and unresponsive
Resp:	Respirations are 32 per minute and shallow; trachea is midline; no external signs of trauma
CVS:	Both the radial and carotid pulses are present but are rapid and weak; skin is pale and diaphoretic
ABD:	Soft and nontender in all four quadrants; no signs of vomiting; patient has been incontinent of urine
Muscl/Skel:	No injuries detected

Vital Signs

Pulse:	120/min
Resp:	36/min, shallow
BP:	124/82 mm Hg
SpO$_2$:	90 percent
ECG:	Sinus tachycardia
Past Hx:	The teacher states that the patient has epilepsy. She shows paramedics a prescription bottle of Dilantin from the patient's coat pocket. The patient had the first seizure at 0850, and the second started at 0900. She does not know if he has been sick or experienced any recent trauma.

Treatment

One paramedic performs oropharyngeal suction to remove some frothy sputum from the patient's mouth and then ventilates the patient with a bag-valve-mask unit with 100 percent oxygen. Following contact with the base hospital, another paramedic is preparing to give lorazepam (Ativan) IV push. An 18-gauge IV is initiated in the right antecubital fossa and secured in place with tape and kling in case the patient has another seizure. The patient's blood glucose level is checked from the blood in the IV hub, and it is 5.6 mmol/L (100 mg/dL). He then begins to seize, and paramedics administer lorazepam 2–4 mg IV push. If that does not terminate the seizure, a repeat dose of 2-4 mg may be given. Paramedics administer the first dose of lorazepam, and the seizure subsides in 1 minute. Within 5 minutes the patient is in the postictal stage. He is transported to the hospital without incident and without further seizure. At the hospital the patient's Dilantin level is checked to see if it was too low. The Dilantin level obtained from the blood is 3.4 mg/L (therapeutic level is 10 to 20 mg/L). IV Dilantin is administered, and the patient admitted to the intensive care unit. He does well, with no additional seizures, and is released with an increased daily dosage of Dilantin.

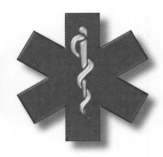

chapter 11

Drugs Used in the Treatment of Obstetrical and Gynecological Emergencies

OBJECTIVES

After completing this chapter, the reader should be able to

1. List three obstetrical and gynecological emergencies that require intervention with pharmacological agents.

2. Define the following terms: *abruptio placenta, eclampsia, ectopic pregnancy, placenta previa, postpartum hemorrhage, preeclampsia,* and *spontaneous abortion.*

3. Describe and list the indications, contraindications, and dosages for oxytocin.

4. List the signs and symptoms of hypertensive disorders of pregnancy.

5. Distinguish among pregnancy-induced hypertension, preeclampsia, and eclampsia.

6. Describe and list the indications, contraindications, and dosages for magnesium sulfate.

7. Describe the management of a patient in preterm labor.

8. Describe and list the indications, contraindications, and dosages for terbutaline.

INTRODUCTION

Prehospital care for most obstetrical and gynecological emergencies is supportive. There are three complications, however, that necessitate intervention with pharmacological agents. These are the hypertensive disorders of pregnancy, severe vaginal bleeding, and preterm labor. *Magnesium sulfate* has proved effective in controlling the convulsions associated with eclampsia. *Pitocin*, a drug chemically identical to the hormone oxytocin, is effective in causing uterine contraction and will control many cases of postpartum vaginal bleeding. *Terbutaline*, B_2-antagonist, is effective in the suppression of preterm labor.

SEVERE VAGINAL BLEEDING

Vaginal bleeding that occurs during the first trimester of pregnancy is usually due to spontaneous abortion or ectopic pregnancy. During the third trimester of pregnancy, vaginal bleeding is most frequently caused by either abruptio placenta or placenta previa.

Bleeding following childbirth is common. Hypovolemic shock can develop when blood loss is in excess of 500 mL. Severe vaginal bleeding can be a life-threatening emergency, necessitating immediate therapy. The management of severe vaginal bleeding is similar to that employed with any other type of severe hemorrhage. Initial treatment should include airway maintenance, administration of supplemental oxygen, and infusion of intravenous volume expanders. In addition, the intravenous (IV) administration of Pitocin in postpartum hemorrhage can be effective in controlling severe vaginal bleeding.

℞ OXYTOCIN (PITOCIN)

Class: Hormone and uterine stimulant

Description

Oxytocin is a naturally occurring hormone that is secreted by the posterior pituitary.

Mechanism of Action

Oxytocin causes contraction of uterine smooth muscle and lactation. Oxytocin is used to induce labor in selected cases and is also effective in inducing uterine contractions following delivery, thereby controlling postpartum hemorrhage. When a baby is placed on the breast, the sucking action causes the posterior pituitary to release oxytocin. It is important to remember this inherent mechanism whenever confronted by a patient suffering moderate to severe postpartum bleeding.

Indication

Oxytocin is used for postpartum hemorrhage.

Contraindications

In the prehospital setting, oxytocin should be administered only to patients suffering severe postpartum bleeding. Before administration it is essential to verify that the baby *and the placenta* have been delivered and that there is not an additional fetus in the uterus.

Precautions

Excess oxytocin can cause overstimulation of the uterus and possible uterine rupture. Hypertension, cardiac arrhythmia, and anaphylaxis have been reported in conjunction with the administration of oxytocin. Vital signs and uterine tone should be monitored.

Side Effects

Oxytocin can cause hypotension, arrhythmias, tachycardia, seizures, coma, nausea, and vomiting in the mother. When administered prior to delivery, oxytocin can cause fetal hypoxia, fetal asphyxia, fetal arrhythmias, and possibly fetal intracranial bleeding.

Interactions

Oxytocin can cause hypertension when administered in conjunction with vasoconstrictors such as norepinephrine.

Dosage

Following are two regimens for the administration of oxytocin in the management of patients with postpartum hemorrhage: (1) 3 to 10 units can be administered intramuscularly following delivery of the placenta or (2) 10 to 20 units can be placed in either 500 or 1000 mL of D_5W, 0.9 percent normal saline, or lactated Ringer's solution. This should be titrated according to the severity of the bleeding and the uterine response. Oxytocin should only be administered intramuscularly or by slow IV infusion.

How Supplied

Pitocin is supplied in 0.5 and 1 mL ampules containing 10 mg/mL. A 1 mL prefilled syringe containing the same concentration is also available.

HYPERTENSIVE DISORDERS OF PREGNANCY

In addition to vaginal bleeding, paramedics should be aware of several pregnancy-associated problems known collectively as *hypertensive disorders of pregnancy* (formerly called *toxemia of pregnancy*). These disorders are characterized by hypertension, weight gain, edema, protein in the urine, and, in late stages, seizures. Hypertensive disorders of pregnancy occur in approximately 5 percent of pregnancies. They are thought to be caused by abnormal vasospasm in the mother, which results in increased blood pressure and other associated symptoms. The hypertensive disorders of pregnancy generally include the following:

Pregnancy-induced hypertension (PIH). PIH is characterized by a blood pressure of 140/90 level or greater in pregnancy in a patient who was previously normotensive. PIH is the early stage of the disease process. It is important to remember that blood pressure usually drops in pregnancy, and a blood pressure reading of 130/80 may be elevated.

Preeclampsia. Preeclamptic patients are those who have hypertension, abnormal weight gain, edema, headache, protein in the urine, epigastric pain, and, occasionally, visual disturbances. If untreated, preeclampsia may progress to the next stage, eclampsia.

Eclampsia. Eclampsia is the most serious manifestation of the hypertensive disorders of pregnancy. It is characterized by grand mal seizure activity. Eclampsia is often preceded by visual disturbances, such as flashing lights or spots before the eyes. Also, the development of epigastric pain or pain in the right upper abdominal quadrant often indicates impending seizure. Eclampsia can be distinguished from epilepsy by the history and physical appearance of the patient. Patients who become eclamptic are usually edematous and have markedly elevated blood pressure, whereas epileptics usually have a prior history of seizures and are taking anticonvulsant medications.

The hypertensive disorders of pregnancy tend to occur most often with a woman's first pregnancy. They also appear to occur more frequently in patients with preexisting hypertension. Diabetes mellitus is also associated with an increased incidence of this disease process.

Patients who develop PIH and preeclampsia are at increased risk for cerebral hemorrhage, the development of renal failure, and pulmonary edema. Patients who are preeclamptic have intravascular volume depletion, because a great deal of their body fluid is in the third space. If eclampsia develops, death of the mother and fetus frequently results. Eclampsia must be treated aggressively. *Magnesium sulfate* is the drug of choice for controlling the convulsions associated with eclampsia. In addition, it may be necessary to administer an antihypertensive agent, such as those discussed in Chapter 7, to prevent the complications of hypertensive crisis. The decision to administer an antihypertensive in the prehospital phase of emergency medical care rests with the base station physician. Each case should be treated individually.

MAGNESIUM SULFATE

Class: Electrolyte

Description

Magnesium sulfate is a salt that dissociates into the magnesium cation (Mg^{2+}) and the sulfate anion when administered. Magnesium is an essential element in numerous biochemical reactions that occur within the body.

Mechanism of Action

Magnesium sulfate is a central nervous system depressant effective in the management of seizures associated with eclampsia. It is used for the initial therapy of convulsions associated with pregnancy. After cessation of seizure activity, other anticonvulsant agents may be administered.

Indications

Magnesium sulfate is used in eclampsia (seizures accompanying pregnancy) and preterm labor.

Contraindications

Magnesium sulfate should not be administered to any patient with heart block. It should not be administered to patients who are in shock; who have persistent, severe hypertension; who routinely undergo dialysis; or who are known to have a decreased calcium level (hypocalcemia).

Precautions

Magnesium sulfate, like other central nervous system depressants, can cause hypotension, circulatory collapse, and depression of cardiac and respiratory function. The most immediate danger is respiratory depression. Calcium chloride should be readily available for IV administration as an antidote in case respiratory depression occurs. Magnesium sulfate should be administered slowly to minimize side effects. Any patient receiving intravenous magnesium sulfate should have continuous cardiac monitoring as well as frequent monitoring of vital signs. If possible, the knee and biceps deep tendon reflexes should be checked prior to and during magnesium therapy.

Side Effects

Magnesium sulfate can cause flushing, sweating, bradycardia, decreased deep tendon reflexes, drowsiness, respiratory depression, arrhythmias, hypotension, hypothermia, itching, and rash.

Interactions

Magnesium sulfate can cause cardiac conduction abnormalities if administered in conjunction with digitalis.

Dosage

The standard dosage for the management of convulsions associated with eclampsia is 2 to 4 g slow IV over 25 min. If an IV cannot be started, magnesium sulfate can be administered intramuscularly. Because of the volume of the drug (5 to 10 mL), the dose should be divided in half and each half administered intramuscularly at a separate site (usually each gluteus).

How Supplied

Magnesium sulfate is supplied in prefilled syringes containing 5 and 10 mL of a 50 percent solution.

PRETERM LABOR

Preterm labor is labor that begins before the age of fetal maturity, usually before 36 weeks. If labor begins early, obstetricians often try to suppress it to allow more time for intrauterine fetal development.

There are three approaches to suppressing preterm labor. The first approach is to sedate the mother. Often, labor begins in response to maternal stress or exhaustion. In these cases, a sedative such as Seconal is given. Alternatively, morphine sulfate can be administered (intramuscularly) for sedation.

The second approach to suppressing preterm labor is administration of a fluid bolus. The hormone oxytocin is manufactured and released from the posterior pituitary. Antidiuretic hormone (ADH) is also manufactured and released from the posterior pituitary. ADH causes the kidneys to retain water. In cases of preterm labor, a fluid bolus (1 to 2 L of lactated Ringer's solution or normal saline) is administered. ADH production and release are inhibited through feedback systems. Because ADH and oxytocin come from the same area of the posterior pituitary, suppression of ADH release also suppresses oxytocin release and thus can help suppress preterm labor.

Finally, labor can be suppressed by the use of tocolytics. Although many tocolytics are available, β_2-agonists are frequently used. Stimulation of uterine β_2-receptors causes uterine relaxation and suppression of preterm labor. Common β_2-agonists include terbutaline and ritodrine (Yutopar). Terbutaline is used more frequently in the emergency setting. Magnesium sulfate, previously discussed, is also effective in suppressing preterm labor.

℞ TERBUTALINE

Class: Sympathetic agonist and tocolytic

Description

Terbutaline is a synthetic sympathomimetic that is selective for β_2-adrenergic receptors.

Mechanism of Action

Terbutaline, because of its effects on β_2-adrenergic receptors, causes immediate bronchodilation with minimal cardiac effects. It is also used to suppress preterm labor. Stimulation of β_2-adrenergic receptors in the uterus causes uterine relaxation and can suppress labor.

Indication

Terbutaline is used for preterm labor.

Contraindications

Terbutaline should not be administered to any patient with a history of hypersensitivity to the drug.

Precautions

As with any sympathomimetic, the patient's vital signs must be monitored. Caution should be used when administering terbutaline to elderly patients and those with cardiovascular disease or hypertension.

Side Effects

Terbutaline can cause palpitations, anxiety, dizziness, headache, nervousness, tremor, hypertension, arrhythmias, chest pain, nausea, and vomiting.

Interactions

The possibility of developing unpleasant side effects increases when terbutaline is used with other sympathetic agonists. β-blockers may blunt the pharmacological effects of terbutaline.

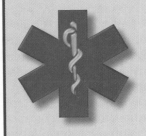

CASE PRESENTATION

An ALS ambulance is called to a rural hospital to transport a maternity patient to a larger city hospital 1 hour away. Paramedics are asked to bring the monitor in with the stretcher. On arrival at the hospital the nurse attending the patient gives the following information: The patient is an 18-year-old female, gravida 1, para 0, in her third trimester of pregnancy. She came to the hospital by private car after suffering a grand mal seizure at home. She had no prior history of seizures, and her pregnancy had been uneventful to date. She evidently was not in labor prior to the seizure. At present the patient is lying on a hospital bed and is not having contractions, as based on the external fetal monitor. The fetal heart rate is stable. The hospital diagnosis is eclampsia.

On Examination

CNS: The patient is conscious but lethargic

Resp: Respirations are 24 per minute and shallow; symmetrical chest wall movement with clear bilateral breath sounds

CVS: Both carotid and radial pulses are present and strong; a systolic flow murmur can be heard; minimal blood loss is noted from the vagina; neck veins are not distended; skin color is normal, warm, and diaphoretic to touch; patient is very edematous

ABD: Obviously pregnant with no contractions noted

Muscl/Skel: No apparent injuries

Extremities: Pedal and finger edema noted

Vital Signs

Pulse: 100/min, regular

Resp: 24/min

BP: 166/112 mm Hg

SpO$_2$: 95 percent

ECG: Normal sinus rhythm

Hospital Treatment

The patient is receiving high-flow oxygen. A large-bore IV was started in the left forearm. Magnesium sulfate is being infused at a rate of 1 g/hr. The receiving hospital was notified and is expecting the patient.

Treatment

The patient is moved to the ambulance stretcher and moved to the ambulance. Oxygen is administered at 12 L/min by nonrebreathing mask. The pulse oximeter is applied and shows an SpO$_2$ of 96 percent. The cardiac monitor shows a regular sinus rhythm and is quently by the paramedics who are watching for any ECG changes. The IV of magnesium sulfate initiated in the hospital is continued at 1 g/hr. The interior ambulance lights are dimmed to help prevent additional seizure activity. A prefilled syringe of Valium is removed from the lock box in case the patient suffers another seizure.

During transport the patient is continually assessed, with special attention to the IV of magnesium sulfate. Deep tendon reflexes are periodically checked to ensure the magnesium effect is not excessive. The trip to the hospital is uneventful. On arrival at the receiving facility, an emergency sonogram is obtained. It shows a fetal age of 37 weeks ($\pm$ 2 weeks). Labor is induced, and the patient delivers a healthy female infant 18 hours later.

Dosage

Terbutaline should be administered initially by subcutaneous injection. The initial dose should be 0.25 mg administered subcutaneously. This dose can be repeated in 30 minutes to 1 hour as required. A terbutaline drip can be used to provide ongoing suppression of labor. It can be prepared by placing 5 mg of terbutaline in 500 mL of lactated Ringer's solution or normal saline. The drip should be started at 30 mL/hr ($5\mu g$/min). This can be slowly increased to a maximum dose of 80 μg/min as required.

How Supplied

Terbutaline is supplied in vials containing 1 mg of the drug in 1 mL of solvent.

SUMMARY

Most obstetrical and gynecological emergencies are not managed in the field. Prehospital treatment should include stabilization of the airway, administration of supplemental oxygen, and replacement of intravascular volume. In severe postpartum bleeding, the administration of Pitocin is often effective. In the hypertensive disorders of pregnancy, magnesium sulfate may be used during the prehospital phase of emergency medical care to control convulsions. The definitive treatment of preeclampsia and eclampsia is delivery of the fetus.

KEY WORDS

abruptio placenta. A premature separation of the placenta from the uterus before birth. Because it often results in severe bleeding, it is considered to be a serious condition.

eclampsia. The most serious manifestation of the hypertensive disorders of pregnancy. It is characterized by grand mal seizure activity. Eclampsia is often preceded by visual disturbances, such as flashing lights or spots before the eyes. Also, the development of epigastric pain or pain in the right upper abdominal quadrant often indicates impending seizure.

Patients who become eclamptic are usually edematous and have markedly elevated blood pressure.

ectopic pregnancy. The implantation of a developing fetus outside the uterus, often in the fallopian tube.

placenta previa. A condition in which the placenta partly or completely covers the opening of the cervix. It is the most common cause of painless bleeding in the third trimester.

postpartum hemorrhage. The loss of 500 mL or more blood in the first 24 hours following delivery.

preeclampsia. A manifestation of the hypertensive disorders of pregnancy characterized by hypertension, abnormal weight gain, edema, headache, protein in the urine, epigastric pain, and, occasionally, visual disturbances. If untreated, preeclampsia may progress to the next stage, eclampsia.

spontaneous abortion. A fetal loss, also called a miscarriage, that occurs of its own accord. Most spontaneous abortions occur before the 12th week of pregnancy. Many occur 2 weeks after conception and are mistaken for menstrual periods.

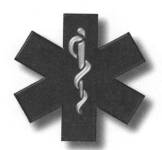

chapter 12

TOXICOLOGICAL EMERGENCIES IN PREHOSPITAL CARE

OBJECTIVES

After completing this chapter, the reader should be able to

1. Discuss the importance of toxicological emergencies in prehospital care.

2. Discuss the role of regional poison centers in the management of the poisoned patient.

3. Describe the key historical information required in the management of a toxicological emergency.

4. Describe the various routes of exposure to toxic substances.

5. Define the term *toxidrome* and describe the common toxidromes encountered in prehospital care.

6. Describe the general management of the patient exposed to a toxin, including decontamination and elimination.

7. Describe the signs, symptoms, and management (including antidotes where appropriate) of the following toxic exposures and overdoses: acetaminophen, beta-blockers, calcium channel blockers, carbon monoxide, cyanide, digoxin/digitalis, ethylene glycol, iron, isopropyl alcohol, methanol, narcotics and narcotic antagonists, organophosphates and carbamates, salicylates, selective serotonin reuptake inhibitors (SSRIs), and tricyclic antidepressants.

INTRODUCTION

Toxicology is a rapidly evolving science that can provide the prehospital care provider with a fascinating window into the field of pharmacology and pharmacokinetics. Management of toxin exposures and overdoses represents an important and constantly expanding aspect of prehospital care. Maintaining clinical competence in managing this patient population is a significant challenge because there is a continuous introduction of new medications, each of which has its own unique toxicological potential. The approach to the poisoned or overdosed patient can be likened to a form of detective work. The clinical clues required to manage these patients optimally are often subtle, and providers must be aware that virtually any patient presentation may be directly or indirectly related to a toxicological problem. Without suspicion, even the most obvious clinical clues can go unnoticed. In this chapter the discussion focuses not only on prescription drugs but also on nonprescription toxins that may be encountered in prehospital care. The format includes both a review of general principles of toxicology and a focused review of some of the commonly encountered toxins.

REGIONAL POISON CENTERS

Once the possibility of a poisoning or overdose has been identified, several resources are available to assist in patient management. Traditionally, hospital-based medical control has provided guidance and direction for the management of toxicological emergencies. In recent years the emergence of toxicology as a distinct discipline has led to the development of regional poison centers whose role is to provide information and advice to caregivers encountering poisoned patients. Poison information specialists are typically nurses and pharmacists with specialized training in toxicology. They are generally available 24 hours per day to provide telephone advice to prehospital care providers, laypeople, and hospital medical staff. They can serve as an extremely valuable resource to care providers, particularly in rural settings where the decision to transfer a patient to a larger center can be a difficult one. The prehospital care provider should not overlook the potential benefit of consultation with a regional poison center.

PATIENT HISTORY

The history constitutes an essential part of the initial approach to the toxicology patient. Like all detective work, suspicion is the foundation for discovering the truth; the truth in this case is the identity, quantity, and time of exposure to the toxic substance. Despite its importance, the history is frequently confusing and inconsistent in this patient population. The problem is related to factors such as illicit drug use, associated psychiatric illnesses, and in some cases a lack of awareness on the part of both the patient and the care provider that an exposure has actually occurred.

A thorough history includes *what* agent the patient was exposed to, *how much* of the agent, *when* the exposure occurred (time), *how* the exposure occurred *(route of exposure), where* (location) the exposure occurred, and any *treatment* the patient may have received prior to the arrival of the prehospital care provider.

The importance of identifying the agent in question is obvious. Knowing which agent is involved can allow the care provider to plan decontamination, provide initial treatment, and anticipate problems before they actually occur. With some toxic agents immediate management is required in the field, whereas others can have therapy initiated in the emergency department. In the latter cases, it is extremely useful to provide hospital staff with all available information so that they can prepare for the patient's arrival. Some agents have antidotes that can be lifesaving if used appropriately. In circumstances in which the toxic agent cannot be identified or an antidote is not available, management may be limited to supportive care. Searching the scene for pill bottles, poisons, evidence of drug abuse, venomous plants, and animals is paramount. Whenever possible, toxicological evidence, especially pill bottles and medication dispensers, should be transported to the hospital for review by a physician.

The dose or amount of toxin can be very helpful in predicting the occurrence or severity of clinical symptoms. It may also help to determine the need for decontamination procedures and antidote treatment. Making note of the date on prescription medication containers and the number of pills still present can assist in quantifying the dosage.

The time of exposure is important for several reasons. First, it allows an estimation of the degree of toxicity (however, many toxins have delayed symptom onset). Second, it allows some planning for decontamination and management. Finally, some agents (salicylates and acetaminophen) require blood levels to determine the need for treatment. Interpretation of these blood levels often requires knowledge of the time of ingestion. Reviewing the patient's recent activities and time of symptom onset with family members or friends can be very helpful.

Potential routes of exposure include *oral ingestion, inhalation, dermal exposure, injection* (*intra-* or *extravascular*) and *mucosal absorption*. The route of exposure guides treatment (e.g., gastric decontamination would not be indicated in a patient who has had dermal exposure).

The location of the exposure can be helpful in identifying the agent (e.g., an agricultural worker who develops symptoms shortly after spraying organophosphate pesticides on a wheat field). The route of exposure can be crucial in ensuring the safety of the care provider because some toxins can be airborne (e.g., carbon monoxide) or spread through patient contact (e.g., organophosphate pesticides).

Identifying any treatment provided prior to medical attention is also important. The occurrence of vomiting is relevant because it suggests some emptying of residual gastric toxins has already occurred. Although no longer widely used and potentially dangerous, syrup of ipecac is still available and may be administered by laypeople. If administered, the prehospital care provider must anticipate vomiting and take steps to prevent aspiration of gastric contents.

GENERAL APPROACH TO THE POISONED PATIENT

As emphasized earlier, the foundation of managing the poisoned patient is a clinical suspicion supplemented by clues present at the scene and in the presentation of the patient. The initial approach to the poisoned patient includes early attention to *airway, breathing,* and *circulation*. Airway control should occur early where indicated, followed by establishment of vascular access. Because vomiting is a frequent occurrence in the poisoned patient, aspiration is a significant risk and should be anticipated and prevented wherever possible. *Vital signs* must be recorded early because they can provide clues to both the type of toxin and the severity of the overdose. *Cardiac monitoring* is crucial because many toxic exposures are associated with serious arrhythmias. In the setting of tricyclic antidepressant overdose, the presence of a wide QRS complex may guide treatment, as discussed in greater detail later in the chapter. *Blood glucose level* should be measured in all patients with altered level of consciousness because hypoglycemia can often be misinterpreted as an intoxicated state. As discussed previously, both the patient and care providers must be protected from further exposure to the toxin. Discussion of physical exam findings is deferred to the later review of specific toxidromes.

Decontamination and enhancing *elimination* of toxins in the poisoned patient may have a role in prehospital care. Traditional approaches include *syrup of ipecac, gastric lavage,* and *activated charcoal* with or without a cathartic agent (an agent that enhances bowel motility and speeds transit through the gut). Syrup of ipecac acts by inducing vomiting and thereby decreasing further absorption of remaining toxins from the gastrointestinal tract. Its usage has largely fallen out of favor recently due to a lack of evidence for improved patient outcome as well as significant concerns regarding its safety. The largest safety concern relates to the fact that altered level of consciousness is relatively common in toxic ingestions, and combining reduced consciousness with induced emesis creates considerable risk of airway compromise and aspiration. Gastric lavage remains a relatively commonly utilized method of in-hospital gastric decontamination. Although its efficacy remains somewhat unproven, it is occasionally utilized in cases of recent ingestion or in agents known to slow gastric emptying. Gastric lavage is impractical for most prehospital settings because it requires multiple personnel and may be associated with significant complications such as aspiration and esophageal rupture. Activated charcoal has been shown to be effective in decreasing the toxicity in certain oral ingestions and in agents with enterohepatic circulation. Charcoal is by no means effective for all orally ingested toxins. Its use is relatively safe; the largest risk is aspiration in the event that vomiting ensues and the patient is unable to protect his or her airway. It is sometimes combined with a cathartic agent such as sorbitol or magnesium citrate to help speed passage of toxins through the small and large bowel and thereby limit absorption. Although cathartic agents may improve elimination somewhat, the resultant frequent and voluminous bowel movements can create a suboptimal patient care environment in the back of an ambulance. To summarize, activated charcoal likely represents the only truly safe and efficacious method of enhancing toxin elimination in the prehospital setting.

TOXIDROMES

A toxidrome is a set of clinical signs that are considered diagnostic of certain toxins or classes of toxins. Although not all toxins have their own unique toxidrome, an ability to recognize the common toxidromes can greatly enhance toxin identification and thereby aid patient care in certain circumstances. The clinical reliability of toxidromes is limited in cases of mixed overdoses, for which physical findings can be contradictory.

Perhaps the most common toxidrome encountered in prehospital care is that of the narcotized patient (*narcotic* or *opiate toxidrome*). Whether self-induced or iatrogenic, the classic triad of decreased level of consciousness, respiratory depression, and constricted pupils (miosis) is seen with frequency and, when present, can guide therapy. Although this triad generally holds for the common narcotics, including morphine, heroin, and codeine, it is important to remember that not all narcotics cause pupillary constriction. Meperidine (Demerol), propoxyphene (Darvon), pentazocine (Talwin), and others may not demonstrate miosis.

Another relatively common toxidrome is that of *anticholinergic* toxicity, as commonly seen with dimenhydrinate and tricyclic antidepressant overdoses. These patients commonly display both central signs and peripheral antimuscarinic signs. Peripheral signs are typically more common and include dry skin and mucous membranes, thirst, dysphagia, blurred vision, fixed dilated pupils, tachycardia, fine red (scarlatiniform) rash, hyperthermia, abdominal distention with decreased or absent bowel sounds, and urinary urgency or retention. Central signs include lethargy, confusion, restlessness, delirium, hallucinations, ataxia, seizures, and in severe cases cardiopulmonary collapse. Agents that can cause this toxidrome include dimenhydrinate and cyclic antidepressants. A common mnemonic for remembering the clinical signs of anticholinergic syndrome is "*hot* as a Hades, *blind* as a bat, *dry* as a bone, *red* as a beet, *mad* as a hatter."

The *cholinergic toxidrome*, as is classically seen with organophosphate pesticide poisoning, can present with a complex cascade of signs that include muscarinic, nicotinic, and central nervous system (CNS) signs and symptoms. Once again, the multiple clinical signs can be simplified through the use of a mnemonic. The muscarinic symptoms are described by the mnemonic *DUMBELS*, in which the signs include defecation, urination, miosis, bronchorrhea, excitation (muscular), lacrimation, and salivation or seizures. The nicotinic symptoms can be summarized by a mnemonic based on the days of the week, *MTWtHF*, which stands for muscle weakness and paralysis, tachycardia, weakness, hypertension, and fasiculations.

The *sympathomimetic syndrome* can present with various symptoms depending on which class of agents is involved. Alpha-adrenergic agents include phenylephrine, methoxamine, and phenylpropanolamine and typically present with hypertension (HTN) and reflex bradycardia secondary to vasoconstriction of resistance vessels. Beta-adrenergic agents include theophylline, caffeine, and metoproterenol and typically present with tachycardia with or without hypotension (secondary to excessive stimulation of the sinus node or vascular smooth muscle dilatation).

SPECIFIC TOXIC AGENTS ENCOUNTERED IN PREHOSPITAL CARE

The following sections summarize some of the commonly encountered toxins in prehospital care. The list of agents discussed is by no means comprehensive but emphasizes those that may require specific treatment.

Acetaminophen

Acetaminophen is found in many over-the-counter medications and, as such, is a commonly encountered overdose. The primary concern in this overdose is the potential for irreversible hepatic injury. Therapy is aimed at preventing hepatotoxicity. A specific antidote, N-acetylcysteine, is available but is generally reserved for use in the hospital.

Route of Exposure	Oral.
Mechanism of Toxicity	Metabolism is primarily hepatic; the production of toxic metabolites results in direct hepatic toxicity. Ninety percent is conjugated with glucuronic or sulfuric acid in the liver to form nontoxic compounds that are excreted in the urine. An additional 2 percent is excreted unchanged in the urine. A toxic by-product formed by this process is normally conjugated with hepatic glutathione and subsequently excreted in the urine. When glutathione stores are depleted, as in a massive overdose, hepatotoxicity occurs.
Toxic Dose	Acute ingestion: Doses greater than 7.5 g or 140 mg/kg are predictive of hepatotoxicity in an adult. Hepatotoxicity is rare in children. Certain drugs such as cimetidine and ethanol are protective in acute overdose because they compete with acetaminophen.
	Chronic ingestion: Variable toxicity can occur at low doses, especially in chronic alcoholics who have higher levels of acetaminophen and thus develop toxic metabolites more readily.
	Toxicity can be accurately predicted using serum (assuming the time of ingestion is known).
Signs and Symptoms	Signs and symptoms are classified into stages (see Table 12–1).
Prehospital Management	Supportive care should be provided, including airway support as indicated and activated charcoal where permitted by medical control guidelines.
In-Hospital Management	Treatment with N-acetylcysteine (NAC) either orally or intravenously is the mainstay of therapy in cases of confirmed toxicity. Lavage is sometimes used if the patient presents

TABLE 12–1

Stage	Time Postingestion	Characteristics
I	1/2 to 24 hours[a]	Anorexia, nausea, vomiting, malaise, pallor, and diaphoresis
II	24 to 48 hours	Abdominal pain, liver tenderness, elevated liver enzymes, and oliguria
III	72 to 96 hours	Peak liver enzyme abnormalities, jaundice, hypoglycemia, coagulopathies, and encephalopathy
IV	4 days to 2 weeks	Resolution of hepatotoxicity or progressive hepatic failure

[a]Some patients may be completely asymptomatic during Stage I.

within 2 hours of ingestion. Toxicity and the need for NAC therapy are determined by measurement of serum levels. These serum levels are most useful if measured 4 hours postingestion but can be used up to 25 hours postingestion. The level is plotted on the Rumack-Matthew nomogram for acetaminophen poisoning. Hepatotoxicity can be prevented with NAC therapy but once present is generally irreversible. NAC therapy is most effective if initiated within 8 hours of ingestion but in some circumstances is used even later. Liver transplant has been performed as a lifesaving measure in rare cases.

Anticholinergics

Anticholinergic properties can be found in many agents including both prescription drugs and drugs of abuse. Drugs with anticholinergic properties include tricyclic antidepressants, antihistamines, phenothiazines, and antiparkinsonian drugs. Dimenhydrinate, an antiemetic, is a drug with anticholinergic properties that is commonly used recreationally, especially among adolescents. Some plants and mushrooms (including the hallucinogenic varieties that are used recreationally) also have anticholinergic properties.

Route of Exposure	Oral, intravenous (IV), or dermal.
Mechanism of Toxicity	As described previously, cholinergic blockade occurs both centrally and peripherally and involves both muscarinic and nicotinic receptors. Different agents have different degrees of effect on the two receptor types and, as such, can have slightly different presentations.
Toxic Dose	Variable.
Signs and Symptoms	See earlier description of anticholinergic toxidrome. (Remember: hot as Hades, blind as a bat, dry as a bone, red as a beet, mad as a Hatter.)
Prehospital Management	Conservative supportive care is the mainstay of therapy. Monitoring of airway, breathing, and circulation supplemented with IV access and cardiac monitoring is indicated in all but the most minor overdoses. Activated charcoal may be useful.
In-Hospital Management	Supportive care should be provided as in prehospital management. Lavage may be indicated even late in overdose because of the effects that anticholinergics have on delaying gastric emptying. Seizures and agitation are treated with benzodiazepines. Arrhythmias can be treated with conventional therapy with the exception that Class Ia drugs (quinidine, disopyramide,

and procainamide) should be avoided because of the quinidine-like effects of some anticholinergics. The use of physostigmine, a reversible acetylcholinesterase inhibitor, remains controversial. It may aggravate arrhythmias and seizures, and as such its use is limited to severe toxicity unresponsive to conventional therapy. Indications may include uncontrollable agitation, hemodynamically unstable arrhythmias, and coma with respiratory depression, malignant hypertension, or refractory hypotension. Physostigmine can potentiate toxicity in tricyclic antidepressant overdose and should be avoided. Toxic symptoms of anticholinergics are generally evident within 4 to 6 hours of ingestion, and patients asymptomatic at that point can generally be safely discharged.

Neuroleptics

Neuroleptics are a broad class of agents which include the antipsychotics and some tranquilizers. The two most commonly encountered neuroleptic classes are the butyrophenones (such as haloperidol and droperidol) and the phenothiazines (such as chlorpromazine). These agents are typically prescribed to patients with significant psychiatric illness and, as such, are frequently seen in overdose settings. Significant adverse reactions can occur to these agents even when taken at normally prescribed dosages.

Route of Exposure	Oral, IV or IM.
Mechanism of Toxicity	Act by blocking neurotransmission involving dopaminergic, adrenergic, muscarinic and histaminic receptors. Therapeutic and toxicologic effects vary from agent to agent depending on the degree of blockage of each receptor subtype.
Toxic Dose	Variable.
Signs and Symptoms	Adverse reactions are common and may occur even in the setting of normal therapeutic dosages. These reactions include the following;
	Dystonic reaction which features involuntary muscle spasm including torticollis, facial grimacing, opisthotonos (flexion adduction of the arms), oculogyric crisis, and laryngeal spasm. Treatment is diphenhydramine or benztropine.
	Akathisia which features restlessness, jittery feeling, and insomnia. May be treated with benztropine, amantidine, or propranolol.
	Parkinsonism featuring resting tremor, rigidity, and masked facies. May be treated with benztropine or amantidine.
	Tardive dyskinesia which features lip smacking, tongue protrusion, grimacing, and chew-

ing motion.

Neuroleptic malignant syndrome (NMS) which is a life-threatening condition (10% mortality rate) featuring hyperthermia, rigidity, altered mental status, and autonomic instability.

Symptoms of acute overdose are highly variable and can include any of the previously described conditions as well as CNS depression (ranging from sedation to coma), respiratory depression, hypo or hyperthermia, pinpoint pupils (especially phenothiazines), anticholinergic symptoms, hypotension with reflex tachycardia, cardiac dysrhythmias, and prolongation of the PR and QT intervals (with resultant ventricular dysrhythmias such as torsade de pointes).

Prehospital Management ABCs, cardiac monitoring, nalaxone, and chemstrip if altered LOC. Treat hypotension with crystalloid (normal saline) and norepinephrine or phenylephrine as needed. Ventricular dysrhythmias should be treated initially with bicarbonate (1–2 mEq/kg IV bolus) followed by lidocaine or phenytoin. Torsade de pointes should be treated initially with magnesium, followed by isoproterenol or overdrive pacing as needed. Seizures should be treated using standard methods including benzodiazapines, phenytoin, or phenobarbital.

In-Hospital Management Consists of supportive care including all the aforementioned methods. Gastrointestinal decontamination should be performed using activated charcoal and gastric lavage if the patient is intubated and a short interval has elapsed since the time of ingestion. Class 1A antiarrhythmics such as quinidine and procainamide should be avoided as they may exacerbate the cardiac toxicity. Cooling or warming techniques may be needed to control extremes of temperature. Management of NMS includes muscle relaxation using benzodiazepines and, if necessary, neuromuscular blockade. Dantrolene and bromocriptine, a dopamine agonist, have been used with mixed results in the treatment of NMS.

 # FLUMAZENIL (ANEXATE, ROMAZICON)

Class: Benzodiazepine antagonist

Description

Flumazenil is a benzodiazepine antagonist. It is used to reverse the sedative effects of benzodiazepines, especially respiratory depression.

Mechanism of Action

Flumazenil antagonizes the actions of the benzodiazepines in the central nervous system. Particularly, it inhibits their actions on the gamma-aminobutyric acid–benzodiazepine complex. It is used to reverse the sedative effects of the benzodiazepines.

Indications

Fumazenil is used for complete and partial reversal of CNS and respiratory depression caused by benzodiazepines including the following agents: Valium, Versed, Ativan, Halcion, Restoril, Dalmane, Tranxene, Serax, Klonopin, Ambien, Doral, ProSom, Centrax, and Xanax. Flumazenil should *not* be used as a diagnostic agent for benzodiazepine overdose in the manner naloxone is used for narcotic overdose. The potential of inducing a life-threatening benzodiazepine withdrawal reaction in patients addicted to benzodiazepines with flumazenil is not worth the perceived benefits.

Contraindications

Flumazenil is contraindicated in patients with a known hypersensitivity to the drug or to benzodiazepines. It should not be administered to patients who have received benzodiazepines to control life-threatening conditions such as status epilepticus. It should not be used in patients with tricyclic antidepressant overdoses.

Precautions

Flumazenil should be administered with caution to patients dependent on benzodiazepines. Benzodiazepine withdrawal can be life-threatening. Signs and symptoms of benzodiazepine withdrawal include tachycardia, hypertension, anxiousness, confusion, and seizures. The effects of flumazenil can wear off, resulting in the return of sedation. Following administration, patients should be monitored for signs of resedation and respiratory depression.

Side Effects

Flumazenil can cause fatigue, headache, agitation, nervousness, dizziness, flushing, confusion, convulsions, arrhythmias, nausea, and vomiting.

Interactions

There are few interactions in the emergency setting.

Dosage

The standard dose of flumazenil is 0.2 mg intravenously administered over 30 seconds. This dose can be repeated, as required, up to a maximum dose of 1.0 mg. Flumazenil should only be given intravenously in the emergency setting.

How Supplied

Flumazenil (Romazicon) is supplied in 5 and 10 mL multidose vials containing 0.1 mg/mL.

Beta-Blockers

Although intentional overdose on beta-blockers is relatively rare, toxic symptoms occur frequently. True overdoses are often life-threatening and difficult to manage because of the profound hemodynamic effects. Glucagon is the primary antidote and is often the only useful treatment modality.

Route of Exposure	Generally oral; occasionally ocular.
Mechanism of Toxicity	Beta-blockers cause blockade of both β_1- and β_2-receptors in the adrenergic nervous system. This blockade can affect several organ systems, most notably the cardiovascular (bradycardia, atrioventricular [AV] block, or vasodilation) and respiratory (bronchospasm or congestive heart failure).
Toxic Dose	The toxic dose is highly variable. Toxicity is more likely in setting of underlying heart disease.
Signs and Symptoms	Bradycardia, AV blockade, and hypotension are common. Tachycardia has been reported with some β-blockers such as practolol, pindolol, and sotalol. Hypotension is a result of negative chronotropy (bradycardia) and negative inotropy (decreased cardiac contractility). Changes in mental status, ranging from confusion to seizures or coma, have been described. Bronchospasm and congestive heart failure can occur. Beta-blockers can mask the normal adrenergic signs and symptoms of hypoglycemia. In addition, they can impair recovery from hypoglycemia.
Prehospital Management	Supportive care, including airway management, is provided where indicated. Activated charcoal may be indicated. Symptomatic patients with abnormal vital signs may respond to atropine or catecholamines (epinephrine) but more frequently require glucagon therapy. Glucagon acts by augmenting heart rate, AV conduction, and myocardial contractility. The required dose for glucagon therapy in this setting is typically 3 to 10 mg given as a bolus. This dosage is frequently problematic in that few emergency medical services (EMS) vehicles carry these quantities of glucagon in the field. Cases unresponsive to these pharmacological interventions may be supported with fluid therapy and/or transcutaneous pacing. Seizures can be treated with benzodiazepines (diazepam or lorazepam) or in refractory cases phenytoin or phenobarbital. Bronchospasm can be treated with β_2-agonists and in severe cases aminophylline.

In-Hospital Management	Supportive care should be provided as in prehospital management. Patients often require intensive care unit (ICU) support including continuous glucagon infusion with or without pressor therapy (dopamine or epinephrine).

Calcium Channel Blockers

The clinical presentation of calcium channel blocker overdose can be extremely variable depending on the agent involved but is often clinically similar to beta-blocker toxicity. Although calcium therapy can be useful, major overdoses are often dependant on inotrope therapy (epinephrine or dopamine) and occasionally glucagon.

Route of Exposure	Oral, sublingual, or intravenous.
Mechanism of Toxicity	Virtually any cell utilizing calcium can be affected, most notably myocardium, the sinoatrial (SA) and AV nodes, and the AV nodal conduction pathway. Metabolism occurs in the liver.
Toxic Dose	The toxic dose is variable. The effects are generally more severe in the presence of underlying cardiovascular disease.
Signs and Symptoms	Hypotension, bradycardia, and AV conduction blocks are common. The extent of these effects is dependent on the specific agent ingested. Nonspecific features include lethargy, slurred speech, nausea, vomiting, coma, and respiratory depression.
Prehospital Management	Supportive care is provided as required. Activated charcoal may be indicated. In cases of severe toxicity, calcium chloride or calcium gluconate may be given intravenously in a dosage of 10 cc of a 10 percent solution. Calcium therapy is occasionally but not universally effective. Other therapeutic options for cardiac toxicity include atropine, isoproterenol, and transcutaneous pacing. Intravenous glucagon therapy has also been tried with some success in cases unresponsive to calcium and pressors. Hypotension may be partially responsive to IV fluids and inotropes (dopamine and norepinephrine).
In-Hospital Management	Supportive care should be provided as in prehospital management. Decontamination may include gastric lavage as well as the use of activated charcoal. Prolonged toxicity is common, and observation for extended periods is often required. Severe cases may require ICU admission with assisted ventilation and inotropic therapy.

Carbon Monoxide

Carbon monoxide (CO) exposure, both intentional and accidental, is a common toxicological problem. Death is not infrequent, and long-term neurological sequelae are also common. Oxygen is the mainstay of therapy, and hyperbaric oxygen therapy may be indicated in severe cases.

Route of Exposure	Inhalation is the most common route of exposure and is caused by blocked ventilation of furnace, chimney, or automobile exhaust system. Carbon monoxide exposure is also common in smoke inhalation and can be seen with ingestion or inhalation of paint thinners (containing methylene chloride, which can be metabolized to CO).
Mechanism of Toxicity	CO binds hemoglobin to form carboxyhemoglobin, thereby reducing the availability of hemoglobin to carry oxygen and thus inducing hypoxemia. It may also impair cellular oxygenation by competing with oxygen for binding sites of enzymes on the cytochrome chain. The affinity of hemoglobin for CO is 250× that of O_2. CO also binds directly to both cardiac and skeletal myoglobin, thereby decreasing contractility. In the CNS, CO can induce cerebral edema and necrosis of white matter.
Toxic Dose	Variable.
Signs and Symptoms	Signs and symptoms depend on levels:

<10 percent:	Generally asymptomatic; smokers often run levels up to 10 percent
10–20 percent:	Headache and dyspnea
20–30 percent:	Headache, fatigue, and visual disturbance
40–50 percent:	Tachycardia and altered level of consciousness; may precipitate angina
>60 percent:	Coma, seizures, and cherry red skin

Levels can only be measured via blood testing in the hospital. At levels greater than 40 percent, virtually any organ system can be affected. Pulmonary effects include noncardiogenic pulmonary edema, congestive heart failure, and aspiration. CNS effects include ataxia, nystagmus, hearing loss, tinnitus, papilledema, retinal hemorrhages, coma, and seizures. Cardiovascular system (CVS) effects include dysrhythmias, ST and T wave changes on electrocardiogram (ECG), and occasionally ischemia or infarction. Renal effects include rhabdomyolysis or myoglobinuria and acute renal failure. Although the occurrence of cherry red skin is commonly described in the presence of CO poisoning, it is actually a rare finding and its absence does not rule out CO poisoning. Pallor or cyanosis is seen relatively frequently in CO poisoning.

Prehospital Management   Supportive care supplemented by O_2 (via 100 percent nonrebreather mask) and airway management should be provided as required. Oxygen acts to decrease the half-life of CO:

$t_{1/2}$ room air = 320 minutes

$t_{1/2}$ 100 percent O_2 = 60–80 minutes

$t_{1/2}$ hyperbaric O_2 = 20–30 minutes

The measured O_2 saturation is unreliable in the setting of CO poisoning because the unit cannot differentiate between carboxyhemoglobin and oxyhemoglobin. As such it gives a falsely high saturation reading. The difference between an accurately measured O_2 saturation and the falsely elevated oximetry measurement is known as the saturation gap and is characteristic of CO poisoning. Unfortunately, accurate measurement of the O_2 saturation requires the use of arterial blood gases and therefore is generally not possible in a prehospital care setting.

In-Hospital Management   Supportive care should be provided as in prehospital management. Use of hyperbaric oxygen therapy remains controversial but may offer benefit in patients with severe symptoms and neurological deficits. Indications for hyperbaric O_2 therapy include patients with significant neurological abnormalities, patients with cardiovascular abnormalities, or symptomatic pregnant patients. Some studies suggest symptomatic patients with levels >20 to 25 percent warrant hyperbaric O_2 therapy. Long-term neurological sequelae occur, and some centers routinely use psychometric testing to monitor neurological function.

Cyanide

Cyanide is a substance with a somewhat notorious history commonly found in many industrial products, medications, and plants. It is found in many manufacturing plants and laboratories and is produced in the burning of some plastics, wool, silk, and furniture. It is found in plant material, including apricot, peach, and cherry pits, and in some poisons. It is an uncommon but potentially deadly toxin; patients who have been exposed to it can be treated using a specific antidote kit that may be life-saving if used early.

Route of Exposure	Inhalation, ingestion, intravenous, or dermal contact.
Mechanism of Toxicity	Cyanide binds a key cellular enzyme, cytochrome oxidase, causing cellular asphyxia and thus affecting virtually all organ systems.
Toxic Dose	Highly variable.
Signs and Symptoms	Most commonly present very quickly postexposure as unconscious, noncyanosed patients with hypotension and bradycardia; death occurs in seconds to minutes. In less severe cases or very early postexposure, the patient may have headache, dyspnea, confusion, or seizures with hypotension. Permanent neurological sequelae can occur in survivors. A bitter almond odor may be detected by care providers.
Prehospital Management	Recognition of cyanide exposure is the key to management because the window for implementing therapy is extremely short. As always, initial supportive care, including airway breathing and circulation, is paramount. A specific antidote, known as the Lilly Cyanide Antidote Kit, is available and is often kept on-site at industrial sites using cyanide products. Some EMS systems, particularly in rural settings, carry the antidote kit. The kit contains three different products, amyl nitrite pearls for inhalation, sodium nitrite solution for intravenous use, and sodium thiosulfate for intravenous use. The amyl nitrite pearls are meant to be broken and inhaled by the victim immediately, and the sodium nitrite is meant to be given immediately on establishment of IV access. Both nitrite products work by inducing methemoglobinemia—a form of hemoglobin that scavenges cyanide. Sodium thiosulfate works by converting cyanide to thiocyanate, a much less toxic compound that is gradually excreted in the urine. If the symptoms are relatively mild, sodium thiosulfate should be used alone, because methemoglobinemia can itself be dangerous and is only valuable in truly life-threatening cases of cyanide poisoning. Base physician contact or poison center consultation should come early in the course of managing cyanide poisoning.
In-Hospital Management	Supportive care should be provided as in prehospital management. Inhalational exposures related to closed-space combustion can often present with concurrent cyanide and carbon monoxide toxicity, and both must be treated

aggressively. In cases requiring nitrite therapy, methemoglobin levels must be closely monitored. Intravenous hydroxycobalamin (vitamin B_{12a}) can be a useful adjunct because it combines with cyanide to form a nontoxic cyanocobalamin that is excreted renally. Hyperbaric oxygen has no proven role in cyanide poisoning, although it may be indicated in cases of concurrent CO poisoning. For oral cyanide ingestion, charcoal may be beneficial.

Cyclic Antidepressants (Tricyclics)

Despite the introduction of various new classes of antidepressant agents in recent years, tricyclics continue to be widely prescribed. Unfortunately, the clinical benefit of these agents is often offset by their lethal potential in the setting of overdose. Cardiac toxicity, predominantly in the form of lethal arrhythmias, is the clinical hallmark, and intravenous bicarbonate therapy continues to be an essential part of management. Examples of agents in this class include amitriptyline and nortriptyline.

Route of Exposure	Oral.
Mechanism of Toxicity	Multiple physiological effects lead to clinical toxicity. Blockage of norepinephrine, dopamine, and serotonin reuptake at the presynaptic receptor leads to eventual norepinephrine depletion. Tricyclics also possess some anticholinergic activity, calcium channel blocking activity, and alpha-blocking activity. Cardiac toxicity is related to antagonism of cardiac fast sodium channels (quinidine-like effects), resulting in prolonged QRS complexes, as well as blockade of potassium efflux, resulting in QT interval prolongation. Metabolism is almost entirely hepatic, with a half-life of approximately 24 hours at therapeutic doses. In the setting of overdose, the half-life can be as much as 72 hours.
Toxic Dose	Highly variable.
Signs and Symptoms	Symptoms include dizziness, confusion, blurred vision, and dry mouth. Signs can be classified into three categories—cardiovascular, CNS, and anticholinergic. Cardiovascular signs include conduction blocks, hypotension, arrhythmias, and cardiac arrest. CNS signs include delirium, agitation, extrapyramidal signs, myoclonus, seizures, and coma. Anticholinergic signs occur as described previously and include tachycardia, mydriasis, decreased bowel sounds, urinary retention, and hyper- or hypothermia. The earliest and most sensitive sign of cyclic antidepressant overdose is

	tachycardia. Life-threatening arrhythmias are generally preceded by prolongation of the QRS complex.
Prehospital Management	Supportive care, including airway support, should be provided as indicated. Multidose activated charcoal is indicated. Intravenous access and fluid therapy are indicated if hypotension is present. Sodium bicarbonate remains a mainstay of therapy and has the following specific indications: hypotension, ventricular dysrhythmias, seizure activity (bicarbonate is not therapeutic for the seizure itself, but seizure activity is considered predictive of impending cardiac arrhythmias, which may be averted with bicarbonate therapy), and wide QRS complexes on cardiac monitor (the QRS interval requiring bicarbonate therapy remains somewhat controversial—some authors advocate 0.10 seconds, whereas others advocate that it be reserved for complexes >0.16 seconds; base physician contact is generally indicated where possible).
	Several mechanisms have been postulated for the therapeutic effects of bicarbonate, including increased protein binding of tricyclic antidepressant (TCA) in an alkaline environment (thus less free TCA to induce cardiac toxicity), alkalinization increasing the amount of unionized TCA, which appears to be less able to bind the sodium channel, and alkalinization causing free TCA to be pulled out of cardiac tissue. Additionally, some evidence suggests that the sodium in sodium bicarbonate helps to overcome the sodium channel blockade.
	Hypotension unresponsive to bicarbonate and IV fluid may require inotrope therapy. Seizure activity unresponsive to bicarbonate therapy may be treated with benzodiazepines such as diazepam or lorazepam. Mechanical hyperventilation may be of some value in reducing cardiac and CNS toxicity.
In-Hospital Management	Supportive care should be provided as in prehospital management. Gastric lavage may be indicated if less than 2 hours postingestion. Cases of suspected toxicity require an observation period of at least 6 hours to rule out serious sequelae.

Digoxin and Digitalis

Although not as widely used as it once was, digoxin remains a relatively common drug that can cause severe illness and death in the setting of overdose.

A specific antidote, digitalis-specific Fab fragments, is available but is not commonly used in the prehospital setting. Digoxin has a relatively narrow therapeutic window, and EMS providers should maintain a high index of suspicion for toxicity in cases in which a patient is known to be taking the drug. It is found in several sources, including prescription medications, plants (most notably foxglove), and certain toad venom.

Route of Exposure	Generally oral; can be related to plant exposure (digitalis is derived from plants, most notably the foxglove plant).
Mechanism of Toxicity	Digoxin and digitalis inhibit the sodium-potassium ATPase, causing potassium efflux and sodium and calcium influx into cells. Toxicity is enhanced in hypokalemia, hypomagnesemia, hypercalcemia, and alkalosis.
Toxic Dose	The toxic dose is highly variable. Patients with underlying heart disease, renal failure, hypothyroidism, and hypoxemia and those using nonsteroidal anti-inflammatory drugs (NSAIDs) are more prone to toxicity.
Signs and Symptoms	Symptoms are nonspecific and include fatigue, anorexia, disorientation, confusion, delerium, hallucinations, gastrointestinal upset, visual halos (green or yellow), slowed conduction in SA and AV nodes, increased PR interval, shortened QT intervals, AV block, asystole, ST-T wave scooping, junctional rhythms, and hemodynamic instability. Virtually any cardiac arrhythmia can be seen.
Prehospital Management	Supportive care, including fluids and pressor agents for the treatment of hypotension, should be provided. Multidose activated charcoal may be useful. Calcium, which will worsen digoxin toxicity, should *not* be given.
In-Hospital Management	Supportive care should be provided as in prehospital management. Electrolyte abnormalities, including hyperkalemia, should be corrected. Calcium should *not* be given. Magnesium therapy may lessen cardiac toxicity. Phenytoin or dilantin may be helpful for ventricular dysrhythmias. Atropine and pacing may be required for symptomatic bradycardias. Procainamide and quinidine are contraindicated because they may worsen conduction and contractility problems. Digibind (digoxin Fab fragments) can be lifesaving in severe overdose. It acts by directly binding and inactivating digoxin, thereby allowing for rapid excretion by the kidneys. Digibind is indicated in ingestions that are potentially lethal based on the amount of ingested drug (generally 10 mg in an adult), high serum levels (>12.8 to 19.2 mmol/L), marked hyperkalemia, malig-

nant dysrhythmias, resistant bradycardias, and hypotension. Clinical response to Digibind can occur as early as 20 to 30 minutes after administration.

Ethylene Glycol

The toxic alcohols include ethylene glycol, methanol, and isopropyl alcohol. In the case of ethylene glycol, which is most commonly found in antifreeze, ingestion is often accidental and may not be recognized until severe toxicity has occurred. Ethylene glycol poisoning is frequently misdiagnosed as ethanol intoxication, often resulting in suboptimal outcomes. Ethanol therapy helps to avert toxicity, but in severe cases dialysis may be required.

Route of Exposure	Generally oral.
Mechanism of Toxicity	Toxic metabolites are formed, causing acidosis and renal damage. Ethylene glycol is metabolized by alcohol dehydrogenase into several toxic metabolites including glycoaldehyde, glycolic acid, glyoxylic acid, and oxalate. These products take some time to accumulate, and thus signs and symptoms may not appear until 6 to 12 hours after the ingestion. This delay is even more pronounced if ethanol is also ingested because ethanol competes for alcohol dehydrogenase and thereby slows the development of toxic metabolites.
Toxic Dose	The minimal toxic dose is 1 to 2 mL/kg.
Signs and Symptoms	Toxicity is sometimes divided into three phases.

Phase I is from 1 to 12 hours postingestion and typically presents with signs of intoxication without the smell of ethanol (which prehospital care providers should be able to recognize). CNS symptoms may include ataxia, seizures, and nystagmus. Nausea and vomiting are common in Phase I.

Phase II occurs from 12 to 36 hours postingestion and consists of cardiopulmonary toxicity including hypertension, tachycardia, and tachypnea. In severe poisoning pulmonary edema, congestive heart failure, and shock may develop.

Phase III occurs from 24 to 72 hours postingestion and is associated with acute renal toxicity consisting of flank pain, cerebrovascular accident (CVA) tenderness, decreased urine output, and acute renal failure.

Not all patients go through these phases; some can present critically ill early postingestion (i.e., within 12 hours). The fluorescent additive in antifreeze can sometimes be seen excreted in the urine.

Prehospital Management	Supportive care, including airway management, should be provided as required. Intravenous fluid therapy is indicated because dehydration is common and renal perfusion may be compromised. Ethanol therapy is indicated as a means of preventing metabolism to toxic metabolites. Although not widely used in a prehospital care setting, some circumstances (such as long transport times) may warrant the use of oral or IV ethanol therapy. Patients who have been coingesting ethanol have the benefit of having initiated their own therapy.
In-Hospital Management	Supportive care should be provided as in prehospital management. Metabolism to toxic metabolites is limited by administering ethanol as a competitive inhibitor of alcohol dehydrogenase. In this way ethanol allows for excretion of unchanged ethylene glycol without metabolism. The half-life of ethylene glycol is 5 hours, whereas with therapeutic ethanol levels it is increased to approximately 17 hours. Serum ethanol levels are used to determine the need for ethanol therapy, which is usually given intravenously but can be given orally in unusual circumstances. Hemodialysis is indicated in cases of renal failure, in severe metabolic acidosis, or as determined by blood levels. Hypocalcemia can occur and, when present, requires treatment. Magnesium is a cofactor in the conversion to nontoxic metabolites, and magnesium supplementation is sometimes required. Bicarbonate is used in cases of profound acidosis. Pyridoxine is used to help promote conversion of glyoxylic acid to its nontoxic metabolite, glycine.

Iron

Iron overdose is relatively common and tends to be seen most frequently in the pediatric population. Symptoms are highly variable, depending on the time since ingestion. A specific antidote, deferoxamine, is available but is generally reserved for use in the hospital.

Route of Exposure	Oral.
Mechanism of Toxicity	Iron has a direct corrosive effect on gastric and intestinal mucosa that can lead to hemorrhage or perforation. Fluid loss from the gastrointestinal (GI) tract and vasodilation can cause hypotension. Iron is also an intracellular toxin that causes uncoupling of ox-

idative phosphorylation, leading to impaired generation of ATP and cellular death.

Toxic Dose

The toxic dose is somewhat dependent on the form of iron ingested because it is the elemental amount of iron present that is relevant. Ferrous sulfate tablets contain only 20 percent elemental iron per weight, whereas ferrous fumarate contains 33 percent iron by weight. Taking this into account, 20 to 60 mg/kg of elemental iron has moderate risk of toxicity, whereas >60 mg/kg has high risk for toxicity.

Signs and Symptoms

Some authors describe four distinct stages of iron toxicity, and others describe five. The classification based on four stages is presented here.

Stage 1 (1/2 to 2 hours postingestion): Severe vomiting and diarrhea (often with blood), lethargy, coma, pallor, tachycardia, hypotension, acidosis, hyperglycemia, hypovolemia, shock, renal failure, and death.

Stage 2 (2 to 12 hours postingestion): Relatively asymptomatic period.

Stage 3 (12 to 48 hours postingestion): Recurrence of GI symptoms including bloody emesis and diarrhea, GI perforation, coma, seizures, shock, hepatorenal failure, coagulation defects, hypoglycemia, and severe metabolic acidosis.

Stage 4 (beyond 48 hours postingestion): Pyloric (gastric outlet) strictures. In this stage either death or recovery occurs.

Prehospital Management

Treatment is limited to supportive care including airway support and fluid resuscitation in cases of volume depletion.

In-Hospital Management

Supportive care should be provided as in prehospital management. Iron levels are helpful but do not completely rule out iron toxicity, particularly in the later stages. Levels generally peak 3 to 5 hours postingestion, and levels drawn outside this window may be misleading. Iron tablets can often be seen on X ray, and, as such, abdominal X rays may be helpful. Charcoal does not bind iron and is therefore not indicated. Gastric lavage is of limited value because iron can form concretions or bezoars, which are too large to fit in lavage tubing. Whole-bowel irrigation is the decontamination method of choice. Patients with toxic levels or clinical signs and symptoms are treated with deferoxamine, which works by binding with iron to form a water-soluble compound, ferrioxamine, which is renally excreted. A deferoxamine challenge test is sometimes used in which deferoxamine is administered and a change in urine color (vin-rose) is considered diagnostic of a toxic iron ingestion. Charcoal hemoperfusion and exchange transfusions have been used occasionally with some success. Symptomatology always takes precedence over laboratory values in managing cases of suspected iron overdose.

Isopropyl Alcohol

Isopropyl alcohol, commonly known as rubbing alcohol, is a commonly abused toxic alcohol. Although it is far less toxic than methanol or ethylene glycol, in high doses it can induce hypotension unresponsive to conventional therapy and cardiac ischemia.

Route of Exposure	Oral, skin contact, or inhalation.
Mechanism of Toxicity	Isopropyl alcohol is a CNS depressant and vasodilator. In the liver it is metabolized to acetone, which is subsequently excreted by the kidneys.
Toxic Dose	Toxic dose is 0.5 to 1 mL/kg of 70 percent isopropanol (typical concentration).
Signs and Symptoms	Signs of intoxication and CNS depression may appear. It is twice as potent a CNS depressant as ethanol. In severe overdose, hypotension secondary to vasodilation that is largely unresponsive to fluids and pressor therapy can occur. Cardiac ischemia or infarction can occur.
Prehospital Management	Supportive care, including airway management, assisted ventilation, and fluid therapy, should be provided as needed. Gastric lavage and activated charcoal may be indicated for recent ingestions. Ethanol therapy is not indicated.
In-Hospital Management	Supportive care should be provided as in prehospital management. Vasopressor therapy, though of limited value, may be tried. Dialysis is rarely required but may be indicated in cases involving severe, unresponsive hypotension.

Lithium

Lithium is a relatively common medication used in the treatment of certain psychiatric disorders such as bipolar (manic-depressive) disorder. Although overdose is not common, it can be serious. No specific antidote is available, and therapy is generally aimed at enhancing elimination and providing supportive care.

Route of Exposure	Oral.
Mechanism of Toxicity	Lithium replaces sodium, thereby altering cellular processes, membrane structures, response to hormones, and utilization of energy

at a cellular level. In the CNS these effects can result in permanent neurological damage. Lithium is excreted almost entirely by the kidneys. Because it decreases renal function, lithium tends to decrease its own clearance and can in fact enhance its own reabsorption by the kidney.

Toxic Dose
The toxic dose is highly variable depending on whether it is an acute or chronic ingestion. Overdose in the setting of chronic ingestion tends to be more severe because serum lithium levels are already high, allowing lithium to enter cells (predominantly CNS) more readily. Toxicity is generally more severe in the setting of poor underlying renal function, diuretic use, and dehydration.

Signs and Symptoms
Signs and symptoms are variable depending on levels.

Low (serum levels less than 1.5 mEq/L): GI symptoms including nausea, vomiting, and diarrhea.

Moderate (serum levels 1.5 to 3.0 mEq/L): Polyuria followed by urinary and fecal incontinence, muscle weakness (which can progress to myoclonic twitches and muscle rigidity with choreoathetoid movements), and neurological symptoms (which can include restlessness, vertigo, slurred speech, blurred vision, and coma).

Severe (serum levels >3.0 mEq/L): Seizures, coma, cardiac arrhythmias, hypotension with peripheral vascular collapse, muscle twitching, and spasticity.

Prehospital Management
Supportive care should be provided as indicated. Virtually all patients with lithium overdoses are volume depleted, and aggressive fluid resuscitation using normal saline is indicated. It remains unclear whether the administration of sodium chloride aids elimination.

In-Hospital Management
Lavage may be helpful if less than 1 hour has elapsed from the time of ingestion. Whole-bowel irrigation has also been shown to be beneficial. Correction of volume depletion is essential and can take several hours. Hemodialysis is indicated in cases of renal failure, of severe cardiovascular or neurological abnormalities, or with high serum levels.

Methanol

Methanol is found in many solutions including wood alcohol, window washer fluid, paint solvent, and industrial solvents. Ingestion is generally accidental, and small doses can be fatal. Although virtually any organ system can be involved, visual disturbances including blindness remain the clinical hallmark. Toxicity is dependent on the formation of toxic metabolites, and thus toxicity is generally delayed for several hours.

Route of Exposure	Generally oral but can be dermal or by inhalation.
Mechanism of Toxicity	Toxic metabolites, predominantly formaldehyde and formic acid, are formed through the metabolism of methanol by alcohol dehydrogenase. These toxic metabolites have direct toxic effects at a cellular level and result in a profound acidosis that can further accelerate toxicity. Methanol is metabolized by alcohol dehydrogenase to form formaldehyde, which in turn is converted to fomic acid by aldehyde dehydrogenase. Up to 5 percent of ingested methanol may be excreted unchanged by the kidneys and via respiration.
Toxic Dose	Death has been reported with as little as 15 to 30 mL (1 to 2 tablespoons).
Signs and Symptoms	An initial latent period ranging from 6 to 30 hours consists of signs of intoxication and gastrointestinal irritation. Some patients may have a prolonged asymptomatic period, particularly if ethanol has been coingested. Caution must be used, because a lack of symptoms early on does not preclude toxicity.
	As toxic metabolites are formed, nausea, vomiting, abdominal pain, and CNS symptoms (ranging from headache and confusion to coma) occur. Ocular toxicity is the hallmark of methanol overdose and can manifest as decreased visual acuity (haziness or "snowfield blindness").
	Death is generally related to profound acidosis and severe CNS effects including cerebral edema. Gastrointestinal bleeding secondary to gastritis can occur.
Prehospital Management	Supportive care, including airway management, should be provided as indicated. As with ethylene glycol, oral or IV ethanol therapy has been utilized in some prehospital care settings. Gastric lavage is sometimes used in recent ingestions. Charcoal is not helpful.
In-Hospital Management	Diagnosis can be difficult because blood levels are not always available or reliable at the time of presentation. Laboratory investigation generally reveals an anion gap metabolic acidosis, as well as an osmolar gap. Supportive care augmented by intravenous ethanol therapy is the mainstay of therapy. Hemodialysis is indicated in the presence of visual symptoms,

severe acidosis, high serum levels, or an ingestion of greater than 30 mL. Bicarbonate is reserved for cases of profound acidosis. Folate is a cofactor for the conversion of formate to nontoxic by-products and has a role in therapy.

Narcotics and Opioids

Narcotics and opioids are widely used for both medicinal and therapeutic purposes. Overdoses are common, especially in large urban centers. Recognition of these overdoses is important, because a specific antidote (naloxone) is available in most prehospital settings. In hospital settings, Revex, a long-acting opioid antagonist, may be given.

Route of Exposure	Oral, intravenous, intramuscular, or dermal.
Mechanism of Toxicity	Narcotics and opioids act directly on opiate receptors within the CNS, causing CNS depression. Some opioids have mixed agonist and antagonist properties.
Signs and Symptoms	The classic triad of opioid overdose consists of miosis, respiratory depression, and decreased level of consciousness. Certain types of opioids (e.g., meperidine, morphine, propoxyphene, and pentazocine) can present with mydriasis rather than miosis. Occasionally seizures, hypotension and ventricular arrhythmias can be seen.
Prehospital Management	Supportive care, including airway management, takes priority over naloxone therapy. Track marks (IV) are helpful diagnostically when present and should always be examined. Following assessment and initial stabilization, early use of naloxone (Narcan) may avert the need for invasive airway control. Patients with opioid overdose can rapidly become combative and violent when given naloxone, and precautions need to be taken to ensure that both the patient and care providers are adequately protected from injury. This may include prophylactic use of restraints. Response to naloxone is often effective for diagnosis as well as treatment.
In-Hospital Management	Supportive care and naloxone therapy are provided as described earlier. Long periods of observation are often required to ensure that sedation does not recur. The duration of action of intravenous naloxone is typically 20 to 60 minutes, which is considerably shorter than the duration of action of most opioids (typically 3 to 6 hours). In cases of severe, prolonged opioid toxicity, continuous naloxone infusion may be indicated.

NALOXONE (NARCAN)

Class: Narcotic antagonist

Description

Naloxone is an effective narcotic antagonist. It has proved effective in the management and reversal of overdoses caused by narcotics or synthetic narcotic agents.

Mechanism of Action

Naloxone is chemically similar to the narcotics. However, it has only antagonistic properties. Naloxone competes for opiate receptors in the brain. It also displaces narcotic molecules from opiate receptors. It can reverse respiratory depression associated with narcotic overdose.

Indications

Naloxone is used for the complete or partial reversal of depression caused by narcotics including the following agents: morphine, Demerol, heroin, paregoric, Dilaudid, codeine, Percodan, fentanyl, and methadone. It is also used for the complete or partial reversal of depression caused by synthetic narcotic analgesic agents including the following drugs: Nubain, Talwin, Stadol, and Darvon. Naloxone may be used in the treatment of coma of unknown origin.

Contraindications

Naloxone should not be administered to a patient with a history of hypersensitivity to the drug.

Precautions

Naloxone should be administered cautiously to patients who are known or suspected to be physically dependent on narcotics. Abrupt and complete reversal by naloxone can cause withdrawal-type effects. This includes newborn infants of mothers with known or suspected narcotic dependence.

Side Effects

Side effects associated with naloxone are rare. However, hypotension, hypertension, ventricular arrhythmias, nausea, and vomiting have been reported.

Interactions

Naloxone may cause narcotic withdrawal in the narcotic-dependent patient. In cases of suspected narcotic dependence, only enough of the drug to reverse respiratory depression should be administered.

Dosage

The standard dosage for suspected or confirmed narcotic or synthetic narcotic overdoses is 1 to 2 mg administered IV. If unsuccessful, then a second dose may be administered 5 minutes later. Failure to obtain reversal after two to three doses indicates another disease process or overdosage on nonopioid drugs. Larger than average doses (2 to 5 mg) have been used in the management of Darvon overdoses and alcoholic coma. An intravenous infusion can be prepared by placing 2 mg of naloxone in 500 mL of D_5W. This gives a concentration of 4 µg/mL; 100 mL/hr should be infused, thus delivering 0.4 mg/hr. In the emergency setting, naloxone should be administered intravenously only. When an IV line cannot be established, intramuscular or subcutaneous administration can be performed. Naloxone can be administered endotracheally. The dose should be increased to 2.0 to 2.5 times the intravenous dose. Furthermore, naloxone should be diluted in enough normal saline to provide a total of 10 mL of fluid.

How Supplied

Naloxone is supplied in ampules and prefilled syringes containing 2 mg in 2 mL of solvent. In addition, vials containing 10 mL of the 1 mg/mL concentration are also available.

NALMEFENE (REVEX)

Class: Opioid antagonist

Description

Revex is an opioid antagonist used for the reversal (partial or complete) of opioid effects, including respiratory and CNS depression.

Mechanism of Action

Revex completely blocks the effects of opioids, including CNS and respiratory depression, without producing any agonist (opioid-like) effects.

Indications

Revex is used for reversal of opioid effects and management of known or suspected opioid overdose.

Contraindications

Revex should be avoided in patients with known hypersensitivity.

Precautions

Overdose of long-acting opioids may require repeat dosing. Revex should be used with caution in pregnant patients and patients known to be dependent on opioid agents.

Side Effects

Side effects include dysphoria, headache, hypertension, hypotension, tachycardia, vasodilation, abdominal cramps, nausea, joint pain, myalgia, chills, fever, and postoperative pain.

Interactions

No significant interactions have been noted.

Dosage

Adults are administered 0.5 μg/70 kg IV followed by incremental doses of 1.0 μg/70 kg every 2 to 5 minutes (up to a total dose of 1.5 μg/kg).

How Supplied

Revex is supplied as 100 μg/mL (blue label) and 1 mg/mL (green label).

Organophosphates and Carbamides

Organophosphates and carbamides are commonly found in commercial insecticides. Although rare, toxic exposure to these agents is generally serious and often fatal. Diagnosis is frequently difficult because of the subtle nature of many exposures and generalized symptoms. A contaminated piece of clothing may prolong exposure over several days, further confusing the diagnosis. Atropine is widely used and can be highly effective for treatment of poisoning secondary to these agents.

Route of Exposure	Dermal, oral, ocular, or by inhalation.
Mechanism of Toxicity	Organophosphates and carbamides inhibit acetylcholinesterase activity, leading to increased acetylcholine at nerve synapses and an initial overstimulation followed by disruption of transmission in the CNS, parasympathetic nerve endings and some sympathetic nerve endings, somatic nerve endings, and autonomic ganglia.
Toxic Dose	Highly variable; toxicity can occur with minimal exposure. Recurrent exposure secondary to contaminated clothing is common.
Signs and Symptoms	The CNS symptoms include agitation, drowsiness, seizures, cardiorespiratory depression, coma, and death. The mnemonic DUMBELS can be used to describe the muscarinic signs and symptoms of cholinergic excess, and the mnemonic MTWtHF is used to describe the nicotinic features (see description under "Toxidromes") earlier in this chapter. Miosis is typically present, but in 10 percent of cases mydriasis is present. The history is not always clear in identifying an exposure. A garlic odor may be present.
Prehospital Management	As with all toxicological emergencies, supportive care must be provided immediately. Atropine in doses of 0.5 to 1 mg every 2 to 5 minutes (maximum of 100 mg) reverses the cholinergic symptoms. End points for atropine therapy include drying of secretions, reversal of bradycardia, and pupillary mydriasis. It is important to monitor ventilation closely because diaphragmatic weakness is not treated by atropine.

Extreme care must be taken to avoid contamination of care providers by removal of contaminated clothing and use of gloves and gowns (where available). Contaminated clothing should be removed as soon as practically possible.

In-Hospital Management | Supportive care should be provided as in prehospital management. Additional therapies include the use of pralidoxime (2-PAM), which acts to regenerate acetylcholinesterase. Charcoal and lavage may be indicated for oral ingestions.

Salicylates

Salicylate (ASA) overdose is commonly encountered and can be fatal if not treated appropriately. These agents are found in a variety of over-the-counter medications and are frequently confused with other analgesics such as ibuprofen and acetaminophen. The clinical presentation is variable depending on the time since ingestion. Although a specific antidote is not available, therapy is aimed at enhancing elimination and thereby preventing long-term sequelae.

Route of Exposure	Oral; occasionally dermal.
Mechanism of Toxicity	Salicylates cause cellular toxicity through the uncoupling of oxidative phosphorylation and induce anion gap metabolic acidosis.
Metabolism	Salicylates are extensively metabolized by the liver; inactive metabolites are excreted by the kidneys.
Toxic Dose	Acute:
	150 to 300 mg/kg = mild to moderate toxicity
	>300 mg/kg = moderate to severe toxicity
	Chronic: Variable
Signs and Symptoms	Mild to moderate: Tachypnea, vomiting, diaphoresis, tinnitus, and acid-base disturbances. The tachypnea is typically early in the course of overdose and can result in an early respiratory alkalosis.
	Severe: CNS abnormalities ranging from confusion and delirium to coma secondary to cerebral edema, hypoglycemia (rare), pulmonary edema, coagulopathies and platelet dysfunction, and occasionally hyperthermia. An anion gap metabolic acidosis is the classic acid-base disturbance in the later stages of toxicity. Renal failure is possible.
Prehospital Management	Supportive care, including airway management, should be provided as required. Activated charcoal may be used. Hypoglycemia should be ruled out (especially in children).

In-Hospital Management	Toxicity is determined both by clinical criteria and by plotting blood levels taken at least 6 hours postingestion on the Done nomogram. The nomogram is a guideline only and is not useful for chronic toxicity. A single serum salicylate value is not always conclusive, and repeat levels aimed at determining half-lives are sometimes required. When toxicity is suspected by history and physical exam, therapy is initiated regardless of availability of serum levels. Gastric lavage is utilized in early presentations. Multidose activated charcoal has been shown to decrease absorbtion and toxicity. Renal excretion of salicylate is enhanced by inducing an alkaline diuresis. This is typically accomplished using an IV solution consisting of sodium bicarbonate mixed in D_5W. Potassium supplementation is often required. Hemodialysis is indicated in severe toxicity associated with renal failure, severe CNS or cardiac dysfunction, or severe acidosis not responsive to the alkaline diuresis.

SSRIs

Selective serotonin reuptake inhibitors (SSRIs) are the newest generation of antidepressant agents and are currently prescribed more frequently than more traditional antidepressants such as tricyclics. The popularity of these agents is largely attributable to their improved safety profile, particularly in the setting of overdose. Prototypical agents include fluoxetine (Prozac), trazadone, sertraline, and paroxetine.

Route of Exposure	Oral.
Mechanism of Toxicity	SSRIs block reuptake of serotonin at the presynaptic junction.
Toxic Dose	The toxic dose is variable, but the SSRIs are generally well tolerated even in large overdoses. If used in combination with a monoamine oxidase inhibitor (MAOI) the serotonin syndrome, which is potentially fatal, can occur.
Signs and Symptoms	Overdose with SSRIs is often asymptomatic. Symptoms and signs include agitation, insomnia, CNS excitation, tachycardia, hypertension, and ST depression. Serotonin syndrome can occur when the drug is used in combination with MAOIs. Serotonin syndrome can include hyperthermia, shivering, tremor, myoclonus, seizures, delirium, agitation, rigidity or hypertonia, autonomic instability, coma, and death.
Prehospital Treatment	Only supportive care is provided; no specific treatment is available.

| In-Hospital Treatment | Supportive care is supplemented by activated charcoal and lavage (if less than 1 hour postingestion). |
| | Serotonin syndrome may require aggressive airway management, assisted ventilation, and pharmacological therapy including IV Dantrolene or oral cyproheptadine. Seizures are treated with benzodiazepines, and hypertension can be treated with calcium channel blockers such as nifedipine. |

SUMMARY

Paramedics must be diligent in the assessment and treatment of suspected overdose without a high index of suspicion, even the most obvious clues can go unnoticed. By reviewing the general principles of toxicology, the paramedic will be better prepared to treat these emergencies.

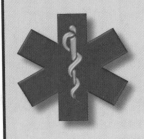

CASE PRESENTATION

Paramedics are dispatched at 14:30 hours on a weekday to a residence in an older neighborhood. Enroute the call taker provides further information. The patient is a 4-year-old female who is unconscious. On arrival a woman in her late 60s runs out of the house carrying a flaccid, unresponsive 4-year-old child.

On Examination

CNS: The child is unresponsive. Her pupils are dilated and unresponsive to light. She is unresponsive to voice and pain.

Resp: Respirations are agonal at 4 per minute and shallow. Her lungs are clear bilaterally with equal air entry. The trachea is midline and there are no signs of trauma.

CVS: The carotid pulse is present, but weak. The radial pulse is absent. Her skin is pale, with cyanotic/gray color to face. Skin is cool, and dry.

ABD: Soft and non-tender in all 4 quadrants. There are no signs of vomiting or diarrhea.

Musc/Skel: No injuries are noted.

Vital Signs:

Pulse: 40 per minute

Resp: 4 per minute and shallow

B/P: 30/?? mmHg

SpO$_2$: error

ECG: 3rd degree block

Past Hx: The grandmother states that she put her granddaughter down for a nap around 14:00 hours. At about 14:30 she checked on her granddaughter and found her on the floor of the grandmother's bedroom. The girl was unconscious and unresponsive with an open bottle of heart pills beside her. The grandmother called 911. The prescription is for Isoptin (verapamil) 120 mg. There are 10–12 pills on the floor. The bottle of 60 is empty.

The granddaughter has no previous illnesses and is in good health. She is not taking any medications, nor does she have any allergies.

Treatment

An OPA is inserted and the patient's respirations are assisted by a bag-valve-mask device with 100% oxygen via a reservoir bag. The patient is placed on a cardiac monitor, which shows a third degree block. A weak pulse is still present. An intravenous line is initiated with a 20 gauge catheter in the ante cubital fossa.

At the earliest moment, paramedics contact the poison control center for advice.

The patient is given fluid bolus of 20 mL/kg. The patient is approximately 25 kg so a bolus of 500mL is administered. If perfusion does not improve with the bolus the paramedics will, in consultation with poison control, administer calcium chloride 10% at 10–25 mg/kg diluted to 50 mL and given over 5 minutes. If calcium was not available, paramedics would consider epinephrine 0.01 mg/kg administered slow IV push.

The patient is prepared for transcutaneous pacing. Since this patient weighs more than 15 kg, the adult pads should work. Although this is unusual in children, the paramedics feel it is indicated because of the profound symptoms and may be required if the patient does not respond to medications. The paramedics realize that atropine does not work on third degree heart blocks.

Outcome

The patient responded to medications and her heart rate increased to 100 with a junctional rhythm. She was transferred to ICU where she battled an aspiration pneumonia and liver failure (secondary to verapamil). She was eventually discharged from hospital with no complications.

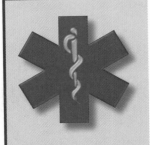

CASE PRESENTATION

Early one evening Waterville EMS is called to a residence in an up-scale area of the city. Dispatch reports that they are responding to a "man down," unconscious, unresponsive, and not breathing. On arrival a woman in her 20s meets the paramedics and states that her boyfriend is not breathing. Paramedics are led to the living room, where they find a male in his mid-20s lying supine on the floor. There is emesis near the patient.

On Examination

CNS: The patient is unresponsive; Glasgow Coma Scale score is 3; both pupils are pinpoint yet equal

Resp: Respirations are 6 per minute and very shallow; the airway has residue from vomiting

CVS: The carotid pulse is slow and weak; the radial pulse is absent; skin is pale; lips are blue

ABD: Soft and nontender in all four quadrants; the patient has vomited

Muscl/Skel: No apparent injuries; no pitting edema

Vital Signs

Pulse: 56/min

Resp: 6/min

B/P: 70/52 mm Hg

SpO$_2$: 72 percent

ECG: Sinus bradycardia

Past Hx: Initially the patient's girlfriend states that she does not know what happened. She states that her boyfriend is very healthy, has no medical problems, and does not take any medication. Paramedics specifically ask about alcohol or recreational drugs. The girlfriend emphatically states, "No."

Treatment

Police backup is requested. The initial treatment begins with the ABCs. The airway is suctioned, and an oropharyngeal airway is placed. Ventilation by bag-valve-mask device and 100 percent oxygen by reservoir bag is initiated at 24 breaths per minute. Airway compliance is good. An IV of normal saline is prepared and paramedics perform venipuncture with a 16-gauge catheter. Blood is drawn for a red-top tube, and the hub of the needle is used to obtain a blood sample for glucose testing. The IV of normal saline is connected to the catheter, and the fluid is administered at 100 mL/hr.

As one paramedic starts the IV, she looks for previous needle marks and does not find any. The absence of needle marks does not change the paramedic's assessment. Based on the age of the patient (a male in his mid-20s does not just stop breathing), the slow respirations, and the pinpoint pupils, the paramedic is fairly certain that the patient has taken a narcotic or some designer drug.

The patient's girlfriend is questioned once again as to whether her boyfriend uses any drugs. The paramedic tells her that her boyfriend's condition is very serious and that she must be absolutely honest. Finally the girlfriend states that her boyfriend uses heroin. She found him on the floor when she came home and then called for the ambulance after she hid the drugs and syringes.

At this point the police arrive and assist the paramedics. The patient is moved to the stretcher and restrained. The paramedics are concerned for their safety because the patient may be aggressive or violent as he comes out of the coma. His airway is still patent, and intubation is not required at this time. Narcan is administered intravenously in 1.0 mg dosages. The paramedics carefully titrate the dose to increase the respiratory rate. The stretcher and patient are moved to the ambulance, and a police officer agrees to accompany the paramedics to the hospital. The patient is not fighting against the bag-valve-mask device or straining against the restraints. The patient's girlfriend gives the paramedics the rest of the drugs and the syringe.

En route to the hospital a paramedic monitors the patient's vital signs closely. Respirations increase to 20 per minute, and the patient is placed on oxygen by nonrebreather mask at 12 L/min. The pulse rate increases to 112 per minute, and blood pressure increases to 124/82 mm Hg. The blood glucose reading is 125 mg/dL (7.0 mmol/L). The half-life of Narcan is likely to be less than that of the narcotic. Thus, the patient's level of consciousness may decrease. On arrival at the hospital, the patient is conscious and verbally abusive and has stable vital signs. While awaiting the results of laboratory tests, the patient gets up, sneaks out the back door, and leaves the emergency department unseen.

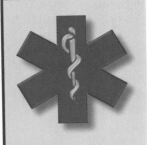

CASE PRESENTATION

Paramedics are called to meet the police at a local motel, where they have found an unconscious person in one of the motel suites. On arrival, several police officers escort paramedics to the room, where they find a 42-year-old male lying supine on the bed. He appears to have been alone in the room, and there is an empty bottle of whiskey lying on the floor next to the bed.

On Examination

CNS: The patient is unresponsive; his pupils are pinpoint and unresponsive to light

Resp: Respirations are 4 per minute and shallow; lungs are clear bilaterally, with equal air entry; trachea is midline; no signs of trauma

CVS: The carotid pulse is present but weak; the radial pulse is absent; skin is pale, cool, and dry, with dry mucous membranes

ABD: Soft and nontender in all four quadrants; no signs of vomiting or diarrhea

Muscl/Skel: No injuries are noted

Vital Signs

Pulse: 124/min

Resp: 4/min and shallow

BP: 70/40 mm Hg

SpO$_2$: 80 percent

ECG: Sinus tachycardia

Past Hx: The police state that the patient had called his wife earlier in the evening and had threatened to kill himself. His wife then called the police, who managed to track the patient down to this motel. The patient's wife told the police that the patient had been suffering from depression for the past couple of months and had recently begun to drink heavily. The police found two empty pill bottles in the bathroom. One bottle contained amitriptyline (Elavil), and the other contained meperidine (Demerol). Both prescriptions had been filled recently.

Treatment

An OPA is inserted, and the patient's respirations are assisted by a bag-valve-mask device with 100 percent oxygen via a reservoir bag. The patient is placed on a cardiac monitor, which shows a sinus tachycardia with widened QRS complexes at 0.16 mm width. An intravenous line is initiated with a 16-gauge catheter, and a solution of normal saline is run wide open (20 mL/kg fluid bolus); 100 mEq sodium bicarbonate is administered along with 2 mg naloxone. The patient is prepared for transport to the hospital with the assistance of the police. Following the administration of the sodium bicarbonate, the QRS complexes eventually narrow to 0.12 mm. However, the patient's level of consciousness does not change. Once in the ambulance, the patient is intubated. The patient's condition remains unchanged during transport to the hospital. On arrival at the hospital, the patient is treated with gastric lavage and activated charcoal and then admitted to ICU.

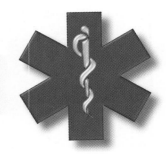

chapter 13

Drugs Used in the Treatment of Behavioral Emergencies

OBJECTIVES

After completing this chapter, the reader should be able to

1. Define the term *behavioral emergency.*
2. List the intrapsychic causes of altered behavior.
3. Explain interpersonal and environmental causes of behavioral emergencies.
4. Explain organic causes of behavioral emergencies.
5. Describe and list the indications, contraindications, and dosages for the following drugs used in behavioral emergencies: haloperidol, droperidol, chlorpromazine, diazepam, and hydroxyzine.

INTRODUCTION

Behavioral emergencies rarely require pharmacological intervention during the prehospital phase of emergency medical care. There are situations, however, in which emergency personnel may be called on to administer a sedative or similar agent. Among these are acute anxiety reactions and paranoid psychoses. Occasionally, it may be necessary to administer a sedative to friends or family of a patient who has been severely injured or who has recently died.

UNDERSTANDING BEHAVIORAL EMERGENCIES

A *behavioral emergency* is an intrapsychic, environmental, situational, or organic alteration that results in behavior that cannot be tolerated by the patient or other members of society. It usually requires immediate attention.

Intrapsychic Causes

Intrapsychic causes of altered behavior arise from problems within the person. Such behavior usually results from an acute stage of an underlying psychiatric condition. A wide range of behaviors can be manifested, including depression, withdrawal, catatonia, violence, suicidal acts, homicidal acts, paranoid reactions, phobias, hysterical conversion, disorientation, and disorganization. In the field, behavioral emergencies resulting from intrapsychic causes are less common than those resulting from other causes, such as alcohol or drug abuse.

Interpersonal and Environmental Causes

Interpersonal and *environmental causes* of behavioral emergencies result from reactions to stimuli outside the person. They often result from overwhelming and stressful incidents, such as the death of a loved one, rape, or a disaster. The change in behavior can frequently be linked to a specific incident or series of incidents. The range of behavior manifested is broad, and a patient's specific symptoms often relate to the type of incident that precipitated them.

Organic Causes

An *organic cause* of altered behavior results from a disturbance in the patient's physical or biochemical state. Such disturbances include drug or substance abuse, alcohol abuse, trauma, medical illness, and dementia. The area of the brain affected by the disturbance determines the type of behavior change.

It is important to consider the possibility of organic disease in *all* behavioral emergencies. As a result, physical assessment of patients with aberrant behavior is extremely important. It may uncover unsuspected causes of the altered behavior, such as drug or alcohol abuse, hypoxia, hypoglycemia, head injury, or meningitis. Common agents used in the acute treatment of behavioral emergencies include haloperidol (Haldol), chlorpromazine (Thorazine), diazepam (Valium), and hydroxyzine (Vistaril).

HALOPERIDOL (HALDOL)

Class: Antipsychotic and neuroleptic

Description

Haloperidol is a frequently used major tranquilizer.

Mechanism of Action

Haloperidol is a major tranquilizer that has proved effective in the management of acute psychotic episodes. It has pharmacological properties similar to those of the phenothiazine class of drugs (e.g., Thorazine). Haloperidol appears to block dopamine receptors in the brain associated with mood and behavior. However, its precise mechanism of action is not clearly understood. Haloperidol has weak anticholinergic properties.

Indication

Haloperidol is used in acute psychotic episodes.

Contraindications

Haloperidol should not be administered in cases in which other drugs, especially sedatives, may be present. It should not be used in the management of dysphoria caused by Talwin because it may promote sedation and anesthesia.

Precautions

Haloperidol may impair mental and physical abilities. Occasionally, orthostatic hypotension may be seen in conjunction with haloperidol use. Caution should be used when administering haloperidol to patients taking anticoagulants. Extrapyramidal or dystonic reactions have been known to occur following the administration of haloperidol, especially in children. Diphenhydramine (Benadryl) should be readily available.

Side Effects

Haloperidol can cause extrapyramidal symptoms (EPS), insomnia, restlessness, drowsiness, seizures, respiratory depression, dry mouth, constipation, hypotension, and tachycardia.

Interactions

Antihypertensive medications may increase the likelihood of a patient developing hypotension with haloperidol administration. Haloperidol should be used with caution in patients taking lithium, because irreversible brain damage (encephalopathic syndrome) has been reported when these two drugs are used together.

Dosage

Doses of 2 to 5 mg administered intramuscularly are fairly standard in the management of an acute psychotic episode with severe symptoms. Haloperidol should be given intramuscularly only.

How Supplied

Haloperidol is supplied in 1 mL ampules containing 5 mg of the drug.

DROPERIDOL (INAPSINE)

Class: Tranquilizer and general anesthesia

Description

Droperidol produces marked tranquilization and sedation. It allays anxiety and provides a mental state of detachment and indifference while maintaining a state of reflex alertness. The effects of droperidol are rapid in onset and of relatively short duration; the onset of action of single intramuscular (IM) and intravenous (IV) doses is from 3 to 10 minutes following administration, although the peak effect may not be apparent for up to 30 minutes. Tranquilizing and sedative activity diminishes within 2 to 4 hours, although alteration of consciousness may persist up to 12 hours and extrapyramidal symptoms occasionally last up to 24 hours. Droperidol potentiates other central nervous system (CNS) depressants.

Mechanism of Action

Droperidol produces mild alpha-adrenergic blockade, peripheral vascular dilatation, and reduction of the pressor effect of epinephrine. It can produce hypotension and decrease peripheral vascular resistance. It is a butyrophenone neuroleptic similar to haloperidol (Haldol), reduces anxiety and produces a state of mental detachment, and has antiemetic and antinauseant properties. Onset of action ranges from 3 to 10 minutes (IM) and lasts from 2 to 4 hours, although an altered level of consciousness may persist for up to 12 hours.

Indications

Droperidol is used in rapid tranquilization (chemical restraint) and anesthesia for premedication, induction, and maintenance.

Contraindications

Droperidol is contraindicated in patients with hypotension, known allergies to butyrophenones, and known anticholinergic poisoning.

Precautions

Patients' blood pressure and respiratory status should be monitored frequently. Patients should be restrained in a fashion that allows careful observation and the ability to breathe normally.

Side Effects

Extrapyramidal or dystonic reactions have been known to occur following the administration of droperidol, especially in children. Diphenhydramine (Benadryl) should be readily available. Droperidol can cause restlessness, drowsiness, hallucination, depression, shivering, laryngospasm, bronchospasm, and tachycardia.

Interactions

Antihypertensive medications may increase the likelihood of a patient developing hypotension with haloperidol administration.

Dosage

Patients 14 to 60 years of age should receive 5 mg IM with or without 2 mg midazolam IM in the same syringe; the dose of droperidol can be repeated once in 15 minutes as needed. Patients over age 60 years of age should receive 2.5 mg IM with or without 2 mg midazolam in the same syringe; the dose of droperidol can be repeated once in 15 minutes as needed.

How Supplied

Droperidol is supplied as 2.5 mg/mL in 2 mL brown glass vials.

Notes: Rapid tranquilization has been shown to be effective and safe for controlling patients who are agitated, potentially assaultive, destructive, or overly violent.

Droperidol is administered IM at a gluteal site. It may be given directly through the patient's clothing in situations of restraint when undressing the patient is not possible.

CHLORPROMAZINE (THORAZINE, LARGACTIL)

Class: Antipsychotic and neuroleptic

Description

Chlorpromazine is an antipsychotic and neuroleptic used in the management of severe psychotic episodes.

Mechanism of Action

Chlorpromazine is a member of the phenothiazine class of drugs. Phenothiazine drugs are thought to block dopamine receptors in the brain that are associated with behavior and mood. Chlorpromazine is also effective in the management of mild alcohol withdrawal and intractable hiccoughs. It is also effective in treating nausea and vomiting, although more appropriate agents are available.

Indications

Chlorpromazine is used in acute psychotic episodes, mild alcohol withdrawal, intractable hiccoughs, and nausea and vomiting.

Contraindications

Chlorpromazine should not be administered to patients in comatose states or who have recently taken a large amount of sedatives. Chlorpromazine should not be administered to patients who may have recently taken hallucinogens because it tends to promote seizures.

Precautions

Chlorpromazine may impair mental and physical abilities. Occasionally, orthostatic hypotension may be seen in conjunction with chlorpromazine use. Extrapyramidal or dystonic reactions have been known to occur following the administration of chlorpromazine, especially in children. Diphenhydramine should be readily available.

Side Effects

Chlorpromazine can cause dry mouth, constipation, blurred vision, dry eyes, sedation, headache, drowsiness, hypotension, and tachycardia.

Interactions

Antihypertensive medications may increase the likelihood of a patient developing hypotension with chlorpromazine administration.

Dosage

The standard dose of chlorpromazine in the management of an acute psychotic episode is 25 to 50 mg administered intramuscularly. Intractable hiccoughs will usually respond to a 25 mg dose of chlorpromazine. Chlorpromazine should only be administered intramuscularly by paramedics.

How Supplied

Chlorpromazine is supplied in 1 and 2 mL ampules containing 25 mg/mL.

 ## DIAZEPAM (VALIUM)

Class: Sedative, anticonvulsant, and antianxiety agent

Description

Diazepam is a benzodiazepine that is frequently used as a sedative, hypnotic, and anticonvulsant.

Mechanism of Action

Diazepam, one of the most frequently prescribed medications in the United States, is used in the management of anxiety and stress. It is effective in treating the tremors and anxiety associated with alcohol withdrawal. It is also an effective skeletal muscle relaxant, which makes it an effective adjunct in orthopedic injuries. It is a good premedication for minor operative procedures and cardioversion because it induces amnesia, which diminishes the patient's recall of such procedures. In emergency medicine, diazepam is principally used for its anticonvulsant properties. It suppresses the spread of seizure activity through the motor cortex of the brain. It does not appear to abolish the abnormal discharge focus, however.

Indications

Diazepam is used in acute anxiety states, as a premedication before cardioversion, as a skeletal muscle relaxant, in major motor seizures, and in status epilepticus.

Contraindications

Diazepam should not be administered to any patient with a history of hypersensitivity to the drug.

Precautions

Because diazepam is a relatively short-acting drug, seizure activity may recur. In such cases, an additional dose may be required. Flumazenil

(Romazicon), a benzodiazepine antagonist, should be available to use as an antidote if required. Injectable diazepam can cause local venous irritation. To minimize irritation, it should only be injected into relatively large veins and should not be given faster than 1 mL/min.

Side Effects

Diazepam can cause hypotension, tachycardia, drowsiness, headache, amnesia, hallucinations, respiratory depression, blurred vision, nausea, and vomiting.

Interactions

Diazepam is incompatible with many medications. Whenever diazepam is given intravenously in conjunction with other drugs, the IV line should be adequately flushed. The effects of diazepam can be additive when used in conjunction with other CNS depressants and alcohol.

Dosage

In acute anxiety reactions, the standard dosage is 2 to 5 mg administered intramuscularly or intravenously. To induce amnesia prior to cardioversion, a dosage of 5 to 15 mg of diazepam is given intravenously. Peak effects are seen in 5 to 10 minutes. Diazepam should be given intravenously by slow IV push. It can be injected intramuscularly, but absorption via this route is variable. When an IV line cannot be started, parenteral diazepam can be administered rectally with a similar onset of action. In the management of seizures, the usual dose of diazepam is 5 to 10 mg administered IV. In many instances it may be necessary to give diazepam directly into the vein, because the seizure activity will prevent the insertion of an indwelling catheter. When given directly into a vein, it is essential that a large vein, preferably in the antecubital fossa, be used.

How Supplied

Valium is supplied in ampules and prefilled syringes containing 10 mg in 2 mL of solvent.

HYDROXYZINE (VISTARIL, ATARAX)

Class: Antianxiety agent and sedative

Description

Hydroxyzine is an antianxiety and sedative agent with sedative properties. It is a versatile drug used frequently in emergency medicine.

Mechanism of Action

Hydroxyzine is chemically unrelated to the phenothiazines. Because of its antihistamine properties, hydroxyzine has been shown to exert a calming effect during acute psychotic states. It is an effective antiemetic and muscle relaxant. When administered concurrently with many analgesics, it tends to potentiate their effects.

Indications

Hydroxyzine is used to potentiate the effects of narcotics and synthetic narcotics, for nausea and vomiting, and for anxiety reactions.

Contraindications

Hydroxyzine should not be administered to any patient with a history of hypersensitivity to the drug.

Precautions

Hydroxyzine is given by intramuscular injection only. When administered concomitantly with analgesics, the potentiating effects of hydroxyzine should be kept in mind, and the total analgesic dose should be adjusted accordingly.

Side Effects

Hydroxyzine can cause sedation, dizziness, headache, dry mouth, and seizures.

Interactions

The sedative effects of hydroxyzine can be potentiated by CNS depressants such as narcotics, other antihistamines, sedatives, hypnotics, and alcohol.

Dosage

The standard dosage of hydroxyzine in the management of an acute anxiety reaction is 50 to 100 mg administered intramuscularly. The standard antiemetic dose is 25 to 50 mg. Hydroxyzine should be administered by intramuscular injection. Localized burning is a common complaint following an injection of hydroxyzine.

How Supplied

Hydroxyzine is supplied in single-dose vials containing 25 or 50 mg in 1 mL. Because the vials resemble each other, it is important to recheck the label to ensure the correct dose is delivered to the patient.

SUMMARY

It is important to consider and rule out physical causes for bizarre behavior before determining that a patient's disorder is of psychiatric origin. Diabetes, head injury, and alcohol intoxication can cause bizarre behavior easily mistaken for psychosis. The psychotic patient is best handled in an emergency department by personnel skilled in psychiatric intervention. However, some patients may require pharmacological intervention before transport is possible.

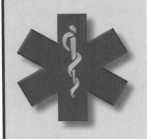

CASE PRESENTATION

Early on a Saturday morning paramedics are dispatched to a local residence for a 40-year-old male patient who is acting violently toward his family members. On arrival paramedics are met by the patient's wife and son, who state they were having breakfast when the patient suddenly "snapped." They state that he keeps talking about how everyone is out to get him and that he seems to think that everyone is part of a conspiracy to "frame" him. His wife and son have tried unsuccessfully to calm him down, but he is getting more aggressive toward them with each attempt to talk to him. Just prior to the arrival of the ambulance, he punched his son and told him "they" would have to kill him before he would leave his house. The police are on the way to back the paramedics up. When the police arrive a few minutes later, paramedics approach the patient. He is standing in the kitchen yelling at everyone to get out before he "kills" them.

On Examination

Paramedics are unable to physically assess the patient at this time. A visual survey reveals the following:

CNS: The patient is conscious, able to speak, and appears in good physical health

Resp: His respirations are 28 per minute; no obvious signs of trauma

CVS: His skin is flushed in color

ABD: Unable to assess

Muscl/Skel: No injuries noticed

Vitals Signs

Paramedics are unable to assess the man's vital signs.

Past Hx: Over the past couple of weeks, the patient has had several episodes in which he would start raving about being persecuted by everyone around him. Usually they would only last for several minutes and then he would return to normal without any memory of what had just occurred. This time it has been over 30 minutes. This is the worst episode yet and is the first time he has been physically violent toward his family.

Treatment

The paramedics realize that there are several factors to recognize here. First, the patient is 40 years old and appears to be in good physical health. An attempt to physically restrain him could be dangerous for both the patient and the ambulance crew. Second, there is a history of violence, although paramedics are unsure of the extent of that violence. Medical control was contacted and gave an order for 5 mg of droperidol (Inapsine) and 2 mg of lorazepam (Ativan) mixed together in the same syringe and then given IM. Advice from the medical director was for the paramedics and police to restrain the patient long enough to give the Inapsine-Ativan mixture and then release the patient and give the medication time to work. The patient was then to be brought to the hospital, with vital signs monitored en route.

A paramedic explained the situation to the police officers, and with a coordinated effort they were able to restrain the patient and give the medications. Ten minutes later the patient had calmed down significantly and was placed on the stretcher and restrained with straps as a precaution. An uneventful trip to the hospital followed. At the hospital he was admitted to the psychiatric service, where he was treated and then released several days later on medications to help prevent further outbursts.

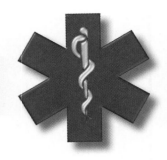

chapter 14

Drugs Used in the Treatment of Gastrointestinal Emergencies

OBJECTIVES

After completing this chapter, the reader should be able to

1. Define the term *antiemetic.*
2. Describe and list the indications, contraindications, and dosages for promethazine, dimenhydrinate, prochlorperazine, metoclopramide, and trimethobenzamide.

GASTROINTESTINAL MEDICATIONS

Although there are many medications for use in the treatment of gastrointestinal problems, few are used in prehospital care. The majority of gastrointestinal drugs used in prehospital care are antiemetics. These drugs are effective in treating nausea and vomiting. Many of these medications are used concomitantly with narcotics, both to potentiate their effects and to reduce the likelihood of the side effects commonly associated with narcotic usage. Antiemetics commonly used in emergency medicine include promethazine

(Phenergan), dimenhydrinate (Gravol, Dramamine), prochlorperazine (Compazine), hydroxyzine (Vistaril), metoclopramide (Reglan), and trimethobenzamide (Tigan). Hydroxyzine was discussed in Chapter 13.

The major antiemetics include antihistamines, phenothiazines, and serotonin receptor agonists. Antihistamine antiemetics are absorbed well from the gastrointestinal (GI) tract when administered orally.

PROMETHAZINE (PHENERGAN)

Class: Antihistamine and antiemetic

Description

Promethazine is a phenothiazine derivative with potent antihistamine properties and anticholinergic properties.

Mechanism of Action

Promethazine possesses sedative, antihistamine, antiemetic, and anticholinergic properties. It competitively blocks histamine receptors. The duration of action of promethazine is 4 to 6 hours. It is an effective and frequently used antiemetic. Promethazine, unlike hydroxyzine, can be given intravenously. It is often administered with analgesics, particularly narcotics, to potentiate their effect.

Indications

Promethazine is used for nausea and vomiting, motion sickness, and sedation and to potentiate the effects of analgesics.

Contraindications

Promethazine is contraindicated in patients in comatose states and in those who have received a large amount of depressants. Also, it should not be administered to any patient with a history of hypersensitivity to the drug.

Precautions

Promethazine may impair mental and physical abilities. Care must be taken to avoid accidental intra-arterial injection. It should never be administered subcutaneously. Extrapyramidal symptoms (EPS) have been reported following promethazine use. Diphenhydramine (Benadryl) should be available.

Side Effects

Promethazine can cause drowsiness, sedation, blurred vision, tachycardia, bradycardia, and dizziness.

Interactions

The depressant effect on the central nervous system (CNS) of narcotics, sedatives or hypnotics, and alcohol is potentiated by promethazine. An increased incidence of extrapyramidal symptoms has been reported when promethazine is administered to patients taking monamine oxidase inhibitors (MAOIs).

Dosage

The standard dosage of promethazine in the management of nausea and vomiting is 12.5 to 25 mg administered either intravenously (IV) or intramuscularly (IM). The standard dosage in adjunctive use with analgesics is 25 mg. Promethazine should be given by IV or deep intramuscular injection only. Care must be taken to avoid accidental intra-arterial injection.

How Supplied

Promethazine is supplied in ampules and Tubex syringes containing 25 mg of the drug in 1 mL of solvent.

℞ DIMENHYDRINATE (GRAVOL, DRAMAMINE)

Class: Antiemetic

Description

Dimenhydrinate belongs to the antihistamine class of drugs, although it is not commonly used for this action. Its site and action are not precisely known.

Mechanism of Action

The mechanism of action of dimenhydrinate is not precisely known. There is evidence that it acts to depress hyperstimulated labyrinthine functions or associated neural pathways. It is an effective and frequently used antiemetic in Canada. It is often used with analgesics, particularly narcotics.

Indications

Dimenhydrinate is used for the prevention or relief of nausea and vomiting, motion sickness, and drug-induced nausea and vomiting (particularly narcotics).

Contraindications

There are no significant contraindications in the emergency setting.

Precautions

Dimenhydrinate should be used with caution in patients with seizure disorders and asthma. Those who are administered the drug should be cautioned against operating motor vehicles or dangerous machinery because of drowsiness associated with the drug.

Side Effects

Dimenhydrinate can cause drowsiness, dizziness, blurred vision, dry mouth, dry nose and bronchi, and tinnitus.

Interactions

The CNS-depressant effect of narcotics, sedatives or hypnotics, and alcohol is potentiated by dimenhydrinate.

Dosage

The standard dose of dimenhydrinate in the management of nausea and vomiting is 12.5 to 25 mg (diluted) slow IV or 50 to 100 mg IM or by mouth. This dose can be repeated every 4 hours as needed.

How Supplied

Dimenhydrinate is supplied as 50 mg in 5 mL vials or ampules (10 mg/mL), 50 mg/mL ampule, and 50 mg/2 mL (25 mg/mL).

PROCHLORPERAZINE (COMPAZINE)

Class: Antiemetic

Description

Prochlorperazine is a phenothiazine derivative. It is highly effective in the treatment of severe nausea and vomiting.

Mechanism of Action

Prochlorperazine is an effective and frequently used antiemetic. It does not prevent vertigo and motion sickness, as do many of the other phenothiazines. Prochlorperazine blocks dopaminergic receptors in the brain. It also has weak anticholinergic properties.

Indications

Prochlorperazine is used in severe nausea and vomiting and acute psychosis.

Contraindications

Prochlorperazine should not be used in patients with a history of hypersensitivity to the drug or the phenothiazine class of medications. It should not be administered to comatose patients or those who have received large amounts of CNS depressants.

Precautions

Prochlorperazine may impair mental and physical abilities. It should never be administered subcutaneously because of local tissue irritation. The incidence of EPS appears to be higher with prochlorperazine than with many of the other phenothiazines. Diphenhydramine (Benadryl) should be available.

Side Effects

Prochlorperazine can cause drowsiness, sedation, blurred vision, tachycardia, bradycardia, dizziness, and hypotension.

Interactions

The CNS-depressant effect of narcotics, sedatives or hypnotics, and alcohol is potentiated by prochlorperazine.

Dosage

The standard dose of prochlorperazine is 5 to 10 mg administered intramuscularly or intravenously. The intravenous route is preferred with severe nausea and vomiting because the onset of action is much more rapid. Often, 10 mg of prochlorperazine is placed into 1 L of normal saline or lactated Ringer's solution and administered.

How Supplied

Prochlorperazine (Compazine) is supplied in 2 mL vials containing 5 mg/mL of the drug.

METOCLOPRAMIDE (REGLAN)

Class: Antiemetic

Description

Metoclopramide is a medication used in the treatment of gastroesophageal reflux and nausea and vomiting.

Mechanism of Action

Metoclopramide is an effective antiemetic. It stimulates motility of the upper gastrointestinal tract and promotes emptying of the stomach. It increases the tone of the valve between the esophagus and the stomach (lower esophageal sphincter), which reduces reflux of stomach contents into the distal esophagus. Metoclopramide's antiemetic effects appear to result from its blockade of central and peripheral dopamine receptors.

Indications

Metoclopramide is used in severe nausea and vomiting and gastroesophageal reflux.

Contraindications

Metoclopramide should not be used in patients with possible gastrointestinal hemorrhage, bowel obstruction, or perforation. It is also contraindicated in patients with a history of hypersensitivity to the drug.

Precautions

Metoclopramide may impair mental and physical abilities. Mental depression has occurred in patients with and without a prior history of depression following metoclopramide therapy. EPS can occur following metoclopramide administration. Diphenhydramine (Benadryl) should be available.

Side Effects

Metoclopramide can cause drowsiness, fatigue, sedation, dizziness, mental depression, hypertension, hypotension, tachycardia, bradycardia, and diarrhea.

Interactions

The effects of metoclopramide on gastric motility can be antagonized by anticholinergic drugs such as atropine. The CNS-depressant effect of narcotics, sedatives or hypnotics, and alcohol can be potentiated by metoclopramide. Hypertension can result when metoclopramide is administered to patients receiving MAOIs.

Dosage

The standard dose of metoclopramide is 10 to 20 mg administered intramuscularly. Metoclopramide can be administered intravenously for severe or intractable nausea and vomiting. The standard intravenous dose is 10 mg administered by slow IV push over 1 to 2 minutes. Alternatively, 10 mg of metoclopramide can be diluted in 50 mL of normal saline and administered over 15 minutes. The intravenous route is preferred in severe nausea and vomiting because the onset of action is much more rapid.

How Supplied

Metoclopramide (Reglan) is supplied in 2 mL vials containing 5 mg/mL of the drug.

TRIMETHOBENZAMIDE (TIGAN)

Class: Antiemetic

Description

Trimethobenzamide is an antiemetic that does not have the sedative effects of other commonly used antiemetic drugs.

Mechanism of Action

The mechanism of action of trimethobenzamide is unclear. It appears to work on the chemoreceptor trigger zone in the medulla oblongata.

Indication

Trimethobenzamide is used for severe nausea and vomiting.

Contraindications

The injectable form of trimethobenzamide should not be used in children. Trimethobenzamide should not be administered to patients with a history of hypersensitivity to the drug.

Precautions

The antiemetic effects of trimethobenzamide may render diagnosis more difficult in conditions such as appendicitis. EPS have been reported following administration of trimethobenzamide; however, their incidence appears to be much less than with other antiemetics. Diphenhydramine (Benadryl) should be available. Trimethobenzamide should not be administered intravenously.

Side Effects

Trimethobenzamide can cause blurred vision, diarrhea, dizziness, headache, muscle cramps, and allergic symptoms.

Interactions

The CNS-depressant effects of alcohol may be potentiated by trimethobenzamide.

Dosage

The standard dose of trimethobenzamide is 200 mg administered intramuscularly. Trimethobenzamide should not be administered intravenously.

How Supplied

Trimethobenzamide (Tigan) is supplied in 2 mL ampules and vials containing 100 mg/mL of the drug.

SUMMARY

Medications are rarely required in the prehospital management of gastrointestinal emergencies. However, many emergency medical services (EMS) systems utilize antiemetics for severe or intractable nausea and vomiting. Prehospital administration of antiemetics decreases the potential for dehydration, improves patient comfort, and reduces exposure of EMS personnel to body fluids. The antiemetics are often used to potentiate the effects of the narcotics. Paramedics are encouraged to be familiar with the antiemetics used in their system.

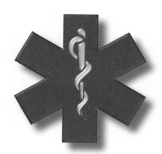

chapter 15

DRUGS USED IN PAIN MANAGEMENT

OBJECTIVES

After completing this chapter, the reader should be able to

1. Discuss the history of pain management in prehospital care.
2. Explain the characteristics of the ideal analgesic agent for prehospital care.
3. Define the terms *analgesic* and *narcotic*.
4. Describe the analgesics available for use in prehospital care.
5. Describe and list the indications, contraindications, and dosages for the following medications used in pain management: morphine sulfate, meperidine, fentanyl citrate, nitrous oxide, nalbuphine, butorphanol, tartrate, and ketorolac.

INTRODUCTION

Emergency medical services (EMS) and the prehospital care of patients have made significant advances over the past decade. The focus of these efforts has been primarily the overall reduction of death and disability in the critically ill or injured patient. However, controversy continues around the extent of prehospital intervention and the influence these efforts have on the outcome of patients. Through these advances, very little attention has been given to the relief of pain and anxiety.

In the early 1970s the focus of prehospital care in the United States and Canada was on the treatment of cardiac arrest and myocardial infarction. Because of the importance of pain relief in the treatment of acute myocardial infarction, a narcotic (usually morphine) was included in the treatment protocol for prehospital advanced life support. However, the use of analgesics for pain relief has not been universally accepted beyond its use in myocardial infarction.

Meanwhile, British clinicians took a different view. Baskett introduced the use of a fixed-ratio mixture (50:50) of nitrous oxide and oxygen to the ambulance service in 1969. During the next decade, use of the gas mixture became widespread for both basic and advanced life support systems in Australia, Canada, and the United States.

However, during the past decade there has been a lack of interest in providing adequate pain relief for patients in the prehospital care setting. "In every medical study of analgesia in hospital settings, pain relief in patients was found to be inconsistent, inadequate, and revealing of serious misconceptions or frank ignorance on the part of the physician or nursing staff. Add to this the fact that the uncontrolled prehospital environment argued against the safe administration of any medication, and there is little wonder that relief of pain in patients got a short shrift." And despite the advances made in prehospital care and medical control over the past decade, very little progress has been made in the area of pain relief. "There has been the suggestion (albeit an old chestnut, seemingly resuscitated) that field analgesics will complicate in-hospital management and confuse diagnosis. This attitude, a variation on the old dictum with origins in the 19th and early 20th centuries, appears to have a new lease on life when applied to the prehospital setting. The availability of newer agents given in appropriate doses by appropriate routes should relegate this formerly sound medical truism to the scrap heap of medical myths."[1]

Is the relief of pain in the prehospital setting important? This question can be put to rest by patients who have suffered in agony while trapped in a motor vehicle or by patients with compound fractures who have been bounced around while being moved out of ditches and transported across rural or urban roads. What about the pain experienced by patients with extensive body surface burns? It is not only humanitarian to provide pain relief in prehospital care, but the relief of pain can be of physiological benefit to seriously ill and injured patients.

Perhaps it is time we paid more attention to managing the most common complaint faced in prehospital care today—pain. The ideal analgesic agent for prehospital care has characteristics that are not easily met by one agent. First, the safety of the analgesic must be of prime concern. Second, it must be rapid in onset and short in duration. Rapidity of onset is the function of the route of administration, and that implies the intravenous route. Third, the ease with which an agent is stored and administered is important in prehospital care. For example, the relative bulk and weight of double- or single-tank nitrous oxide–oxygen mixtures have inhibited their frequent use in the prehospital setting. Perhaps, then, the ideal agent has yet to be discovered.

Still, much can be done in the prehospital care setting to relieve pain and anxiety. Basic measures should consist of gentle handling, splinting, and compassionate caring rapport with the patient. Other factors, such as exposure to the cold, may occur during extrication or other prehospital

[1]R. D. Stewart, "Analgesia in the Field," *Prehospital and Disaster Medicine* 4, no. 1 (1989).

procedures. Exposure may cause shivering and movement of fractures or other painful parts, increasing the patient's discomfort and negating the effect of almost any analgesic agent.

The good news is that pain relief is being reexamined as an important element of prehospital care. This interest is focused not only on agents previously used but also on new drugs and routes of administration. This chapter will prepare paramedics to provide prehospital patients with relief from pain and freedom from fear and anxiety. Many agents appropriate for prehospital care are discussed on the following pages.

ANALGESICS

Drugs that have proved to be effective in alleviating pain are referred to as analgesics. Although they may be administered in many different types of emergencies, they are usually reserved for the treatment of emergencies involving the cardiovascular system, especially myocardial infarction.

As a rule, undiagnosed pain is usually not treated. Early administration of analgesics to these patients may alter physical findings and impair subsequent evaluation by the emergency physician. Some types of pain may be easy to distinguish and are sometimes treated in the prehospital setting. These include chest pain associated with acute myocardial infarction, pain from severe burns, and pain associated with kidney stones.

Analgesics used in prehospital care include the following:

- Morphine sulfate
- Meperidine (Demerol)
- Fentanyl (Sublimaze)
- Nitrous oxide (Nitronox)
- Nalbuphine (Nubain)
- Butorphanol tartrate (Stadol)
- Ketorolac (Toradol)

Morphine is derived from the opium plant. It has impressive analgesic and hemodynamic effects. Meperidine, although similar to morphine in its analgesic effects, is considerably different chemically and is synthetically derived. Nalbuphine (Nubain) is also a potent synthetic analgesic. It does not have the hemodynamic effects that morphine does, yet it is often used in emergency medicine because it does not cause respiratory depression and has a low tendency for abuse. Stadol, another of the new breed of synthetic analgesics, is similar to Nubain but is rarely used in treating cardiovascular emergencies. Nitronox, a 50 percent mixture of oxygen and nitrous oxide that can be easily inhaled by the patient, is entirely different from the other analgesic agents discussed. Its analgesic effects are also very potent yet disappear within a few minutes after the cessation of administration. Thus, Nitronox can be given for many types of pain in the field without fear of impairing subsequent physical examination in the emergency department. In addition to its analgesic effects, Nitronox delivers oxygen to the patient, which makes it useful in cardiac emergencies. Ketorolac (Toradol) is the first injectable nonsteroidal anti-inflammatory agent. It is often used in emergency medicine as an analgesic because it does not affect the patient's mental status.

MORPHINE SULFATE

Class: Narcotic analgesic

Description

Morphine is a central nervous system depressant and a potent analgesic. Although morphine sulfate is one of the most potent analgesics known to humans, it also has hemodynamic properties that make it extremely useful in emergency medicine.

Mechanism of Action

Morphine sulfate is a central nervous system depressant that acts on opiate receptors in the brain, providing both analgesia and sedation. It increases peripheral venous capacitance and decreases venous return. This effect is sometimes called a chemical phlebotomy. Morphine also decreases myocardial oxygen demand. This action is due to both the decreased systemic vascular resistance and the sedative effects of the drug. Patient apprehension and fear can significantly increase myocardial oxygen demand and in some cases can conceivably increase the size of myocardial infarction. The hemodynamic properties of morphine make it one of the most important drugs used in the treatment of pulmonary edema. Morphine is frequently administered to patients with signs and symptoms of pulmonary edema who are not having chest pain.

Indications

Morphine sulfate is used for severe pain associated with myocardial infarction, kidney stones, and so forth and pulmonary edema either with or without associated pain.

Contraindications

Because of the hemodynamic effects described earlier, morphine should not be used in patients who are volume depleted or severely hypotensive. Morphine should not be administered to any patient with a history of hypersensitivity to the drug or to patients with undiagnosed head injury or abdominal pain.

Precautions

Morphine is a narcotic derivative of opium. It has a high tendency for addiction and abuse and is thus covered under the Controlled Substances Act of 1970. It is classified as a Schedule II drug. Consequently, special considerations are involved in the handling of the drug. Many EMS systems have opted to use the synthetic analgesics, such as nalbuphine and pentazocine, instead of morphine and meperidine because of these problems. Morphine causes severe respiratory depression in higher doses. This is especially true in patients who already have some form of respiratory impairment. The narcotic antagonist naloxone (Narcan) should be readily available whenever the drug is administered.

Side Effects

Morphine can cause nausea, vomiting, abdominal cramps, blurred vision, constricted pupils, altered mental status, headache, and respiratory depression.

Interactions

The CNS depression associated with morphine can be enhanced when administered with antihistamines, antiemetics, sedatives, hypnotics, barbiturates, and alcohol.

Dosage

There are many different approaches to the administration of morphine. An initial dose in the range of 2 to 10 mg administered intravenously is standard. This dose can be augmented with additional doses of 2 mg every few minutes and can be continued until the pain is relieved or until signs of respiratory depression occur.

Intramuscular injection usually requires 5 to 15 mg, based on the patient's weight, to attain desired effects. However, morphine is routinely given intravenously in emergency medicine and is often administered with an antiemetic agent such as promethazine (Phenergan). These agents help prevent the nausea and vomiting that often accompany morphine administration. The antiemetics also tend to potentiate morphine's effects. Morphine can also be given intramuscularly and subcutaneously.

How Supplied

Morphine comes in tamperproof ampules and Tubex prefilled cartridges. To ease administration, the 10 mg/mL in 1 mL dilution is preferred.

MEPERIDINE (DEMEROL)

Class: Narcotic analgesic

Description

Meperidine is a central nervous system depressant and a potent analgesic. It is used extensively in medicine in the treatment of moderate to severe pain. It is less potent than morphine sulfate; 60 to 80 mg of meperidine are roughly equivalent in action to 10 mg of morphine.

Mechanism of Action

Meperidine is a central nervous system depressant that acts on opiate receptors in the brain, providing both analgesia and sedation. It does not have the same hemodynamic properties as morphine but has the same tendency for physical dependence and abuse. Because it causes respiratory depression, naloxone should be available whenever meperidine is administered. The rate of onset is slightly faster than morphine, yet its effects are much shorter in duration. Like morphine, meperidine is a Schedule II drug regulated under the Controlled Substances Act of 1970.

Indication

Meperidine is used for moderate to severe pain.

Contraindications

Meperidine should not be administered to patients with known hypersensitivity to the drug. In addition, it should not be administered to patients with undiagnosed abdominal pain or head injury, or to patients who are receiving, or who have recently received, monoamine oxidase inhibitors (e.g., Nardil, Parnate, and Eutron). Therapeutic doses of meperidine have occasionally caused severe, and sometimes fatal, reactions in patients receiving these agents.

Precautions

Meperidine can cause respiratory depression. Naloxone (Narcan) should always be available to reverse the effects of the drug if respiratory depression ensues. Like morphine, meperidine should be kept in a secure, locked box.

Side Effects

Meperidine can cause nausea, vomiting, abdominal cramps, blurred vision, constricted pupils, altered mental status, hallucinations, headache, and respiratory depression.

Interactions

Meperidine should not be administered to patients who are receiving, or who have recently received, monoamine oxidase inhibitors (e.g., Nardil, Parnate, and Eutron). These agents are used for certain types of depression and behavioral disorders. Therapeutic doses of meperidine have occasionally caused severe, and sometimes fatal, reactions in patients receiving these agents.

Dosage

The usual dose used in the treatment of severe pain is 25 to 50 mg administered intravenously. When administered intramuscularly, 50 to 100 mg is a standard dose. Meperidine is often administered with an antiemetic agent such as promethazine (Phenergan). These agents help prevent the nausea and vomiting that often accompany meperidine administration. Meperidine can be administered either intravenously or intramuscularly.

How Supplied

Meperidine (Demerol) is supplied in ampules and Tubex prefilled cartridges containing 25, 50, or 100 mg of the drug in 1 mL of solvent.

FENTANYL CITRATE (SUBLIMAZE)

Class: Narcotic analgesic

Description

Fentanyl, although chemically unrelated to morphine, produces pharmacological effects and a degree of analgesia similar to those of morphine. On a weight basis, however, fentanyl is 50 to 100 times more potent than morphine, but its duration of action is shorter than that of meperidine or morphine. A parenteral dose of 100 µg of fentanyl is approximately equivalent in analgesic activity to 10 mg of morphine or 75 mg of meperidine.

Mechanism of Action

The principal actions of therapeutic value are analgesic and sedation. Fentanyl is a narcotic analgesic with a rapid onset and a short duration of action. Alterations in respiratory rate and alveolar ventilation, associated with narcotic analgesics, may last longer than the analgesic effect. Large doses may produce apnea. Fentanyl appears to have less emetic activity than other narcotic analgesics.

Indications

Fentanyl is used for maintenance of analgesia, as an adjunct in rapid-sequence induction intubation, and for severe pain.

Contraindications

Contraindications include severe hemorrhage, shock, and known hypersensitivity.

Precautions

Vital signs should be monitored routinely. Fentanyl may produce bradycardia, which may be treated with atropine. However, fentanyl should be used with caution in patients with cardiac bradydysrhythmias.

Fentanyl should be administered with caution to patients with liver and kidney dysfunction because of the importance of these organs in the metabolism and excretion of drugs. As with other CNS depressants, patients who have received fentanyl should have appropriate surveillance. Resuscitation equipment and a narcotic agonist such as naloxone should be readily available to manage apnea.

Side Effects

As with other narcotic analgesics, the most common serious reactions reported to occur with fentanyl are respiratory depression, apnea, muscle rigidity, and bradycardia. If these side effects remain untreated, respiratory arrest, circulatory depression, or cardiac arrest could occur.

Interactions

Other drugs with a depressant effect on the central nervous system (CNS) (e.g., barbiturates, tranquilizers, narcotics, and general anesthetics) have an additive or potentiating effect with fentanyl. When patients have received such drugs, the dose of fentanyl required is less than usual. Likewise, following the administration of fentanyl, the dose of other CNS-depressant drugs should be reduced. Severe and unpredictable potentiation by monoamine oxidase inhibitors (MAOIs) has been reported with narcotic analgesics. Because the safety of fentanyl in this regard has not been established, its use in patients who have received MAOIs within 14 days is not recommended.

Dosage

Adult dosages are IV, 25 to 100 μg (0.025 to 0.1 mg); direct IV, slowly over at least 1 minute, preferably over 2 to 3 minutes (not necessary to dilute—may be diluted to facilitate administration); and 100 μg/2 mL diluted in 3 mL of normal saline for a concentration of 20 μg/mL.

Pediatric dosages are 1.7 to 3.3 μg/kg for children 2 to 12 years of age; the dosage should be reduced in very young, elderly, and poor-risk patients.

How Supplied

Fentanyl is supplied in 2 mL ampules containing 50 μg/mL. It should be protected from light during storage.

 # NITROUS OXIDE (NITRONOX, ENTONOX)

Class: Analgesic and anesthetic gas

Description

Nitronox is a blended mixture of 50 percent nitrous and 50 percent oxygen that has potent analgesic effects.

Mechanism of Action

Nitrous oxide is a CNS depressant with analgesic properties. In the prehospital setting it is delivered in a fixed mixture of 50 percent nitrous oxide and 50 percent oxygen. When inhaled, it has potent analgesic effects. These quickly dissipate, however, within 2 to 5 minutes after cessation of administration. The Nitronox unit consists of one oxygen and one nitrous oxide cylinder. The gases are fed into a blender that combines them at the appropriate concentration. The mixture is then delivered to a modified demand valve for administration to the patient. Nitronox must be self-administered. It is effective in treating many varieties of pain encountered in the prehospital setting, including pain from many types of trauma. The high concentration of oxygen delivered along with the nitrous oxide will increase the oxygen tension in the blood, thus reducing hypoxia.

Indications

Nitrous oxide is used for pain of musculoskeletal origin, particularly fractures; burns; suspected ischemic chest pain; and states of severe anxiety, including hyperventilation.

Contraindications

Nitronox should not be used in any patient who cannot comprehend verbal instructions or who is intoxicated with alcohol or other drugs. It should not be administered to any patient with a head injury who exhibits an altered mental status. Nitronox should not be administered to any patient with chronic obstructive pulmonary disease (COPD) because the high concentration of oxygen (50 percent) might result in respiratory depression.

Nitrous oxide tends to diffuse into closed spaces more readily than either carbon dioxide or oxygen. Many COPD patients have air-containing blebs in their lungs, and nitrous oxide can concentrate in these blebs, causing them to swell. Swollen blebs may rupture, causing a pneumothorax. Nitronox should not be administered to patients with a thoracic injury suspicious of pneumothorax, because the gas may accumulate in the pneumothorax, increasing its size. Also, patients with severe abdominal pain and distention suggestive of bowel obstruction should not receive Nitronox. Nitrous oxide can concentrate in pockets of an obstructed bowel, possibly leading to rupture.

Precautions

Nitronox should only be used in areas that are well ventilated. When the gas is used in the patient compartment of an ambulance, a scavenging system should be in place. Nitrous oxide exists in a liquid state inside the gas cylinder. Heat present in the air, in the cylinder wall, or in the various regulators and lines causes the liquid to vaporize. This vaporization process makes the cylinder tank and lines cool to touch. Following prolonged use, frost may develop on the cylinder, regulator, or lines. In very cold environments, generally less than 21 °F (6 °C), the liquid may be slow to vaporize, and administration may be impossible.

Side Effects

A nitrous oxide–oxygen mixture can cause dizziness, light-headedness, altered mental status, hallucinations, nausea, and vomiting.

Interactions

Nitrous oxide can potentiate the effects of other CNS depressants such as narcotics, sedatives, hypnotics, and alcohol.

Dosage

Nitronox should only be self-administered. Continuous administration may take place until the pain is significantly relieved or until the patient drops the mask. The patient care record should document the duration of drug administration.

How Supplied

The nitrous oxide–oxygen mixture is supplied in a cylinder system in which both gases are fed into a blender that delivers a fixed 50 percent/50 percent mixture to the patient. The blender is designed to shut off if the oxygen cylinder becomes depleted. It will allow continued administration of oxygen if the nitrous oxide cylinder becomes depleted.

In several countries (England, Canada, and Australia) the nitrous oxide–oxygen mixture (Entonox and Dolonox) is premixed and supplied in a single cylinder. This setup is much lighter than the system used in the United States.

NALBUPHINE (NUBAIN)

Class: Synthetic analgesic

Description

Nalbuphine is a synthetic analgesic agent with a potency equivalent to morphine on a milligram-to-milligram basis.

Mechanism of Action

Like the narcotics, nalbuphine is a centrally acting analgesic that binds to the opiate receptors in the central nervous system. Its onset of action is considerably faster than that of morphine, occurring within 2 to 3 minutes after intravenous administration. Its duration of effect is reported to be 3 to 6 hours. Although nalbuphine causes some respiratory depression in doses up to 10 mg, these effects do not seem to get worse in doses that exceed 10 mg. Naloxone (Narcan) is an effective antagonist and should be available when nalbuphine is administered.

In addition to its effects on opiate receptors, nalbuphine has antagonistic effects similar to those of naloxone. This feature minimizes the abuse potential of the drug and appears to lessen the chances of significant respiratory depression. At this time, nalbuphine is not regulated under the Controlled Substances Act of 1970. Current studies show that it has a minimal tendency for physical dependence and abuse. This property has made nalbuphine increasingly popular in prehospital care.

Indication

Nalbuphine is used for moderate to severe pain.

Contraindications

Nalbuphine should not be administered to patients with head injury or undiagnosed abdominal pain.

Precautions

The primary precaution in using nalbuphine is in patients with impaired respiratory function. Small doses of nalbuphine may cause significant respiratory depression. Naloxone should be readily available. Nalbuphine also has narcotic antagonistic properties. Thus, it should be administered with caution to patients dependent on narcotics, because it may cause withdrawal effects. The dosage of nalbuphine should be reduced in older patients because the effects are less predictable in this age group. Small repeated boluses are often safer than a single large dose.

Side Effects

Nalbuphine can cause headache, altered mental status, hypotension, bradycardia, blurred vision, rash, respiratory depression, nausea, and vomiting.

Interactions

Nalbuphine can potentiate the CNS depression associated with narcotics, sedatives, hypnotics, and alcohol. Because of its antagonistic properties, nalbuphine can cause withdrawal symptoms in patients addicted to narcotics. Nalbuphine can interfere with certain types of anesthesia (nitrous and narcotic techniques) because of its antagonistic properties.

Dosage

The general regimen for nalbuphine administration is 5 mg intravenously initially. This dose may be augmented with additional 2 mg doses if necessary. Nalbuphine is often administered with an antiemetic agent such as promethazine (Phenergan). These agents help prevent the nausea and vomiting that often accompany nalbuphine administration. Nalbuphine can be administered intravenously or intramuscularly.

How Supplied

Nalbuphine is supplied in 1 mL ampules containing 10 mg of the drug.

℞ BUTORPHANOL TARTRATE (STADOL)

Class: Synthetic analgesic

Description

Butorphanol is a synthetic analgesic used frequently in emergency medicine. It is quite potent; the analgesic effects of 2 mg of butorphanol are roughly equivalent to 10 mg of morphine.

Mechanism of Action

Butorphanol is a centrally acting analgesic that binds to the opiate receptors in the central nervous system, causing CNS depression and analgesia. Like nalbuphine, it has some antagonistic (naloxone-like) properties. Although butorphanol can cause respiratory depression, this effect usually plateaus following administration of approximately 4 mg. Currently, butorphanol is not restricted under the 1970 act. Thus it is quite attractive for use in the prehospital phase of emergency medical care.

Indication

Butorphanol is used for moderate to severe pain.

Contraindications

Butorphanol should not be administered to any patient with a history of hypersensitivity to the drug. Also, it should not be given to patients dependent on narcotics because it may cause some reversal of the narcotic effects. It should not be administered to patients with head injury or undiagnosed abdominal pain.

Precautions

If butorphanol causes marked respiratory depression, then Narcan can be administered to reverse its effects. When administering any potent analgesic, it is possible to mask other signs and symptoms. All analgesics should be administered only after a thorough physical examination. Butorphanol should not be administered to any patient with head injury because it may cause an increase in cerebrospinal pressure. The dosage of nalbuphine should be reduced in older patients because the effects are less predictable in this age group. Small repeated boluses are often safer than a single large dose.

Side Effects

Butorphanol can cause headache, altered mental status, hypotension, bradycardia, blurred vision, rash, respiratory depression, nausea, and vomiting.

Interactions

Like nalbuphine, butorphanol has some narcotic antagonistic properties. Caution should be used when administering butorphanol to patients already dependent on narcotics because it may precipitate withdrawal.

Dosage

The standard dose of butorphanol is 1 mg administered intravenously every 3 to 4 hours. When given intramuscularly, the standard dose is 2 mg. Butorphanol should only be administered intravenously or intramuscularly.

How Supplied

Butorphanol is supplied in 2 mL vials containing 2 mg of the drug.

KETOROLAC (TORADOL)

Class: Nonsteroidal anti-inflammatory agent

Description

Ketorolac is the first injectable nonsteroidal anti-inflammatory drug to become available in the United States. It is useful in treating mild to moderate pain.

Mechanism of Action

Ketorolac is a nonsteroidal anti-inflammatory drug (NSAID). It has analgesic, anti-inflammatory, and antipyretic effects. Unlike narcotics, which act on the central nervous system, ketorolac is considered a peripherally acting analgesic. Consequently, it does not have the sedative properties of the narcotics. Ketorolac has been used concomitantly with morphine and meperidine without adverse effects. In dental studies, ketorolac was found to be quite effective as an analgesic.

Indication

Ketorolac is used for mild to moderate pain.

Contraindications

Ketorolac should not be used in patients with a known hypersensitivity to the drug. It should not be administered to patients who report allergies to aspirin or NSAIDs, or to patients currently taking aspirin or NSAIDs.

Precautions

Gastrointestinal (GI) irritation and hemorrhage can result from therapy with NSAIDs. Long-term usage increases the incidence of serious GI side effects. Ketorolac is cleared through the kidneys. Long-term usage can result in renal impairment.

Side Effects

Ketorolac can cause edema, hypertension, rash, itching, nausea, heartburn, constipation, diarrhea, drowsiness, and dizziness.

Interactions

Ketorolac, when administered with other NSAIDs (including aspirin), can worsen the side effects associated with the use of drugs in this class. Intramuscular ketorolac has been found to reduce the diuretic response to furosemide (Lasix).

Dosage

The typical dose of ketorolac is 30 to 60 mg administered intramuscularly. Half the original dose can be repeated every 6 hours. Ketorolac has recently been approved for IV use by the U.S. Food and Drug Administration (FDA); many emergency departments use ketorolac intravenously to obtain more prompt analgesia. The typical intravenous dose is 30 mg. Some practitioners use 60 mg intravenously. Few adverse reactions have been reported with intravenous ketorolac.

How Supplied

Ketorolac is supplied in prefilled syringes containing 15, 30, and 60 mg of the drug.

SUMMARY

Paramedics can reliably manage most patients who complain of pain. With expanded understanding of pain medications, oversight by medical control, and using critical thinking skills paramedics are ready to relieve the pain many patients suffer.

KEY WORDS

analgesic. A drug used in the relief of pain.

narcotic. A substance that works on the central nervous system to decrease or relieve the sensation of pain. Narcotic pain killers (analgesics) are made from opium or made artificially.

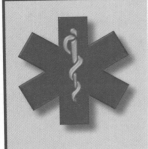

CASE PRESENTATION

At 1430 hours paramedics are called to a football field for a 16-year-old male who has injured his leg playing football. En route the dispatcher tells the paramedics that the 16-year-old male is conscious and breathing, and has a possible fracture of his left leg. On arrival paramedics are directed to the center of the field, where a group of players and coaches are standing. They find their patient lying on the ground with an obviously deformed left ankle. He is wearing football equipment, and first-aid providers have already removed the patient's shoes, socks, and helmet. The patient states that he was running with the ball when he stepped in a small hole in the field. He felt a "pop" in his ankle and then extreme pain. He states he attempted to get up but was unable to because of the pain.

On Examination

CNS: The patient is conscious, alert, and oriented × 4; in extreme pain

Resp: Respirations are 24; trachea is midline; no signs of trauma; lung sounds are clear bilaterally

CVS: Carotid and radial pulses are present and strong; skin is pink and warm

ABD: Soft and nontender

Extremities: Arms and right leg intact with good pulses, sensation, and strength; left leg is deformed at the ankle, with the left foot rotated externally; distal pulse is palpable in left foot, although it is cooler to touch than the right foot

Vital Signs

Pulse: 96/min, regular, strong
Resp: 24/min, shallow
BP: 122/80 mm Hg
SpO$_2$: 99 percent
ECG: Regular sinus rhythm
Hx: The patient is not taking any medications, has no known allergies, and states he is a healthy person.

Treatment

Paramedics examine the patient thoroughly and determine that because of the mechanism of the injury the patient does not need to be spinal immobilized. His left ankle is severely angulated, with obvious external rotation. His left foot is cool to touch but has a strong pulse and is pink in color. During attempts to splint the ankle the patient screams in pain, and therefore paramedics decide to give an analgesic prior to completion of the splinting to make it more bearable for the patient. An IV is initiated using an 18-gauge catheter in the right forearm. The IV of normal saline is run TKVO. Paramedics give the patient 5 mg of morphine IV over 2 minutes as per standing order. The paramedics immobilize the ankle in a pillow splint. The patient is moved to the ambulance. The patient is still in considerable pain, and another 5.0 mg of morphine is administered. The patient's vital signs, especially respirations and blood pressure, are closely monitored. En route to the hospital the patient starts to complain about feeling nauseated and is therefore given 25 mg of dimenhydrinate (Gravol) IV. The rest of the trip to the hospital is uneventful. On arrival at the hospital, the patient is assessed and treated for a severe dislocation fracture of his left ankle.

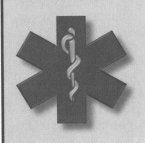

CASE PRESENTATION

At 1900 hours on a fall evening paramedics are called to the high school football stadium for a football player who has injured his shoulder. On arrival they are directed to the sidelines, where the coaches are attending to a player. The player is not wearing shoulder pads and is slouched to his right side.

On Examination

CNS: The patient is conscious, alert, and oriented × 4; in moderate pain

Resp: Respirations are 24; trachea is midline

CVS: Carotid and radial pulses are present; skin is warm and dry

ABD: Soft and nontender

Extremities: Dislocation of right shoulder

Vital Signs

Pulse: 88/min, regular

Resp: 18/min, shallow

BP: 118/72 mm Hg

SpO$_2$: 96 percent

Hx: The patient is not taking any medications, has no known allergies, and states he is a healthy person. The coaches tell the paramedics that the football player is the team quarterback. He was sacked on a play and landed heavily on his shoulder.

Treatment

On assessment paramedics find that the shoulder is dislocated anteriorly. They give the patient nitrous oxide to self-administer. After several minutes of breathing the nitrous oxide, the patient states that the pain is not as intense. Paramedics sling and swathe the arm and shoulder and move the patient to the ambulance. Once in the unit, they administer 75 mg of meperidine IM in the left deltoid. The combination of nitrous oxide and meperidine give the patient almost total pain relief. The transport to the hospital is uneventful.

Glossary of Street Drug Names

CENTRAL NERVOUS SYSTEM STIMULANTS[1]

A
Amp
Bam
Batu (methcathinone)
Beans
Benies
Bennie (Benzidrine)
Black and white
Black beauties
Black birds
Blue angels
Blue beauties
Bombido (injectable amphetamine)
Bombita (Spanish-speaking community)
Candy
Cartwheels
Cat (methcathinone)
Chalk
Chicken powder
Chocolate
Chris

Christine
Christmas eve
Christmas trees
Christy (smokable meth)
Coast to coast
Coke (cocaine)
Copilot
Crack (cocaine)
Crank
Crink
Cris
Crisscross
Crissroads
Croak (method and crack)
Crystal (methamphetamine)
Dexies
Disco pellets
Dominoes
Double cross
Eye openers
Fire (meth and crack)
Flake (cocaine)
Footballs

Glass
Go-fast
Gold dust (cocaine)
Granulated orange
Green and clears
Greenies
Hanyak
Head drugs
Hearts
Hiropon (smokable methamphetamine or methcathinone)
Ice
Inbetweens
Jam
Jelly baby
Jolly baby
Jugs
Kaksonjae
LA (long-acting amphetamines)
LA glass (smokable LA)
LA turnarounds

---

[1]A form of amphetamine unless otherwise stated.

Leapers
Lid poppers
Lid proppers
Little bomb
Max (dissolved gamma
  hydroxy buterate mixed
  with amphetamine)
Meth
Mexican crack
Minibennie
Nugget
Oranges
Peaches

Pep pills
Pink and green
Pinks
Quartz
Rippers
Rock (cocaine)
Rosa (Spanish-speaking
  community)
Roses
Shabu (methcathinone)
Snap
Snow (cocaine)
Speed

Speedball (heroin plus cocaine)
Toot
Truck drivers
Turnarounds
Uppers
Ups
Wake-ups
Whiffledust
Whites
X
XTC
Yellow jackets

PHENCYCLIDINE (PCP)

A Beam me up Scotty (PCP
  and crack)
Ace
Ad
Amoeba
Angel dust
Animal tranquilizer
Aurora
Black acid (PCP and LSD)
Bush
Bust bee
Cheap cocaine
Cosmos
Criptal
Devil's dust
Dipper
DOA
Domex (PCP and ecstasy)
Dummy mist

El Diablito (for combination of
  PCP, marijuana, cocaine,
  and heroin in Spanish-
  speaking community)
Frios (marijuana laced with
  PCP in Spanish-speaking
  community)
Goon
Green
Guerrilla
Hog
Jet
K
Kools (marijuana laced with
  PCP)
Lemon 714
Lovely
Magic dust
Mauve
Mist

Monkey tranquilizers
Mumm dust
Niebla (Spanish-speaking
  community)
Octane (PCP laced with
  gasoline)
Ozone
Peace pill
Purple
Rocket fuel
Shermans
Sherms
Special LA coke
Superacid
Supercoke
Supergrass
Superjoint
Trangs
Tranq[2]
Wack

HEROIN

Black tar
Brown
Chinese white
H
H and stuff

Horse
Junk
Mexican mud
Scat
Shit

Skag
Smack
Snow
Stuff
Tango and Cash

---

[2]Many drugs have the same name.

OTHER ANALGESICS

Black (opium)
Blue velvet (paregoric plus
  amphetamine)
Dollies (methadone)
M (morphine)

Microdots (morphine)
PG or PO (paregoric)
Pinks and grays
  (propaxyphene
  hydrochloride)

Poppy (opium)
Tar (opium)
Terp (terpin hydrate or cough
  syrup with codeine)

CENTRAL NERVOUS SYSTEM DEPRESSANTS[3]

Blue birds
Blue devil
Blue heaven
Blues
Bullets
Dolls
Double trouble
Downs
Goofballs

Green and whites
  (chlordiazepoxide)
Greenies
Ludes
Nembies
Peanuts
Peter (chloral hydrate)
Rainbows
Red Devils

Roaches (chlordiaepoxide)[2]
Seccy
Seggy
T-birds
Toolies
Tranqs[2]
Wallbangers
Yellow jackets
Yellows

HALLUCINOGENS

Acid (LSD)
Blue dots (LSD)
Cactus (mescaline)
Crystal[2]

Cube (LSD)
D (LSD)
Mesc (mescaline)
Mexico mushroom (psilocybin)

Owsleys (LSD)
Pearly gates (morning glory
  seeds)

CANNABINOLS

Acapulco gold
Bhang
Brick
Charas
Colombian
Gage
Ganja
Grass
Hash
Hay
Hemp

J
Jane
Jive
Joint
Key or Kee
Lid
Locoweed
Mary Jane
Mexican
MJ
Muggles

Pot
Reefer
Roach[2]
Rope
Sativa
Stick
Sweet Lucy
Tea
Texas tea
Weed
Yesca

------

[3]Moderate length of action, like secobarbital, unless otherwise noted.

SOLVENTS AND INHALANTS

Air blast
Ames
Amies
Aroma of men
Bang
Boopers
Bullet
Buzz bomb
Climax

Honey oil
Huff
Huffing
Jac aroma
Kicks
Laughing gas (nitrous oxide)
Locker room (isobutyl nitrate)
Medusa
Moon gas

Oz
Pearls (amyl nitrite)
Poppers (isobutyl or amyl nitrite)
Poppers (isobutyl or amyl nitrate)
Rush
Snappers
Sniffers
Whiteout

INHALANTS

Air blast
Ames
Amies
Amys
Aroma of men
Bang
Boppers
Bullet

Buzz bomb
Climax
Honey oil
Huff
Laughing gas (nitrous oxide)
Locker room (isobutyl nitrate)
Medusa
Moon gas

Oz
Pearls (amyl nitrite)
Poor man's pot
Poppers (isobutyl or amyl nitrate)
Whiteout

STREET DRUG LINGO

Abe's cape: $5 bill
Agonies: withdrawal symptoms
All star: user of many types of drugs
Amped out: fatigue after using methamphetamine
Baby habit: occasional user of drugs
Bad go: bad reaction to a drug
Bagging: using inhalants
Batt: hypodermic needle
Bedbugs: fellow addicts
Bender: drug party

Bone: $50 piece of crack
Boulder: $20 worth of crack
Cooker: one who manufactures methamphetamine
Deck: 1 to 15 g of heroin
Demo: sample size of crack
Deuce: $2 worth of drug
Eight ball: 1/8 ounce of any type of drug
Gluey: one who sniffs or inhales glue
Huffer: one who uses inhalants
Hype: an addict, most frequently refers to IV drug

users
Lid: 1 ounce of marijuana
Meth head: regular meth user
Meth monster: one who gets a violent reaction to methamphetamine
Snot: residue left after smoking amphetamines
Snotball: rubber cement rolled into balls and burned so the fumes can be inhaled
Speed freak: regular meth user
Spike: hypodermic needle

EMERGENCY INTRAVENOUS FLUIDS QUICK REFERENCE GUIDE

Plasma Protein Fraction (Plasmanate)

Class	Protein colloid
Action	Plasma volume expander
Indications	Hypovolemic states (especially burn shock)
Contraindications	None when used in the management of life-threatening situations
Precautions	Hypertension
	Short shelf life
Side Effect	Edema
Dosage	Dosage should be titrated according to patient's hemodynamic response; follow accepted resuscitation formulas in the management of burn shock
	Adult: 250–500 mL (12.5–25 g protein) not to exceed 10 mL/min
Route	IV infusion
Pediatric Dosage	10–30 mL/kg at 5–10 mL/min

Dextran

Class	Imitation protein (sugar) colloid
Action	Plasma volume expander
Indication	Hypovolemic shock
Contraindications	Patients with known hypersensitivity to the drug
	Patients receiving anticoagulants
Precautions	Severe anaphylactic reactions have been known to occur
	Monitor for circulatory overload
	Can impede accurate blood typing because dextran molecule coats the erythrocytes; draw tube of blood for blood typing before administering dextran
Side Effects	Nausea
	Vomiting
Dosage	Dosage should be titrated according to patient's hemodynamic response
	500 mL over 15–30 mins
Route	IV infusion
Pediatric Dosage	Same as adult

Hetastarch (Hespan)

Class	Artificial colloid
Action	Plasma volume expander
Indication	Hypovolemic shock
Contraindication	Patients receiving anticoagulants
Precautions	Monitor for circulatory overload
	Large volumes of hetastarch may alter the coagulation mechanism
Side Effects	Nausea
	Vomiting
Dosage	Dosage should be titrated according to patient's hemodynamic response
	500–1000 mL, not to exceed 20 mL/kg/hr; total dose not to exceed 1500 mL in 24 hours
Route	IV infusion
Pediatric Dosage	Safety in children has not been established

Lactated Ringer's Solution

Class	Isotonic crystalloid
Action	Approximates the electrolyte concentration of the blood
Indication	Hypovolemic shock
Contraindications	Congestive heart failure
	Renal failure

Precaution	Monitor for circulatory overload
Side Effects	Rare
Dosage	*Hypovolemic shock (systolic less than 90 mm Hg):* Infuse "wide open" until a systolic of 100 mm Hg is attained; once a systolic of 100 mm Hg has been attained, infusion should be slowed to 100 mL/hr
	Other: As indicated by the patient's condition and situation being treated
Route	IV infusion
Pediatric Dosage	20 mL/kg repeated as required based on hemodynamic response

5 Percent Dextrose in Water (D_5W)

Class	Sugar solution
Action	Glucose nutrient solution
Indications	IV access for emergency drugs
	For dilution of concentrated drugs for IV infusion
Contraindication	Should not be used as a fluid replacement for hypovolemic states
Precautions	Monitor for circulatory overload
	Draw tube of blood before administering to diabetics
Side Effects	Rare
Dosage	Generally administered TKO
Route	IV infusion
Pediatric Dosage	Same as adult

10 Percent Dextrose in Water ($D_{10}W$)

Class	Hypertonic sugar solution
Action	Replaces blood glucose
Indications	Hypoglycemia
	Neonatal resuscitation
	Rarely used as an IV infusion; rather, as a bolus dose as needed.
Contraindication	Should not be used as fluid replacement for hypovolemic states
Precautions	Monitor for circulatory overload
	Draw tube of blood before administering $D_{10}W$ to diabetics
Side Effects	Rare
Dosage	Dependent on patient's condition and condition being treated
Route	IV infusion
Pediatric Dosage	<3 months of age, 2–6 mL/kg IV/IO

0.9 Percent Sodium Chloride (Normal Saline)

Class	Isotonic electrolyte
Action	Fluid and sodium replacement
Indications	Heat-related problems (heat exhaustion and heat stroke)
	Freshwater drowning
	Hypovolemia
	Diabetic ketoacidosis
Contraindication	Congestive heart failure
Precaution	Electrolyte depletion (K^+, Mg^{2+}, Ca^{2+}, among others) can occur following administration of large amounts of normal saline
Side Effect	Thirst
Dosage	Dependent on patient's condition and situation being treated; in freshwater drowning and heat emergencies, the administration is usually rapid
Route	IV infusion
Pediatric Dosage	Dose is dependent on patient's size and condition

0.45 Percent Sodium Chloride (One-Half Normal Saline)

Class	Hypotonic electrolyte
Action	Slow rehydration
Indications	Patients with diminished renal or cardiovascular function for which rapid rehydration is not indicated
Contraindications	Cases in which rapid rehydration is indicated
Precaution	Electrolyte depletion can occur following administration of large amounts of one-half normal saline
Side Effects	Rare
Dosage	Dependent on patient's condition and situation being treated
Route	IV infusion
Pediatric Dosage	Dose is based on patient's size and condition

5 Percent Dextrose in 0.9 Percent Sodium Chloride (D₅NS)

Class	Hypertonic sugar and electrolyte solution
Action	Provides electrolyte and sugar replacement
Indications	Heat-related disorders
	Freshwater drowning
	Hypovolemia
	Peritonitis
Contraindications	Should not be administered to patients with impaired renal or cardiovascular function

Precaution	Draw tube of blood before administering to diabetics
Side Effects	Rare
Dosage	Dependent on patient's condition and situation being treated
Route	IV infusion
Pediatric Dosage	Dose is dependent on patient's size and condition

5 Percent Dextrose in 0.45 Percent Sodium Chloride (D₅1/2NS)

Class	Slightly hypertonic sugar and electrolyte solution
Action	Provides electrolyte and sugar replacement
Indications	Heat exhaustion
	Diabetic disorders
	For use as a TKO solution in patients with impaired renal or cardiovascular function
Contraindications	Situations in which rapid fluid replacement is indicated
Precaution	Draw tube of blood before administering to diabetics
Side Effects	Rare
Dosage	Dependent on patient's condition and situation being treated
Route	IV infusion
Pediatric Dosage	Dose is dependent on patient's size and condition

5 Percent Dextrose in Lactated Ringer's Solution (D₅LR)

Class	Hypertonic sugar and electrolyte solution
Action	Provides electrolyte and sugar replacement
Indications	Hypovolemic shock
	Hemorrhagic shock
	Certain cases of acidosis
Contraindications	Should not be administered to patients with decreased renal or cardiovascular function
Precautions	Monitor for signs of circulatory overload
	Draw tube of blood before administering to diabetics
Side Effects	Rare
Dosage	Dependent on patient's condition and situation being treated
Route	IV infusion
Pediatric Dosage	Dose is dependent on patient's size and condition

Pediatric Fluid Resuscitation

Bolus #1	20 mL normal saline or lactated Ringer's solution
Bolus #2	20 mL normal saline or lactated Ringer's solution
Bolus #3	10 mL/kg of colloid or blood

Quick Drug Reference

INTRODUCTION

This appendix provides a quick reference to the most commonly used emergency medications. The dosages and indications have been taken from the most recent Advanced Cardiac Life Support (ACLS) standards of the American Heart Association. Drugs not covered in ACLS are taken from the American Medical Association's *Drug Evaluation*. It is important to remember that specific drugs, dosages, indications, and routes may vary by area. It is essential that paramedics be familiar with these variations and follow the guidelines established by the medical director of the system in which they work.

Activated Charcoal

Class	Adsorbent
Action	Adsorbs toxins by chemical binding and prevents gastrointestinal adsorption
Indications	Poisoning following emesis or when emesis is contraindicated
Contraindications	None in severe poisoning
Precautions	Should only be administered following emesis in cases in which it is so indicated
	Use with caution in patients with altered mental status
	May absorb ipecac before emesis; if ipecac is administered, wait at least 10 minutes to administer activated charcoal
Side Effects	Nausea and vomiting
	Constipation
Dosage	1 g/kg (typically 50–75 g) mixed with a glass of water to form a slurry
Route	Oral
Pediatric Dosage	1 g/kg mixed with a glass of water to form a slurry

Adenosine (Adenocard)

Class	Antiarrhythmic
Action	Slows atrioventricular conduction
Indication	Symptomatic PSVT
Contraindications	Second- or third-degree heart block
	Sick-sinus syndrome
	Known hypersensitivity to the drug
Precautions	Arrhythmias, including blocks, are common at the time of cardioversion
	Use with caution in patients with asthma
Side Effects	Facial flushing
	Headache
	Shortness of breath
	Dizziness
	Nausea
Dosage	6 mg given as a rapid intravenous (IV) bolus over a 1- to 2-second period; if, after 1–2 minutes, cardioversion does not occur, administer a 12 mg dose over 1–2 seconds
Route	IV; should be administered directly into a vein or into the medication administration port closest to the patient and followed by flushing of the line with IV fluid
Pediatric Dosage	Safety in children has not been established

Albuterol (Proventil)

Class	Sympathomimetic (β_2 selective)
Action	Bronchodilation
Indications	Asthma
	Reversible bronchospasm associated with chronic obstructive pulmonary disease
Contraindications	Known hypersensitivity to the drug
	Symptomatic tachycardia
Precautions	Blood pressure, pulse, and electrocardiogram (ECG) results should be monitored
	Use caution in patients with known heart disease
Side Effects	Palpitations
	Anxiety
	Headache
	Dizziness
	Sweating
Dosage	*Metered-dose inhaler:* One to two sprays (90 μg per spray)

Small-volume nebulizer: 0.5 mL (2.5 mg) in 2.5 mL normal saline over 5–15 minutes

Rotohaler: One 200 μg Rotocap should be placed in the inhaler and breathed by the patient

Route	Inhalation
Pediatric Dosage	0.15 mg/kg (0.03 mL/kg) in 2.5 mL normal saline by small-volume nebulizer

Aminophylline

Class	Xanthine bronchodilator
Actions	Smooth muscle relaxant
	Causes bronchodilation
	Has mild diuretic properties
	Increases heart rate
Indications	Bronchial asthma
	Reversible bronchospasm associated with chronic bronchitis and emphysema
	Congestive heart failure
	Pulmonary edema
Contraindications	Patients with history of hypersensitivity to the drug
	Hypotension
	Patients with peptic ulcer disease
Precautions	Monitor for arrhythmias
	Monitor blood pressure
	Do not administer to patients on chronic theophylline preparations until the theophylline blood level has been determined
Side Effects	Convulsions
	Tremor
	Anxiety
	Dizziness
	Vomiting
	Palpitations
	PVCs
	Tachycardia
Dosages	*Method 1:* 250–500 mg in 90 or 80 mL of D_5W infused over 20–30 minutes (approximately 5–10 mg/kg/hr)
	Method 2: 250–500 mg (5–7 mg/kg) in 20 mL of D_5W infused over 20–30 minutes
Route	Slow intravenous (IV) infusion
Pediatric Dosage	6 mg/kg loading dose to be infused over 20–30 minutes; maximum dose not to exceed 12 mg/kg over 24 hours

Amiodarone HCL (Cordarone)

Class	Antiarrhythmic agent (group III)
Action	Prolongs action potential and refractory period
	Slows the sinus rate; increases PR and QT intervals
	Decreases peripheral vascular resistance
Indications	Life-threatening cardiac arrhythmias such as ventricular tachycardia and ventricular fibrillation
Contraindications	Severe sinus node dysfunction
	Sinus bradycardia
	Second- and third-degree atrioventricular block
	Hemodynamically significant bradycardia
Precautions	Heart failure
Side Effects	Hypotension
	Nausea
	Anorexia
	Malaise, fatigue
	Tremors
	Pulmonary toxicity
	Ventricular ectopic beats
Dosage	*Adults:* Loading dose of 150 mg over 10 minutes (15 mg/min)
	Maintenance dose: 1 mg/min for 6 hours, then 0.5 mg/min until arrhythmia is controlled or oral therapy begins
Route	IV, oral
Pediatric Dosage	5 mg/kg IV or IO; maximum dose: 15 mg/kg.

Amrinone (Inocor)

Class	Cardiac inotrope
Actions	Increases cardiac contractility
	Vasodilator
Indication	Short-term management of severe congestive heart failure
Contraindication	Patients with history of hypersensitivity to the drug
Precautions	May increase myocardial ischemia
	Blood pressure, pulse, and electrocardiogram (ECG) results should be constantly monitored
	Amrinone should only be diluted with normal saline or one-half normal saline; no dextrose solutions should be used
	Furosemide (Lasix) should not be administered into an intravenous (IV) line delivering amrinone
Side Effects	Reduction in platelets
	Nausea and vomiting
	Cardiac arrhythmias

Dosage	0.75 mg/kg bolus given slowly over 2- to 5-minute interval followed by maintenance infusion of 2–15 mg/kg/min
Route	IV bolus and infusion as described earlier
Pediatric Dosage	Safety in children has not been established

Amyl Nitrate

Class	Nitrate
Actions	Causes coronary vasodilation
	Removes cyanide ion via complex mechanism
Indication	Cyanide poisoning (bitter almond smell to breath)
Contraindications	None when used in the management of cyanide poisoning
Precautions	Has tendency for abuse
Side Effects	Headache
	Hypotension
	Reflex tachycardia
	Nausea
Dosage	Inhalant should be broken and inhaled, repeated as needed until patient is delivered to emergency department; effects diminish after 20 minutes
Route	Inhalation
Pediatric Dosage	Inhalant should be broken and inhaled, repeated until patient is delivered to emergency department

Anistreplase (Eminase)

Class	Thrombolytic
Action	Dissolves blood clots
Indication	Acute myocardial infarction
Contraindications	Persons with internal bleeding
	Suspected aortic dissection
	Traumatic cardiopulmonary resuscitation
	Severe persistent hypertension
	Recent head trauma or known intracranial tumor
	History of stroke in the past 6 months
	Pregnancy
Precautions	May be ineffective if administered within 12 months of prior streptokinase or anistreplase therapy
	Antiarrhythmic and resuscitative drugs should be available
Side Effects	Bleeding
	Allergic reactions
	Anaphylaxis
	Fever
	Nausea and vomiting

Dosage	30 units slow intravenously (IV) over 2–5 minutes
Route	IV (slow)
Pediatric Dosage	Not recommended

Aspirin

Class	Platelet inhibitor and anti-inflammatory
Action	Blocks platelet aggregation
Indications	New chest pain suggestive of acute myocardial infarction
	Signs and symptoms suggestive of recent stroke (cerebrovascular accident)
Contraindications	Patients with known hypersensitivity to the drug
Precautions	Gastrointestinal bleeding and upset stomach
Side Effects	Heartburn
	Nausea and vomiting
	Wheezing
Dosage	160 or 325 mg by mouth chewed
Route	Oral
Pediatric Dosage	Not recommended

Atropine

Class	Parasympatholytic (anticholinergic)
Actions	Blocks acetylcholine receptors
	Increases heart rate
	Decreases gastrointestinal secretions
Indications	Hemodynamically significant bradycardia
	Hypotension secondary to bradycardia
	Asystole
	Organophosphate poisoning
Contraindication	None when used in emergency situations
Precautions	Dose of 0.04 mg/kg should not be exceeded except in cases of organophosphate poisonings
	Tachycardia
	Hypertension
Side Effects	Palpitations
	Tachycardia
	Headache
	Dizziness
	Anxiety
	Dry mouth
	Pupillary dilation
	Blurred vision
	Urinary retention (especially in older men)

Dosage	*Bradycardia:* 0.5 mg every 3–5 minutes to maximum of 0.04 mg/kg
	Asystole: 1 mg
	Organophosphate poisoning: 2–5 mg
Routes	Intravenous (IV)
	Endotracheal (endotracheal dose 2 to 2.5 times the IV dose)
Pediatric Dosage	*Bradycardia:* 0.02 mg/kg (minimum dose of 0.1 mg)
	Maximum single dose: child, 0.5 mg; adolescent, 1.0 mg
	Maximum total dose: child, 1.0 mg; adolescent, 2.0 mg

Bretylium Tosylate (Bretylol)

Class	Antiarrhythmic
Actions	Increases ventricular fibrillation threshold
	Blocks the release of norepinephrine from peripheral sympathetic nerves
Indications	Ventricular fibrillation refractory to lidocaine
	Ventricular tachycardia refractory to lidocaine
	PVCs refractory to first-line medications
Contraindications	None when used in the management of life-threatening arrhythmias
Precautions	Postural hypotension occurs in approximately 50 percent of patients receiving bretylium
	Patient must be kept supine
	Dosage is decreased in patients being treated with catecholamine sympathomimetics
Side Effects	Hypotension
	Syncope
	Bradycardia
	Increased frequency of arrhythmias
	Dizziness and vertigo
Dosage	5 mg/kg; may be repeated at dose of 10 mg/kg up to a total dose of 30 mg/kg
Route	Rapid intravenous (IV) bolus
Pediatric Dosage	5 mg/kg

Bumetanide (Bumex)

Class	Potent diuretic
Actions	Inhibits reabsorption of sodium chloride
	Promotes prompt diuresis
	Slight vasodilation
Indications	Congestive heart failure
	Pulmonary edema

Contraindications	Dehydration
	Pregnancy
Precautions	Should be protected from light
	Dehydration
Side Effects	Few in emergency usage
Dosage	0.5–1.0 mg
Routes	Intravenous (IV), intramuscular (IM)
Pediatric Dosage	Safety in children has not been established

Butorphanol (Stadol)

Class	Synthetic analgesic
Actions	Central nervous system depressant
	Decreases sensitivity to pain
Indication	Moderate to severe pain
Contraindications	Patients with a history of hypersensitivity to the drug
	Head injury
	Use with caution in patients with impaired respiratory function
Precautions	Respiratory depression (naloxone should be available)
	Patients dependent on narcotics
Side Effects	Symptoms of withdrawal when administered to persons dependent on narcotics
	Nausea
	Altered levels of consciousness
Dosage	*Intravenous (IV):* 1 mg
	Intramuscular (IM): 2 mg
Routes	IV, IM
Pediatric Dosage	Rarely used

Calcium Chloride

Class	Electrolyte
Action	Increases cardiac contractility
Indications	Acute hyperkalemia (elevated potassium level)
	Acute hypocalcemia (decreased calcium level)
	Calcium channel blocker (e.g., nifedipine, verapamil) overdose
	Abdominal muscle spasm associated with spider bite and Portuguese man-of-war stings
	Antidote for magnesium sulfate
Contraindication	Patients receiving digitalis
Precautions	Intravenous (IV) line should be flushed between calcium chloride and sodium bicarbonate administration
	Extravasation may cause tissue necrosis

Side Effects	Arrhythmias (bradycardia and asystole)
	Hypotension
Dosage	2–4 mg/kg of a 10 percent solution; may be repeated at 10-minute intervals
Route	IV
Pediatric Dosage	5–7 mg/kg of a 10 percent solution

Chlorpromazine (Thorazine, Largactil)

Class	Major tranquilizer
Actions	Blocks dopamine receptors in brain associated with mood and behavior
	Has antiemetic properties
Indications	Acute psychotic episodes
	Mild alcohol withdrawal
	Intractable hiccoughs
	Nausea and vomiting
Contraindications	Comatose states
	Presence of sedatives
	Presence of hallucinogens or phencyclidine-like compounds
Precautions	Orthostatic hypotension
	May cause extrapyramidal reactions (Parkinsonian), especially in children
Side Effects	Physical and mental impairment
	Drowsiness
Dosage	25–100 mg
Route	Intramuscular (IM)
Pediatric Dosage	0.5 mg/kg

Dexamethasone (Decadron, Hexadrol)

Class	Steroid
Actions	Possibly decreases cerebral edema
	Anti-inflammatory
	Suppresses immune response (especially in allergic reactions)
Indications	Cerebral edema
	Anaphylaxis (after epinephrine and diphenhydramine)
	Asthma
	Chronic obstructive pulmonary disease
Contraindications	None in the emergency setting
Precautions	Should be protected from heat
	Onset of action may be 2–6 hours and thus should not be considered to be of use in the critical first hour following an anaphylactic reaction

Side Effects	Gastrointestinal bleeding
	Prolonged wound healing
Dosage	4–24 mg
Routes	Intravenous (IV), intramuscular (IM)
Pediatric Dosage	0.2–0.5 mg/kg

Dextrose (50 Percent)

Class	Carbohydrate
Action	Elevates blood glucose level rapidly
Indication	Hypoglycemia
Contraindications	None in the emergency setting
Precaution	A blood sample should be drawn before administering 50 percent dextrose
Side Effect	Local venous irritation
Dosage	25 g (50 mL)
Route	Intravenous (IV)
Pediatric Dosage	0.5 g/kg slow IV; should be diluted 1:1 with sterile water to form a 25 percent solution

Diazepam (Valium)

Class	Tranquilizer
Actions	Anticonvulsant
	Skeletal muscle relaxant
	Sedative
Indications	Major motor seizures
	Status epilepticus
	Premedication before cardioversion
	Skeletal muscle relaxant
	Acute anxiety states
Contraindication	Patients with a history of hypersensitivity to the drug
Precautions	Can cause local venous irritation
	Has short duration of effect
	Do not mix with other drugs because of possible precipitation problems
	Flumazenil (Romazicon) should be available
Side Effects	Drowsiness
	Hypotension
	Respiratory depression and apnea
Dosage	*Status epilepticus:* 5–10 mg intravenously (IV)
	Acute Anxiety: 2–5 mg intramuscularly (IM) or IV
	Premedication before cardioversion: 5–15 mg IV
Routes	IV (care must be taken not to administer faster than 1 mL/min), IM, rectal
Pediatric Dosage	*Status epilepticus:* 0.1–0.2 mg/kg

Diazoxide (Hyperstat)

Class	Antihypertensive
Actions	Causes decrease in both systolic and diastolic pressures
	Direct peripheral arterial dilation
Indication	Hypertensive emergency
Contraindications	None in the emergency setting
Precautions	Avoid overcorrection of blood pressure
	Blood pressure must be constantly monitored
	Patient should be supine
Side Effects	Hypotension
	Syncope
	Local venous irritation
Dosage	1–3 mg/kg boluses by rapid injection (less than 30 seconds) repeated at 5- to 15-minute intervals up to 150 mg in a single injection
Route	Intravenous (IV) only
Pediatric Dosage	1–3 mg/kg

Digoxin (Lanoxin)

Class	Cardiac glycoside
Actions	Increases cardiac contractile force
	Increases cardiac output
	Reduces edema associated with congestive heart failure
	Slows atrioventricular conduction
Indications	Congestive heart failure
	Rapid atrial arrhythmias, especially atrial flutter and atrial fibrillation
Contraindications	Any patient with signs or symptoms of digitalis toxicity
	Ventricular fibrillation
Precautions	Monitor for signs of digitalis toxicity
	Patients who have recently suffered a myocardial infarction have greater sensitivity to the effects of digitalis
	Calcium should not be administered to patients receiving digitalis
Side Effects	Nausea and vomiting
	Arrhythmias
	Yellow vision
Dosage	0.25–0.50 mg
Route	Intravenous (IV)
Pediatric Dosage	25–40 mg

Diltiazem (Cardizem)

Class	Calcium channel blocker
Actions	Slows conduction through the atrioventricular mode
	Causes vasodilation
	Decreases rate of ventricular response
	Decreases myocardial oxygen demand
Indications	To control rapid ventricular rates associated with atrial fibrillation and flutter
	Angina pectoris
Contraindications	Hypotension
	Wide-complex tachycardia
	Conduction system disturbances
Precautions	Should not be used in patients receiving intravenous β-blockers
	Hypotension
	Must be kept refrigerated
Side Effects	Nausea and vomiting
	Hypotension
	Dizziness
Dosage	0.25 mg/kg bolus (typically 20 mg) intravenous (IV) over 2 minutes, followed by a maintenance infusion of 5–15 mg/hr
Routes	IV, IV drip
Pediatric Dosage	Rarely used

Dimenhydrinate (Gravol, Dramamine)

Class	Antihistamine
Action	Antiemetic
Indications	Nausea and vomiting
	Motion sickness
	To potentiate the effects of analgesics
Contraindications	Comatose states
	Patients who have received a large amount of depressants (including alcohol)
Precautions	Use with caution in patients with seizure disorders
	Asthma
Side Effects	May impair mental and physical ability
	Drowsiness
Dosage	*Slow intravenous (IV):* 12.5–25.0 mg
	Intramuscular (IM) or oral: 50–100 mg
Routes	IV, IM, oral
Pediatric Dosage	Pediatric data unavailable

Diphenhydramine (Benadryl)

Class	Antihistamine
Actions	Blocks histamine receptors
	Has some sedative effects
Indications	Anaphylaxis
	Allergic reactions
	Dystonic reactions due to phenothiazines
Contraindications	Asthma
	Nursing mothers
Precautions	Hypotension
Side Effects	Sedation
	Dries bronchial secretions
	Blurred vision
	Headache
	Palpitations
Dosage	25–50 mg
Routes	Slow intravenous (IV) push, deep intramuscular (IM)
Pediatric Dosage	2–5 mg/kg

Dobutamine (Dobutrex)

Class	Sympathomimetic
Actions	Increases cardiac contractility
	Little chronotropic activity
Indication	Short-term management of congestive heart failure
Contraindication	Should only be used in patients with an adequate heart rate
Precautions	Ventricular irritability
	Use with caution following myocardial infarction
	Can be deactivated by alkaline solutions
Side Effects	Headache
	Hypertension
	Palpitations
Dosage	2.5–20 μg/kg/min
	Method: 250 mg should be placed in 500 mL of D_5W, which gives a concentration of 0.5 mg/mL
Route	Intravenous (IV) drip
Pediatric Dosage	2–20 μg/kg/min

Dopamine (Intropin)

Class	Sympathomimetic
Actions	Increases cardiac contractility
	Causes peripheral vasoconstriction

Indications	Hemodynamically significant hypotension (systolic blood pressure of 70–100 mm Hg) not resulting from hypovolemia
	Cardiogenic shock
Contraindications	Hypovolemic shock in which complete fluid resuscitation has not occurred
	Pheochromocytoma
Precautions	Presence of severe tachyarrhythmias
	Presence of ventricular fibrillation
	Ventricular irritability
	Beneficial effects lost when dose exceeds 20 μg/kg/min
Side Effects	Ventricular tachyarrhythmias
	Hypertension
	Palpitations
Dosage	*Initial dose:* 2–5 μg/kg/min; increase as needed
	Method: 800 mg should be placed in 500 mL of D_5W, giving a concentration of 1600 mg/mL
Route	Intravenous (IV) drip only
Pediatric Dosage	2–20 μg/kg/min

Edrophonium (Tensilon)

Class	Anticholinesterase
Actions	Inhibits action of enzyme cholinesterase, thus potentiating acetylcholine
	Increases parasympathetic tone
Indication	PSVT refractory to vagal maneuvers; considered a second-line agent to verapamil or adenosine
Contraindication	Patients with a history of hypersensitivity to the drug
Precautions	Respirations must be constantly monitored
	Bradycardia
	Hypotension
	Avoid exposure to dextrose solutions
Side Effects	Dizziness
	Syncope
Dosage	5 mg
Route	Intravenous (IV)
Pediatric Dosage	0.1–0.2 mg/kg

Epinephrine 1:1000

Class	Sympathomimetic
Action	Bronchodilation

Indications	Bronchial asthma
	Exacerbation of chronic obstructive pulmonary disease
	Allergic reactions
	Pediatric cardiac arrest (after initial epinephrine dosage)
Contraindications	Patients with underlying cardiovascular disease
	Hypertension
	Pregnancy
	Patients with tachyarrhythmias
Precautions	Should be protected from light
	Blood pressure, pulse, and electrocardiogram (ECG) results must be constantly monitored
Side Effects	Palpitations and tachycardia
	Anxiousness
	Headache
	Tremor
Dosage	0.3–0.5 mg
Route	Subcutaneous
Pediatric Dosage	0.01 mg/kg up to 0.3 mg

Epinephrine 1: 10 000

Class	Sympathomimetic
Actions	Increases heart rate and automaticity
	Increases cardiac contractile force
	Increases myocardial electrical activity
	Increases systemic vascular resistance
	Increases blood pressure
	Causes bronchodilation
Indications	Cardiac arrest
	Anaphylactic shock
	Severe reactive airway disease
Contraindications	Epinephrine 1: 10 000 is for intravenous (IV) or endotracheal use; it should not be used in patients who do not require extensive resuscitative efforts
Precautions	Should be protected from light
	Can be deactivated by alkaline solutions
Side Effects	Palpitations
	Anxiety
	Tremulousness
	Nausea and vomiting
Dosage	*Cardiac arrest:* 0.5–1.0 mg repeated every 3–5 minutes; higher doses may be ordered by medical control
	Severe anaphylaxis: 0.3–0.5 mg (3–5 mL); occasionally an epinephrine drip is required

Routes	IV, IV drip, endotracheal (endotracheal dose 2 to 2.5 times IV dose)
Pediatric Dosage	0.01 mg/kg initially; with subsequent doses, epinephrine 1:1000 should be used at a dose of 0.1 mg/kg

Esmolol (Brevibloc)

Class	Beta-blocker (β_1 selective)
Actions	Decreases heart rate
	Decreases atrioventricular conduction
Indications	Symptomatic supraventricular tachycardia (including atrial fibrillation and atrial flutter) as evidenced by chest pain, palpitations, or dizziness
Contraindications	Sinus bradycardia
	Heart block greater than first degree
	Cardiogenic shock
	Overt congestive heart failure
	Patients with bronchospastic disease (asthma)
Precautions	Hypotension is common and is usually dose related
	Patients with congestive heart failure may have worsening of their symptoms
	May worsen bronchospastic disease
Side Effects	Dizziness
	Diaphoresis
	Hypotension
	Nausea
Dosage	*Preparation:* Place two 2.5 g ampules in 500 mL of D_5W, yielding a concentration of 10 mg/mL
	Loading dose: 500 mg/kg/min for 1 minute, then reduce to maintenance dose
	Maintenance dose: 50 mg/kg/min; if ineffective after 4 minutes, repeat loading dose and increase maintenance dose to 100 mg/kg/min; may repeat as needed until a total maintenance dose of 200 mg/kg/min has been achieved
Route	Intravenous (IV) infusion only
Pediatric Dosage	Safety in children has not been established

Fentanyl Citrate (Sublimaze)

Class	Narcotic
Actions	Central nervous system depressant
	Decreases sensitivity to pain
Indications	Severe pain
	Adjunct to rapid-sequence induction (RSI)
	Adjunct to rapid-sequence sedation (RSS)
	Maintenance of analgesia

Contraindications	Shock
	Severe hemorrhage
	Undiagnosed abdominal pain
	Patients with history of hypersensitivity to the drug
Precautions	Respiratory depression (naloxone should be available)
	Hypotension
	Nausea
Side Effects	Dizziness
	Altered level of consciousness
	Bradycardia
Dosage	25–100 μg
Route	Intravenous (IV)
Pediatric Dosage	2–12 years: 1.7–3.3 μg/kg

Flumazenil (Romazicon)

Class	Benzodiazepine antagonist
Action	Reverses the effects of benzodiazepines
Indication	To reverse central nervous system (CNS) respiratory depression associated with benzodiazepines
Contraindications	Flumazenil should not be used as a diagnostic agent for benzodiazepine overdose in the same manner naloxone is used for narcotic overdose
	Known hypersensitivity to the drug
Precautions	Administer with caution to patients dependent on benzodiazepines because it may induce life-threatening benzodiazepine withdrawal
Side Effects	Fatigue
	Headache
	Nervousness
	Dizziness
Dosage	0.2 mg intravenously (IV) over 30 seconds, repeated as needed to a maximum dose of 1.0 mg
Route	IV
Pediatric Dosage	Pediatric data unavailable

Furosemide (Lasix)

Class	Potent diuretic
Actions	Inhibits reabsorption of sodium chloride
	Promotes prompt diuresis
	Vasodilation
Indications	Congestive heart failure
	Pulmonary edema
Contraindications	Pregnancy
	Dehydration

Precautions	Should be protected from light
	Dehydration
Side Effects	Few in emergency usage
Dosage	40–80 mg
Route	Intravenous (IV)
Pediatric Dosage	1 mg/kg

Glucagon

Class	Hormone (antihypoglycemic agent)
Actions	Causes breakdown of glycogen to glucose
	Inhibits glycogen synthesis
	Elevates blood glucose level
	Increases cardiac contractile force
	Increases heart rate
Indication	Hypoglycemia
Contraindication	Hypersensitivity to the drug
Precautions	Only effective if there are sufficient stores of glycogen within the liver
	Use with caution in patients with cardiovascular or renal disease
	Draw blood for glucose test before administration
Side Effects	Few in emergency situations
Dosage	*Intravenous (IV):* 0.25–0.5 unit
	Intramuscular (IM): 1.0 mg
Routes	IV, IM
Pediatric Dosage	0.03 mg/kg

Haloperidol (Haldol)

Class	Major tranquilizer
Actions	Blocks dopamine receptors in brain responsible for mood and behavior
	Has antiemetic properties
Indication	Acute psychotic episodes
Contraindications	Should not be administered in the presence of other sedatives
	Should not be used in the management of dysphoria caused by Talwin
Precaution	Orthostatic hypotension
Side Effects	Physical and mental impairment
	Parkinson-like reactions have been known to occur, especially in children
Dosage	2–5 mg
Route	Intramuscular (IM)
Pediatric Dosage	Rarely used

Hydralazine (Apresoline)

Class	Antihypertensive (potent vasodilator)
Actions	Relaxes vascular smooth muscle
	Decreases arterial pressure (diastolic greater than systolic)
	Increases cardiac output
Indications	Hypertensive emergency in which a prompt reduction in blood pressure is required
	Hypertension accompanying pregnancy
Contraindications	Patients with a known history of coronary artery disease
	Rheumatic heart disease involving the mitral valve
	History of hypersensitivity to the drug
Precautions	May induce angina
	May cause electrocardiogram (ECG) changes and cardiac ischemia
	Blood pressure, pulse rate, and ECG results should be constantly monitored
Side Effects	Headache
	Nausea
	Vomiting
	Tachycardia
	Palpitations
	Diarrhea
Dosage	20–40 mg given by slow intravenous (IV) bolus; may be repeated, if required
Route	IV
Pediatric Dosage	Safety in children has not been established

Hydrocortisone (Solu-Cortef)

Class	Steroid
Actions	Antiinflammatory
	Suppresses immune response (especially in allergic and anaphylactic reactions)
Indications	Severe anaphylaxis
	Asthma and chronic obstructive pulmonary disease
	Urticaria (hives)
Contraindications	None in the emergency setting
Precautions	Must be reconstituted and used promptly
	Onset of action may be 2–6 hours, and thus the drug should not be expected to be of use in the critical first hour following an acute anaphylactic reaction
Side Effects	Gastrointestinal bleeding
	Prolonged wound healing
	Suppression of natural steroids

Dosage	100–250 mg
Routes	Intravenous (IV), intramuscular (IM)
Pediatric Dosage	30 mg/kg

Hydroxyzine (Vistaril)

Class	Antihistamine
Actions	Antiemetic
	Antihistamine
	Antianxiety
	Potentiates analgesic effects of narcotics and related agents
Indications	To potentiate the effects of narcotics and synthetic narcotics
	Nausea and vomiting
	Anxiety reactions
Contraindication	Patients with a history of hypersensitivity to the drug
Precautions	Orthostatic hypotension
	Analgesic dosages should be reduced when used with hydroxyzine
	Urinary retention
Side Effect	Drowsiness
Dosage	50–100 mg
Route	Deep intramuscular (IM)
Pediatric Dosage	1 mg/kg

Insulin (Humilin, Novolin, Iletin)

Class	Hormone (hypoglycemic agent)
Actions	Causes uptake of glucose by the cells
	Decreases blood glucose level
	Promotes glucose storage
Indications	Elevated blood glucose
	Diabetic ketoacidosis
Contraindications	Avoid overcompensation of blood glucose level; if possible, administration should wait until the patient is in the emergency department
Precautions	Administration of excessive dose may induce hypoglycemia
	Glucose should be available
Side Effects	Few in emergency situations
Dosage	10–25 units regular insulin intravenously (IV) followed by an infusion at 0.1 units/kg/hr
Routes	IV, SQ
Pediatric Dosage	Dosage is based on blood glucose level

Ipecac

Class	Emetic
Actions	Irritates the enteric tract
	Acts on vomiting center in the brain
Indication	Poisoning in conscious patient
Contraindications	Vomiting should not be induced in any patient with impaired consciousness
	Poisonings involving strong acids, bases, or petroleum distillates
	Antiemetic poisonings, especially of the phenothiazine type
Precautions	Monitor and ensure a patent airway
	The risk of aspiration is increased when using ipecac
Side Effects	Rare
Dosage	30 mL (1 oz) followed by 15 mL/kg of warm water
Route	Oral
Pediatric Dosage	*<1 year of age:* 10 mL
	1–12 years of age: 15 mL
	>12 years of age: 30 mL

Ipratropium (Atrovent)

Class	Anticholinergic
Actions	Causes bronchodilation
	Dries respiratory tract secretions
Indications	Bronchial asthma
	Reversible bronchospasm associated with chronic bronchitis and emphysema
Contraindications	Should not be used in patients with history of hypersensitivity to the drug
	Should not be used as primary acute treatment of bronchospasm
Precautions	Monitor vital signs
Side Effects	Palpitations
	Dizziness
	Anxiety
	Headache
	Nervousness
Dosage	500 mg placed in small-volume nebulizer (typically administered with a β-agonist)
Route	Inhaled
Pediatric Dosage	Safety in children has not been established

Isoetharine (Bronkosol)

Class	Sympathomimetic (β_2 selective)
Actions	Bronchodilation
	Increases heart rate
Indications	Asthma
	Reversible bronchospasm associated with chronic bronchitis and emphysema
Contraindication	Patients with history of hypersensitivity to the drug
Precautions	Blood pressure, pulse, and electrocardiogram (ECG) results must be constantly monitored
Side Effects	Palpitations
	Tachycardia
	Anxiety
	Tremors
	Headache
Dosage	*Hand nebulizer:* Four inhalations
	Small-volume nebulizer: 0.5 mL (1:3 with saline)
Route	Inhalation only
Pediatric Dosage	0.25–0.5 mL diluted with 4 mL normal saline

Isoproterenol (Isuprel)

Class	Sympathomimetic
Actions	Increases heart rate
	Increases cardiac contractile force
	Causes bronchodilation
Indications	Bradycardias refractory to atropine (when transcutaneous pacing is unavailable)
	Severe status asthmaticus
Contraindication	Should not be used to increase blood pressure in cardiogenic shock
Precautions	Can cause ventricular irritability
	Can be deactivated by alkaline solutions
	Should be used with caution for recent myocardial infarction
	External pacing, if available, should be used instead of isoproterenol
Side Effects	Tachyarrhythmias
	Tremors
	Palpitations
	Headache
Dosage	1 mg should be placed in 500 mL of D_5W and then slowly infused at 2–10 μg/min and titrated until the desired rate is obtained or until PVCs occur
Route	Intravenous (IV) drip only
Pediatric Dosage	0.1 μg/kg/min

Ketorolac (Toradol)

Class	Nonsteroidal anti-inflammatory agent
Actions	Anti-inflammatory
	Analgesic (peripherally acting)
Indication	Mild to moderate pain
Contraindications	Patients with a history of hypersensitivity to the drug
	Patients allergic to aspirin
Precautions	Gastrointestinal irritation or hemorrhage can occur
Side Effects	Edema
	Rash
	Heartburn
Dosage	*Intravenous (IV):* 15–30 mg
	Intramuscular (IM): 30–60 mg
Routes	IV, IM
Pediatric Dosage	Rarely used

Labetalol (Trandate, Normodyne)

Class	Sympathetic blocker
Actions	Selectively blocks α_1-receptors and nonselectively blocks β-receptors
Indication	Hypertensive crisis
Contraindications	Bronchial asthma
	Congestive heart failure
	Heart block
	Bradycardia
	Cardiogenic shock
Precautions	Blood pressure, pulse, and electrocardiogram (ECG) results must be constantly monitored
	Atropine should be available
Side Effects	Bradycardia
	Heart block
	Congestive heart failure
	Bronchospasm
	Postural hypotension
Dosage	20 mg by slow intravenous (IV) infusion over 2 minutes; doses of 40 mg can be repeated in 10 minutes until desired supine blood pressure is obtained or until 300 mg of the drug has been given
	200 mg placed in 500 mL D_5W to deliver 2 mg/min
Route	IV infusion or slow IV bolus as described earlier
Pediatric Dosage	Safety in children has not been established

Lidocaine (Xylocaine)

Class	Antiarrhythmic
Actions	Suppresses ventricular ectopic activity
	Increases ventricular fibrillation threshold
	Reduces velocity of electrical impulse through conductive system
Indications	Malignant PVCs
	Ventricular tachycardia
	Ventricular fibrillation
	Prophylaxis of arrhythmias associated with thrombolytic therapy
Contraindications	High-degree heart blocks
	PVCs in conjunction with bradycardia
Precautions	Dosage should not exceed 300 mg/hr
	Monitor for central nervous system toxicity
	Dosage should be reduced by 50 percent in patients older than 70 years of age or who have liver disease
	In cardiac arrest, use only bolus therapy
Side Effects	Anxiety
	Drowsiness
	Dizziness
	Confusion
	Nausea and vomiting
	Convulsions
	Widening of QRS complex
Dosage	*Bolus:* Initial bolus of 1.0–1.5 mg/kg; additional boluses of 0.5–0.75 mg/kg can be repeated at 3- to 5-minute intervals until the arrhythmia has been suppressed or until 3.0 mg/kg of the drug has been administered; reduce dosage by 50 percent in patients older than 70 years of age
	Drip: After the arrhythmia has been suppressed, a 2–4 mg/min infusion may be started to maintain adequate blood levels
Routes	Intravenous (IV) bolus, IV infusion
Pediatric Dosage	1 mg/kg

Lorazepam (Ativan)

Class	Tranquilizer
Actions	Anticonvulsant
	Sedative
Indications	Major motor seizures
	Status epilepticus
	Premedication before cardioversion
	Acute anxiety states

Contraindication	Patients with a history of hypersensitivity to the drug
Precautions	Has short duration of effect
	Do not mix with other drugs because of possible precipitation problems
	Flumazenil (Romazicon) should be available
	Dilute with normal saline of D_5W prior to intravenous (IV) administration
Side Effects	Drowsiness
	Hypotension
	Respiratory depression and apnea
Dosage	0.5–2.0 mg IV; may be increased to 1.0–4.0 mg IV
Routes	IV, intramuscular (IM), rectal
Pediatric Dosage	0.05–0.10 mg/kg (maximum dose 4 mg)

Magnesium Sulfate

Class	Anticonvulsant and antiarrhythmic
Actions	Central nervous system depressant
	Anticonvulsant
	Antiarrhythmic
Indications	*Obstetrical:* Eclampsia (toxemia of pregnancy)
	Cardiovascular: Severe refractory ventricular fibrillation or pulseless ventricular tachycardia, post–myocardial infarction as prophylaxis for arrhythmias, and torsade de pointes (multiaxial ventricular tachycardia)
Contraindications	Shock
	Heart block
Precautions	Caution should be used in patients receiving digitalis
	Hypotension
	Calcium chloride should be readily available as an antidote if respiratory depression ensues
	Use with caution in patients with renal failure
Side Effects	Flushing
	Respiratory depression
	Drowsiness
Dosage	1–4 g
Routes	Intravenous (IV), intramuscular (IM)
Pediatric Dosage	Not indicated

Mannitol (Osmotrol)

Class	Osmotic diuretic
Actions	Decreases cellular edema
	Increases urinary output

Indications	Acute cerebral edema
	Blood transfusion reactions
Contraindications	Pulmonary edema
	Patients who are dehydrated
	Hypersensitivity to the drug
Precautions	Rapid administration can cause circulatory overload
	Crystallization of the drug can occur at lower temperatures
	An in-line filter should be used
Side Effects	Pulmonary congestion
	Sodium depletion
	Transient volume overload
Dosage	1.5–2.0 g/kg
Route	Intravenous (IV) slow bolus or infusion
Pediatric Dosage	0.25–0.5 g/kg IV over 60 minutes

Meperidine (Demerol)

Class	Narcotic
Actions	Central nervous system depressant
	Decreases sensitivity to pain
Indication	Moderate to severe pain
Contraindications	Patients receiving monoamine oxidase inhibitors
	Undiagnosed abdominal pain
	Patients with history of hypersensitivity to the drug
Precautions	Respiratory depression (naloxone should be available)
	Hypotension
	Nausea
Side Effects	Dizziness
	Altered level of consciousness
Dosage	*Intravenous (IV):* 25–50 mg
	Intramuscular (IM): 50–100 mg
Routes	IV, IM
Pediatric Dosage	1 mg/kg

Metaproterenol (Alupent)

Class	Sympathomimetic (β_2 selective)
Actions	Bronchodilation
	Increases heart rate
Indications	Bronchial asthma
	Reversible bronchospasm associated with chronic bronchitis and emphysema
Contraindications	Patients with cardiac dysrhythmias or significant tachycardia

Precautions	Blood pressure, pulse, and electrocardiogram (ECG) results must be constantly monitored; occasional nausea and vomiting reported
Side Effects	Palpitations
	Anxiety
	Headache
	Nausea and vomiting
	Dizziness
	Tremor
Dosage	*Metered-dose inhaler:* Two to three inhalations; can be repeated in 3–4 hours if required
	Small-volume nebulizer: 0.2–0.3 mL diluted in 2–3 mL normal saline administered over 5–15 minutes
Route	Inhalation only
Pediatric Dosage	0.05–0.3 mL in 4 mL normal saline

Metaraminol (Aramine)

Class	Sympathomimetic (indirect acting)
Actions	Causes release of endogenous stores of norepinephrine
	Increases cardiac contractile force
	Increases cardiac rate
	Causes peripheral vasoconstriction
Indication	Hemodynamically significant hypotension not due to hypovolemia
Contraindication	Hypotensive states due to hypovolemia
Precautions	Constant monitoring of blood pressure is essential
	Not effective in catecholamine-depleted patients
Side Effects	Palpitations
	Tachycardia
	PVCs
	Hypertension
	Tremor
	Dizziness
Dosage	200 mg should be placed in 500 mL of D_5W; this gives a concentration of 0.4 mg/mL, which should be slowly infused and titrated to blood pressure response
	5–10 mg can be administered intramuscularly (IM) when an intravenous (IV) line cannot be placed
Routes	IV drip, IM
Pediatric Dosage	Safety in children has not been established

Methylprednisone (Solu-Medrol)

Class	Steroid
Actions	Anti-inflammatory
	Suppresses immune response (especially in allergic reactions)
Indications	Severe anaphylaxis
	Asthma and chronic obstructive pulmonary disease
	Possibly effective as an adjunctive agent in the management of spinal cord injury
Contraindications	None in the emergency setting
Precautions	Must be reconstituted and used promptly
	Onset of action may be 2–6 hours, and thus the drug should not be expected to be of use in the critical first hour following an anaphylactic reaction
Side Effects	Gastrointestinal bleeding
	Prolonged wound healing
	Suppression of natural steroids
Dosage	*General usage:* 125–250 mg
	Spinal cord injury: Initial bolus of 30 mg/kg administered over 15-minute period; this is followed by a maintenance infusion of 5.4 mg/kg/hr
Routes	Intravenous (IV), intramuscular (IM)
Pediatric Dosage	30 mg/kg

Metoclopramide (Reglan)

Class	Phenothiazine antiemetic
Actions	Antiemetic
	Reduces gastroesophageal reflux
Indications	Nausea and vomiting
	Gastroesophageal reflux
Contraindications	Gastrointestinal hemorrhage
	Bowel obstruction or perforation
	Patients with a history of hypersensitivity to the drug
Precaution	Extrapyramidal (dystonic) symptoms have been reported
Side Effects	May impair mental and physical ability
	Drowsiness
Dosage	*Intramuscular (IM):* 10–20 mg
	Intravenous (IV): 10 mg by slow IV push over 1–2 minutes
Routes	IV, IM
Pediatric Dosage	Rarely indicated

Metoprolol (Lopressor)

Class	Sympathetic blocker (β_2 selective)
Action	Selectively blocks β_2-adrenergic receptors (cardioprotective)
Indications	Suspected or definite acute myocardial infarction in patients who are hemodynamically stable
Contraindications	Heart rate less than 45 beats per minute
	Systolic blood pressure <100 mm Hg
	Heart block
	Shock
	History of asthma
Precautions	Blood pressure, pulse, and electrocardiogram (ECG) results must be constantly monitored
	Atropine and transcutaneous pacing should be available
Side Effects	Bradycardia
	Heart block
	Congestive heart failure
	Depression
	Bronchospasm
Dosage	Initial bolus of 5 mg slow intravenous (IV) injection
	May repeat 5 mg bolus in 5 minutes if vital signs are stable
	May repeat 5 mg bolus in 10 minutes if vital signs are stable
Route	Slow IV bolus
Pediatric Dosage	Safety in children has not been established

Midazolam (Versed)

Class	Tranquilizer
Actions	Hypnotic
	Sedative
Indications	Premedication before cardioversion
	Acute anxiety states
Contraindications	Patients with a history of hypersensitivity to the drug
	Narrow-angle glaucoma
	Shock
Precautions	Emergency resuscitative equipment must be available
	Flumazenil (Romazicon) should be available
	Dilute with normal saline of D_5W prior to intravenous administration
	Respiratory depression more common with midazolam than with other benzodiazepines

Side Effects	Drowsiness
	Hypotension
	Amnesia
	Respiratory depression and apnea
Dosage	1.0–2.5 mg administered intravenously (IV)
Routes	IV, oral, intranasal
Pediatric Dosage	0.03 mg/kg

Morphine

Class	Narcotic
Actions	Central nervous system depressant
	Causes peripheral vasodilation
	Decreases sensitivity to pain
Indications	Severe pain
	Pulmonary edema
Contraindications	Head injury
	Volume depletion
	Undiagnosed abdominal pain
	History of hypersensitivity to the drug
Precautions	Respiratory depression (naloxone should be available)
	Hypotension
	Nausea
Side Effects	Dizziness
	Altered level of consciousness
Dosage	*Intravenous (IV):* 2–5 mg followed by 2 mg every few minutes until the pain is relieved or until respiratory depression ensues
	Intramuscular (IM): 5–15 mg based on patient's weight
Routes	IV, IM
Pediatric Dosage	0.1–0.2 mg/kg IV

Nalbuphine (Nubain)

Class	Synthetic analgesic
Actions	Central nervous system depressant
	Decreases sensitivity to pain
Indication	Moderate to severe pain
Contraindication	Patients with a history of hypersensitivity to the drug
Precautions	Use with caution in patients with impaired respiratory function
	Respiratory depression (naloxone should be available)
	Patients dependent on narcotics may experience symptoms of withdrawal
	Nausea

Side Effects	Dizziness
	Altered mental status
Dosage	5–10 mg
Routes	Intravenous (IV), intramuscular (IM)
Pediatric Dosage	Rarely used

Naloxone (Narcan)

Class	Narcotic antagonist
Action	Reverses effects of narcotics
Indications	Narcotic overdoses including the following: morphine, Dilaudid, fentanyl, Demerol, paregoric, methadone, heroin, Percodan, and Tylox
	Synthetic analgesic overdoses including the following: Nubain, Stadol, Talwin, Darvon, and alcoholic coma
	To rule out narcotics in coma of unknown origin
Contraindication	Patients with a history of hypersensitivity to the drug
Precautions	May cause withdrawal effects in patients dependent on narcotics
	Short acting; should be augmented every 5 minutes
Side Effects	Rare
Dosage	1–2 mg
Routes	Intravenous (IV), intramuscular (IM), endotracheal (endotracheal dose 2 to 2.5 times IV dose)
Pediatric Dosage	*<5 years old:* 0.1 mg/kg
	>5 years old: 2.0 mg

Nifedipine (Procardia)

Class	Calcium channel blocker
Actions	Relaxes smooth muscle, causing arteriolar vasodilation
	Decreases peripheral vascular resistance
Indications	Severe hypertension
	Angina pectoris
Contraindications	Known hypersensitivity to the drug
	Hypotension
Precautions	Blood pressure should be constantly monitored
	May worsen congestive heart failure
	Nifedipine should not be administered to patients receiving intravenous beta-blockers
Side Effects	Dizziness
	Flushing
	Nausea
	Headache
	Weakness

Dosage	10 mg sublingually; puncture the capsule several times with a needle and place it under the patient's tongue and have him or her withdraw the liquid medication
Routes	Oral, sublingual
Pediatric Dosage	0.25–0.5 mg/kg

Nitroglycerin (Nitrostat)

Class	Antianginal
Actions	Smooth muscle relaxant
	Reduces cardiac work
	Dilates coronary arteries
	Dilates systemic arteries
Indications	Angina pectoris
	Chest pain associated with myocardial infarction
Contraindications	Children younger than 12 years of age
	Hypotension
Precautions	Constantly monitor blood pressure
	Syncope
	Drug must be protected from light
	Expires quickly once bottle is opened
Side Effects	Headache
	Dizziness
	Hypotension
Dosage	One tablet repeated at 3- to 5-minute intervals up to three times
Route	Sublingual
Pediatric Dosage	Not indicated

Nitroglycerin Paste (Nitro-Bid)

Class	Antianginal
Actions	Smooth muscle relaxant
	Decreases cardiac work
	Dilates coronary arteries
	Dilates systemic arteries
Indications	Angina pectoris
	Chest pain associated with myocardial infarction
Contraindications	Children younger than 12 years of age
	Hypotension
Precautions	Constantly monitor blood pressure
	Syncope
	Drug must be protected from light
	Expires quickly once bottle is opened
Side Effects	Dizziness
	Hypotension

Dosage	1/2 to 1 inch
Route	Topical
Pediatric Dosage	Not indicated

Nitroglycerin Spray (Nitrolingual Spray)

Class	Antianginal
Actions	Smooth muscle relaxant
	Decreases cardiac work
	Dilates coronary arteries
	Dilates systemic arteries
Indications	Angina pectoris
	Chest pain associated with myocardial infarction
Contraindication	Hypotension
Precautions	Constantly monitor vital signs
	Syncope can occur
Side Effects	Dizziness
	Hypotension
	Headache
Dosage	One spray administered under the tongue; may be repeated in 3–5 minutes; no more than three sprays in 15-minute period; spray should not be inhaled
Route	Sprayed under tongue on mucous membrane
Pediatric Dosage	Not indicated

Nitrous Oxide (Nitronox, Entonox)

Class	Gas
Action	Central nervous system depressant
Indications	Pain of musculoskeletal origin, particularly fractures
	Burns
	Suspected ischemic chest pain
	States of severe anxiety including hyperventilation
Contraindications	Patients who cannot comprehend verbal instructions
	Patients intoxicated with alcohol or drugs
	Head-injury patients who exhibit an altered mental status
	Chronic obstructive pulmonary disease (COPD): Increased oxygen concentration may cause respiratory depression
	Thoracic injury suspicious of pneumothorax
	Abdominal pain and distension suggestive of bowel obstruction
Precautions	Use only in well-ventilated area
	Gas-scavenging system is recommended
	May not operate properly at low temperatures

Side Effects	Headache
	Dizziness
	Giddiness
	Nausea
	Vomiting
Dosage	Self-administered only using fixed 50 percent nitrous oxide and 50 percent oxygen blender
Route	Inhalation only
Pediatric Dosage	Self-administered only

Norepinephrine (Levophed)

Class	Sympathomimetic
Action	Causes peripheral vasoconstriction
Indications	Hypotension (systolic blood pressure <70 mm Hg refractory to other sympathomimetics)
	Neurogenic shock
Contraindications	Hypotensive states due to hypovolemia
Precautions	Can be deactivated by alkaline solutions
	Constant monitoring of blood pressure is essential
	Extravasation can cause tissue necrosis
Side Effects	Anxiety
	Palpitations
	Headache
	Hypertension
Dosage	0.5–30 mg/min
	Method: 8 mg should be placed in 500 mL of D_5W, giving a concentration of 16 mg/mL
Route	Intravenous (IV) drip only
Pediatric Dosage	0.01–0.5 mg/kg/min (rarely used)

Oxygen

Class	Gas
Action	Necessary for cellular metabolism
Indication	Hypoxia
Contraindications	None
Precautions	Use cautiously in patients with chronic obstructive pulmonary disease (COPD)
	Humidify when providing high-flow rates
Side Effect	Drying of mucous membranes
Dosage	*Cardiac arrest:* 100 percent
	Other critical patients: 100 percent
	COPD: 35 percent (increase as needed)
Route	Inhalation
Pediatric Dosage	24 percent–100 percent as required

Oxytocin (Pitocin)

Class	Hormone (oxytocic)
Actions	Causes uterine contraction
	Causes lactation
	Slows postpartum vaginal bleeding
Indication	Postpartum vaginal bleeding
Contraindications	Any condition other than postpartum bleeding
	Cesarean section
Precautions	Essential to ensure that the placenta has delivered and that there is not another fetus before administering oxytocin
	Overdosage can cause uterine rupture
	Hypertension
Side Effects	Anaphylaxis
	Cardiac arrhythmias
Dosage	*Intravenous (IV):* 10–20 units in 500 mL of D_5W administered according to uterine response
	Intramuscular (IM): 3–10 units
Routes	IV drip, IM
Pediatric Dosage	Not indicated

Pancuronium Bromide (Pavulon)

Class	Neuromuscular-blocking agent (nondepolarizing)
Actions	Skeletal muscle relaxant
	Paralyzes skeletal muscles including respiratory muscles
Indication	To achieve paralysis to facilitate endotracheal intubation
Contraindication	Patients with known hypersensitivity to the drug
Precautions	Should not be administered unless persons skilled in endotracheal intubation are present
	Endotracheal intubation equipment must be available
	Oxygen equipment and emergency resuscitative drugs must be available
	Paralysis occurs within 3–5 minutes and lasts for approximately 60 minutes
Side Effects	Prolonged paralysis
	Hypotension
	Bradycardia
Dosage	0.04–0.1 mg/kg; repeat doses of 0.01–0.02 mg/kg intravenously as required every 20–40 minutes
Route	Intravenous (IV)
Pediatric Dosage	0.1 mg/kg

Phenobarbitol (Luminal)

Class	Barbiturate
Actions	Suppresses spread of seizure activity through the motor cortex
	Central nervous system depressant
Indications	Major motor seizures
	Status epilepticus
	Acute anxiety states
Contraindication	History of hypersensitivity to the drug
Precautions	Respiratory depression
	Hypotension
	Can cause hyperactivity in children
	Extravasation may cause tissue necrosis
Side Effects	Drowsiness
	Children may become hyperactive
Dosage	100–250 mg
Routes	Intravenous (IV) slowly, intramuscular (IM)
Pediatric Dosage	10 mg/kg

Phenytoin (Dilantin)

Class	Anticonvulsant and antiarrhythmic
Actions	Inhibits spread of seizure activity through motor cortex
	Antiarrhythmic
Indications	Major motor seizures
	Status epilepticus
	Arrhythmias due to digitalis toxicity
Contraindications	Any arrhythmia except those due to digitalis toxicity
	High-grade heart blocks
	Patients with history of hypersensitivity to the drug
Precautions	Should not be administered with glucose solutions
	Hypotension
	Electrocardiogram (ECG) monitoring during administration is essential
Side Effects	Local venous irritation
	Itching
	Central nervous system depression
Dosage	*Status epilepticus:* 150–250 mg (10–15 mg/kg) not to exceed 50 mg/min
	Digitalis toxicity: 100 mg over 5 minutes until the arrhythmia is suppressed or until a maximum dose of 1000 mg has been administered or symptoms of central nervous system depression occur
Route	IV (dilute with saline)
Pediatric Dosage	*Status epilepticus:* 8–10 mg/kg intravenously (IV)
	Digitalis toxicity: 3–5 mg/kg IV over 100 minutes

Physotigmine (Antilirium)

Class	Cholinesterase inhibitor
Actions	Inhibits cholinesterase
	Potentiates acetylcholine
Indications	Tricyclic overdoses including the following: Tofranil, Norpramin, Sinequan, Elavil, Adapin, Triavil, and atropine (belladonna) overdoses
Contraindications	Asthma and chronic obstructive pulmonary disease
	Gangrene
	Diabetes
	Cardiovascular disease
Precautions	Monitor for bronchospasm and laryngospasm
	Seizures
Side Effects	Excessive salivation
	Bradycardia
	Emesis
Dosage	0.5–2.0 mg
Route	Intravenous (IV)
Pediatric Dosage	0.5–1.0 mg over 5 minutes

Pralidoxime (2-Pam, Protopam)

Class	Cholinesterase reactivator
Actions	Reactivates cholinesterase in cases of organophosphate poisoning
	Deactivates certain organophosphates by direct chemical reaction
Indications	Severe organophosphate poisoning as characterized by muscle twitching, respiratory depression, and paralysis
Contraindications	Poisonings due to inorganic phosphates
	Poisonings other than organophosphates
Precautions	Always ensure safety and protection of rescue personnel
	Laryngospasm, tachycardia, and muscle rigidity have occurred following rapid administration
	Should only follow atropinization
Side Effects	Excitement
	Manic behavior
Dosage	1–2 g in 250–500 mL of normal saline infused over 30 minutes
Route	Intravenous (IV) drip
Pediatric Dosage	20–40 mg/kg by the same method

Procainamide (Pronestyl)

Class	Antiarrhythmic
Actions	Slows conduction through myocardium
	Elevates ventricular fibrillation threshold
	Suppresses ventricular ectopic activity
Indications	Persistent cardiac arrest due to ventricular fibrillation and refractory to lidocaine
	PVCs refractory to lidocaine
	Ventricular tachycardia refractory to lidocaine
Contraindications	High-degree heart blocks
	PVCs in conjunction with bradycardia
Precautions	Dosage should not exceed 17 mg/kg
	Monitor for central nervous system toxicity
Side Effects	Anxiety
	Nausea
	Convulsions
	Widening of QRS complex
Dosage	*Initial:* 20 mg/min until arrhythmia is abolished, hypotension ensues, QRS complex is widened by 50 percent of original width, or total of 1.7 mg/kg has been given
	Maintenance: 1–4 mg/min
Routes	Slow intravenous (IV) bolus, IV drip
Pediatric Dosage	Rarely used

Prochlorperazine (Compazine)

Class	Phenothiazine antiemetic
Action	Antiemetic
Indications	Nausea and vomiting
	Acute psychosis
Contraindications	Comatose states
	Patients who have received a large amount of depressants (including alcohol)
	Patients with a history of hypersensitivity to the drug
Precaution	Extrapyramidal (dystonic) symptoms have been reported
Side Effects	May impair mental and physical ability
	Drowsiness
Dosage	5–10 mg slow intravenous (IV) or intramuscular (IM)
Routes	IV, IM
Pediatric Dosage	Not recommended

Promethazine (Phenergan)

Class	Antihistamine (H$_1$ antagonist)
Actions	Mild anticholinergic activity
	Antiemetic
	Potentiates actions of analgesics
Indications	Nausea and vomiting
	Motion sickness
	To potentiate the effects of analgesics
	Sedation
Contraindications	Comatose states
	Patients who have received a large amount of depressants (including alcohol)
Precaution	Avoid accidental intraarterial injection
Side Effects	May impair mental and physical ability
	Drowsiness
Dosage	12.5–25.0 mg
Routes	Intravenous (IV), intramuscular (IM)
Pediatric Dosage	0.5 mg/kg

Propranolol (Inderal)

Class	Sympathetic blocker
Action	Nonselectively blocks β-adrenergic receptors
Indications	Ventricular tachyarrhythmias refractory to lidocaine and bretylium
	Recurrent ventricular fibrillation refractory to lidocaine and bretylium
	Tachyarrhythmias due to digitalis toxicity
Contraindications	Asthma and chronic obstructive pulmonary disease
	Patients dependent on sympathetic agonists
	Congestive heart failure
Precautions	Should not be given concurrently with verapamil
	Atropine and transcutaneous pacing should be readily available
Side Effects	Bradycardia
	Heart blocks
	Congestive heart failure
	Bronchospasm
Dosage	1–3 mg diluted in 10–30 mL of D$_5$W given slowly intravenously (IV)
Route	Slow IV bolus
Pediatric Dosage	0.01 mg/kg

Raecemic Epinephrine (MicroNEFRIN)

Class	Sympathomimetic
Actions	Bronchodilation
	Increases heart rate
	Increases cardiac contractile force
Indication	Croup (laryngotracheobronchitis)
Contraindications	Epiglottitis
	Hypersensitivity to the drug
Precautions	Vital signs should be constantly monitored
	Should be used only once in the prehospital setting
Side Effects	Palpitations
	Anxiety
	Headache
Dosage	0.25–0.75 mL of a 2.25 percent solution in 2.0 mL normal saline
Route	Inhalation only (small-volume nebulizer)
Pediatric Dosage	0.25–0.75 mL of a 2.25 percent solution in 2.0 mL normal saline

Rocuronium Bromide (Zemuron)

Class	Nondepolarizing neuromuscular blocker
Action	Prevents neuromuscular transmission by blocking the effect of acetylcholine
	Skeletal muscle paralysis
Indication	Induction of skeletal muscle paralysis
Contraindications	Hypersensitivity to the drug
Precautions	Underlying cardiovascular disease
	Dehydration or electrolyte abnormalities
Side Effects	Bronchospasm
Dosage	*Initial dose rapid-sequence induction:* 600 μg/kg
	Maintenance dose: 100–200 μg/kg continuous infusion
Route	Intravenous (IV), IV drip
Pediatric Dosage	*Initial dose:* 600 μg/kg
	Maintenance dose: 75–125 μg/kg continuous infusion

Salbutamol (Ventolin)

Class	Sympathomimetic (β_2 selective)
Action	Bronchodilation

Indications	Asthma
	Reversible bronchospasm associated with chronic obstructive pulmonary disease
Contraindications	Known hypersensitivity to the drug
	Symptomatic tachycardia
Precautions	Blood pressure, pulse, and electrocardiogram (ECG) results should be monitored
	Use caution in patients with known heart disease
Side Effects	Palpitations
	Anxiety
	Headache
	Dizziness
	Sweating
Dosage	*Metered-dose inhaler:* One to two sprays (90 μg per spray)
	Small-volume nebulizer: 0.5 mL (2.5 mg) in 2.5 mL normal saline over 5–15 minutes
	Rotohaler: One 200 μg Rotocap should be placed in the inhaler and breathed by the patient
Route	Inhalation
Pediatric Dosage	0.15 mg/kg (0.03 mL/kg) in 2.5 mL normal saline by small-volume nebulizer

Sodium Bicarbonate

Class	Alkalinizing agent
Actions	Combines with excessive acids to form a weak volatile acid
	Increases pH
Indications	Late in the management of cardiac arrest, if at all
	Tricyclic antidepressant overdose
	Severe acidosis refractory to hyperventilation
Contraindication	Alkalotic states
Precautions	Correct dosage is essential to avoid overcompensation of pH
	Can deactivate catecholamines
	Can precipitate with calcium
	Delivers large sodium load
Side Effect	Alkalosis
Dosage	1 mEq/kg initially followed by 0.5 mEq/kg every 10 minutes as indicated by blood gas studies
Route	Intravenous (IV)
Pediatric Dosage	1 mEq/kg initially followed by 0.5 mEq/kg every 10 minutes

Sodium Nitroprusside (Nipride, Nitropress)

Class	Potent vasodilator
Actions	Peripheral arterial and venous vasodilator
	Decreases blood pressure
	Increases cardiac output in congestive heart failure
Indication	Hypertensive emergency
Contraindications	None when used in the management of life-threatening emergency
Precautions	Bottle must be wrapped in foil to protect from light
	Should not be administered to children or pregnant women in the prehospital setting
	Reduce the dosage in elderly patients
	Blood pressure, pulse, and electrocardiogram (ECG) results must be diligently monitored
Side Effects	Nausea
	Retching
	Vomiting
	Palpitations
	Diaphoresis
	Tachycardia
	Dizziness
	Side effects often diminish as dosage is reduced
Dosage	0.5 mg/kg/min
Route	Intravenous (IV) infusion only
Pediatric Dosage	Not indicated in prehospital setting

Sotalol HCL (Betapace, Sotacor)

Class	Antiarrhythmic (group II) and beta-adrenergic-blocking agent (nonselective)
Action	Blocks stimulation of β_1 (myocardial) and β_2 (pulmonary, vascular, and uterine) adrenergic receptor sites
	Suppression of arrhythmias
Indication	Management of life-threatening ventricular arrhythmias
Contraindications	Uncompensated congestive heart failure
	Pulmonary edema
	Cardiogenic shock
	Bradycardia or heart block
Precautions	Renal impairment
	Hepatic impairment

Side Effects	Fatigue
	Weakness
	Anxiety
	Dizziness
	Drowsiness
	Insomnia
	Memory loss
	Mental depression
	Mental status changes
	Nervousness
	Nightmares
Dosage	80 mg twice daily; may be gradually increased to 160–320 mg/day in two to three divided doses up to 480–640 mg/day
Route	Oral
Pediatric Dosage	Not indicated

Streptokinase (Strepase)

Class	Thrombolytic
Action	Dissolves blood clots
Indication	Acute myocardial infarction
Contraindications	Persons with internal bleeding
	Suspected aortic dissection
	Traumatic cardiopulmonary resuscitation
	Severe persistent hypertension
	Recent head trauma or known intracranial tumor
	History of stroke in the past 6 months
	Pregnancy
Precautions	May be ineffective if administered within 12 months of prior streptokinase or anistreplase therapy
	Antiarrhythmic and resuscitative drugs should be available
Side Effects	Bleeding
	Allergic reactions
	Anaphylaxis
	Fever
	Nausea and vomiting
Dosage	1.5 million units over 1 hour
Route	Intravenous (IV) drip
Pediatric Dosage	Not recommended

Succinylcholine (Anectine)

Class	Neuromuscular blocking agent (depolarizing)
Actions	Skeletal muscle relaxant
	Paralyzes skeletal muscles including respiratory muscles

Indication	To achieve paralysis to facilitate endotracheal intubation
Contraindication	Patients with known hypersensitivity to the drug
Precautions	Should not be administered unless persons skilled in endotracheal intubation are present
	Endotracheal intubation equipment must be available
	Oxygen equipment and emergency resuscitative drugs must be available
	Paralysis occurs within 1 minute and lasts for approximately 8 minutes
Side Effects	Prolonged paralysis
	Hypotension
	Bradycardia
Dosage	1–1.5 mg/kg (40–100 mg in an adult)
Route	Intravenous (IV)
Pediatric Dosage	1 mg/kg

Terbutaline (Brethine)

Class	Sympathomimetic
Actions	Bronchodilator
	Increases heart rate
Indications	Bronchial asthma
	Reversible bronchospasm associated with chronic obstructive pulmonary disease
	Preterm labor
Contraindication	Patients with known hypersensitivity to the drug
Precautions	Blood pressure, pulse, and electrocardiogram (ECG) results must be constantly monitored
Side Effects	Palpitations
	Tachycardia
	PVCs
	Anxiety
	Tremors
	Headache
Dosage	*Metered-dose inhaler:* Two inhalations, 1 minute apart
	Subcutaneous injection: 0.25 mg; may be repeated in 15–30 minutes
Routes	Inhalation, Subcutaneous injection, intravenous (IV) drip (in preterm labor)
Pediatric Dosage	0.01 mg/kg subcutaneously

Thiamine (Vitamin B$_1$)

Class	Vitamin
Action	Allows normal breakdown of glucose

Indications	Coma of unknown origin
	Alcoholism
	Delirium tremens
Contraindications	None in the emergency setting
Precaution	Rare anaphylactic reactions have been reported
Side Effects	Rare, if any
Dosage	100 mg
Routes	Intravenous (IV), intramuscular (IM)
Pediatric Dosage	Rarely indicated

Tissue Plasminogen Activator (tPA, Activase)

Class	Thrombolytic
Action	Dissolves blood clots
Indication	Acute myocardial infarction
Contraindications	Persons with internal bleeding
	Suspected aortic dissection
	Traumatic cardiopulmonary resuscitation
	Severe persistent hypertension
	Recent head trauma or known intracranial tumor
	History of stroke in the past 6 months
	Pregnancy
Precautions	Antiarrhythmic and resuscitative drugs should be available
Side Effects	Bleeding
	Allergic reactions
	Anaphylaxis
	Fever
	Nausea and vomiting
Dosage	*Front-loaded regimen:* 15 mg intravenous (IV) bolus over 1–2 minutes, followed by infusion of 50 mg over the first hour and 35 mg over the second hour (total dose 100 mg)
	Standard regimen: 10 mg intravenous (IV) bolus over 1–2 minutes, followed by 50 mg over the first hour, 20 mg over the second hour, and 20 mg over the third hour
Route	IV (slow) and IV infusion
Pediatric Dosage	Not recommended

Trimethobenzamide (Tigan)

Class	Antiemetic
Action	Antiemetic with fewer sedative effects than other common antiemetic drugs
Indication	Nausea and vomiting
Contraindications	Children (injectable form only)
	Patients with a history of hypersensitivity to the drug

Precaution	Extrapyramidal (dystonic) symptoms have been reported
Side Effects	May impair mental and physical ability
	Drowsiness
Dosage	200 mg intramuscularly (IM)
Route	IM
Pediatric Dosage	Parenteral administration not recommended

Vecuronium (Norcuron)

Class	Neuromuscular-blocking agent (nondepolarizing)
Action	Skeletal muscle relaxant
	Paralyzes skeletal muscles including respiratory muscles
Indication	To achieve paralysis to facilitate endotracheal intubation
Contraindication	Patients with known hypersensitivity to the drug
Precautions	Should not be administered unless persons skilled in endotracheal intubation are present
	Endotracheal intubation equipment must be available
	Oxygen equipment and emergency resuscitative drugs must be available
	Paralysis occurs within 1 minute and lasts for approximately 30 minutes
Side Effects	Prolonged paralysis
	Hypotension
	Bradycardia
Dosage	0.08–0.1 mg/kg
Route	Intravenous (IV)
Pediatric Dosage	0.1 mg/kg

Verapamil (Isoptin, Calan)

Class	Calcium channel blocker
Actions	Slows conduction through the atrioventricular node
	Inhibits reentry during PSVT
	Decreases rate of ventricular response
	Decreases myocardial oxygen demand
Indication	PSVT
Contraindications	Heart block
	Conduction system disturbances
Precautions	Should not be used in patients receiving intravenous β-blockers
	Hypotension

Side Effects	Nausea
	Vomiting
	Hypotension
	Dizziness
Dosage	2.5–5 mg; a repeat dose of 5–10 mg can be administered after 15–30 minutes if PSVT does not convert; maximum dose is 30 mg in 30 minutes
Route	Intravenous
Pediatric Dosage	*0–1 year:* 0.1–0.2 mg/kg (maximum of 2.0 mg) administered slowly
	1–15 years: 0.1–0.3 mg/kg (maximum of 5.0 mg) administered slowly

COMMON HOME PRESCRIPTION DRUG INFORMATION

The following information pertains to immediate prehospital emergencies. Some of these classifications cover a broad range of drugs. The information provided is very general and is intended only for use as a quick reference.

Classification/Type

Type(s)	Therapeutic classification
Actions	The major mechanism or mechanisms of action and how the drug exerts its therapeutic effects
Indications	Condition or conditions for which the drugs are commonly prescribed
Adverse Effects	Any effect other than those that were therapeutically intended; usually undesirable, specific, and predictable; often a result of too much of the drug; may include any combination of those listed
Interactions	Presence of another drug or drugs may alter the effects of either drug or promote entirely different effects
How Supplied	Most common forms of the drug
Note	Miscellaneous relevant or nice-to-know information.
Common Examples	A few examples (listed by trade name) of drugs in this class; when given, generic names are indicated by boldface type.

Narcotic: Analgesics

Type(s)	Narcotic (opiate) (natural, semisynthetic, synthetic)
Actions	Analgesia (increases pain threshold)
	Decreases anxiety, apprehension, fear
	Central nervous system depressant, sedation
	Cardiovascular (decreased anxiety reduces catecholamine release; vasodilation reduces preload)
Indications	Pain relief
	Cough suppression
	Sedation for anxiety, apprehension, and fear
	Antidiarrheal
Adverse Effects	*Cardiovascular system:* Hypotension, bradycardia, flushing, sweating, and pulmonary edema (noncardiogenic)
	Central nervous system: Respiratory depression, apnea, central nervous system depression, euphoria, drowsiness, dizziness, weakness, excessive sedation, apathy, paradoxical central nervous system, stimulation, nervousness, anxiety, headache, seizure, coma, hallucinations, delusions, and mood change
	Other: N/V, urine retention, may constrict or dilate pupils, and may suppress cough or corneal reflex
Interactions	Central nervous system depressants, tricyclic antidepressants, and monoamine oxidase inhibitors: Potentiate effects
How Supplied	Tablet, capsule, caplet, elixir, suppository, and intravenous
Note	Narcotics have the potential for patient tolerance, abuse, and addiction
	A withdrawal syndrome may result from abrupt cessation after chronic use

Common Examples

Ancasal	Morphine
Atasol	Numorphan
Codeine	Oxycocet
Darvon	Oxycodan
Demerol (meperidine)	Percocet
Dilaudid (hydromorph)	Percodan
Empracet	Talwin
Exdol	Tylenol with codeine (Nos. 1, 2, 3, and 4)

Antianginals

Type(s)	Nitrates and nitrites (primarily) (*see also* Beta-Blockers and Calcium Channel Blockers)

Actions	Nitrates and nitrites (coronary vasodilators)
	Vasodilation
	Decreases myocardial work and reduces MVO_2 by
	Reducing preload and afterload
	Improving coronary perfusion (including collateral)
	May relieve coronary vasospasm
Indications	Angina, acute myocardial infarction, congestive heart failure, and after myocardial infarction
	Coronary artery spasm and SVTs
	To increase exercise tolerance
Adverse Effects	*Cardiovascular system:* Hypotension, bradycardia, paradoxical angina, flushing, feeling of warmth, syncope, reflex tachycardia, palpitation, and possible reperfusion arrhythmias (via relief of coronary vasospasm)
	Central nervous system: Transient or persistent headache, dizziness, weakness, and anxiety
	Other: N/V, may cause slight SL burning sensation
Interactions	Hypotensives, ETOH: May potentiate hypotension
How Supplied	Tablet, ointment or paste, aerosol, and transdermal patch
Note	These patients usually have coronary artery disease
	Tablets may lose potency within a few months
	Aerosols maintain potency for up to 3 years
	Tolerance and dependence may develop after prolonged use
	Paramedics should avoid (prolonged) contact with nitro paste (e.g., during chest compression) because it will be absorbed through their skin
	Canister should *not* be shaken; if it is, that dose is sprayed out and the next dose is administered to the patient
Common Examples	Cardilate Nitrol
	Coronex Nitrolingual spray
	Isordil Nitrong
	Nitrobid Nitrostablin
	Nitrogard Nitrostat

Anxiolytic (Antianxiety)

Type(s)	Primarily benzodiazepines (minor tranquilizers) and carbamates
Actions	Central nervous system depressant, sedation
	Skeletal muscle relaxation

Indications	Excessive anxiety and tension (acute or chronic):
	Stresses of everyday life
	Emotional and physical disorders
	Tension from insomnia
	Anticonvulsant
	Muscle spasms
	Adjunctive management of acute ETOH or opiate withdrawal
Adverse Effects	*Cardiovascular system:* Hypotension and tachycardia
	Central nervous system: Respiratory depression, apnea, excessive central nervous system depression or sedation, coma, drowsiness, dizziness, vertigo, confusion, ataxia, slurred speech, headache, amnesia, fatigue, weakness, occasional paradoxical irritability, excitability, aggression, hallucinations, and delirium
	Other: N/V, pupil dilation
Interactions	Central nervous system depressants, including ETOH: Potentiate effects
How Supplied	Tablet, capsule, and caplet
Note	This is probably the most widely prescribed class of drugs in the world
	There is potential for tolerance, abuse, and addiction
	A withdrawal syndrome may result from abrupt cessation after chronic use

Common Examples

Atarax	Multipax
Ativan (lorazepam)	Serax
Donnatal	Stelzine
Lectopam	Tranxene
Librium (chlordiazepoxide)	Valium (diazepam)
Loftran	Vivol (diazepam)
Mellaril	Xanax

Antiarrhythmics

Type(s)	Various (classes I–IV)
Actions	Various, depends on specific antiarrhythmic:
	(−) chronotropy
	(+) or (−) inotropy
	(−) dromotropy
	Depresses automaticity
	Reduces MVO_2
	Suppresses PVCs
	Suppresses reentry activity
	Vagolytic
	May elevate the threshold for VF

Indications	To maintain NSR (or a controlled or stable abnormal rhythm)
	To prevent chronic rhythm disturbances
Adverse Effects	*Cardiovascular system:* Arrhythmia, conduction disturbances, hypotension, myocardial depression, may induce or exacerbate congestive heart failure or pulmonary edema, and may precipitate angina
	Central nervous system: Headache, central nervous system depression, altered level of consciousness
	Other: N/V
Interactions	Other antiarrhythmics: May potentiate or depress effects
How Supplied	Tablet and capsule
Note	Usually prescribed after some type of cardiac insult
Common Examples	Antiarrhythmics may be classified by their predominant electrophysiological effects (e.g., Vaughn-Williams-Singh Classification).

Class I

Biquin
Dilantin
Mexitil
Norpace
Procan
Pronestyl
Prosedyl
Quinate
Quinidex
Quinine
Rhythmodan
Tonocard
Xylocaine

Class II

Primarily β-Blockers
Betaloc
Biocadren
Corgard
Inderal
Lopressor
Sotacor
Tenormin
Visken

Class III

Bretylate
Bretylol
Cordarone (amiodarone)

Class IV

Calcium channel blockers
Adalat
Cardizem
Isoptin
Cardiac glycosides
Cedilanid
Crystodigin
Digitaline
Lanoxin
Norvasc
Novodigozin

Anticoagulants

Type(s)	Warfarin or Coumadin derivatives
Actions	Decreases the ability of blood to clot:
	Prevents further extension of the clot
	Prolongs blood-clotting time
	May prevent clotting
Indications	Prophylaxis or treatment of blood clotting:
	Venous thrombosis, pulmonary embolism
	Adjunct in the treatment of coronary occlusion and transient ischemic accidents
	Home dialysis
	Recurrent problems with blood clots
	Treatment of embolization in A-fib
	Postthrombolytic therapy
Adverse Effects	Hemorrhage (from any organ or tissue)
	Excessive bleeding from minor cuts, menstruation, or nosebleed
	Melena, petechiae
	N/V/D
Interactions	Salicylates, some antibiotics: May prolong clotting time and increase risk of hemorrhage
How Supplied	Tablet
Note	Also known as "blood thinners"
	Patients on home dialysis may take heparin intravenously
	Antiplatelet (e.g., aspirin Persantine) effects are similar to anticoagulant effects
Common Examples	Coumadin Minihep
	Hepalean Sintrom
	Heparin Warfilone

Anticonvulsants

Type(s)	Benzodiazepines, barbiturates, hydantoins, and succinimides
Actions	Prevents and suppresses the spread of seizure activity in the motor cortex
	Elevates seizure threshold
	Skeletal muscle relaxation
Indications	Epilepsy
	Chronic seizures
	Generalized tonic-clonic (grand mal) seizures
	Absence spells (petit mal) seizures
	Focal, Jacksonian, psychomotor, or myoclonic seizures

Adverse Effects	*Cardiovascular system:* Hypotension and arrhythmia
	Central nervous system: Respiratory depression, apnea, excessive central nervous system depression, ataxia, dizziness, drowsiness, fatigue, weakness, confusion, behavioral disturbances, sedation, coma, amnesia, irritability, nervousness, headache, tremor, and paradoxical seizure (from overdose)
	Other: N/V/D, anorexia, abdominal pain, indigestion, constipation, visual disturbances, and nystagmus
Interactions	Central nervous system depressants: Potentiate effects
How Supplied	Tablet, capsule, and syrup
Note	Many patients are on combination therapy
Common Examples	Celontin Milontin
	Depakene Mogadon
	Dilantin Mysoline
	Epival Rivotril
	Mebaral Tegretol
	Mebroin Zarontin
	Mesantoin

Antidepressants: Monoamine Oxidase Inhibitors

Type(s)	Monoamine oxidase inhibitors (psychotropics)
Actions	Affects mood and behavior:
	Blocks impulse transmission at the synapse
	Inhibits catecholamine breakdown
Indications	Moderate-severe depression (usually refractory to tricyclic antidepressants)
	Atypical depression and phobic disorders (drug of choice)
	Prevention of panic attacks
	Depressive disorders (atypical, neurotic, or reactive)
Adverse Effects	*Cardiovascular system:* Tachycardia, PVCs, VT, hypotension, and sweating
	Central nervous system: Respiratory depression, central nervous system depression, dizziness, headache, irritability, anxiety, paresthesia, tremor, seizure, coma, ataxia, fever, and insomnia
	Other: N/V, urine retention, constipation, stiff neck, and dry mouth
Interactions	Antihypertensives: May potentiate effects
	Sympathomimetics or tyramine-rich foods and drinks: May potentiate effects (may induce hypertensive crisis)
	Central nervous system depressants: May potentiate effects

How Supplied	Tablet
Note	Overdose effects may persist for days
Common Examples	Marplan Parnate
	Nardil

Antidepressants: Tricyclic Antidepressants

Type(s)	Tricyclic antidepressants (psychotropics)
Actions	Mechanism of action is not exactly clear:
	Antidepressant effects
	Mild sedative effects
	Cholinergic blockade
	May inhibit catecholamine breakdown
	Peripheral α blockade
	Impairs cardiac depolarization and conduction
	$(-)$ inotropy
Indications	Severe endogenous depression (drug of choice)
	Prevention of panic attacks
	Pain control (some benefit for patients with fibromyalgia)
Adverse Effects	*Cardiovascular system:* Orthostatic hypotension, bradycardia, (wide complex) tachycardia, arrhythmia, PVCs, conduction defects (widened QRS complex, prolonged PR and QT intervals, ST and T wave abnormalities, and atrioventricular blocks) may precipitate congestive heart failure
	Central nervous system: Initially confusion, anxiety, sweating, ataxia, and vomiting are seen; may precipitate mania and psychosis. Later central nervous system depression, delirium, hallucinations, coma, muscle rigidity, seizure, respiratory depression, and apnea may be present
	Other: Anticholinergic effects (fever, hot flushed skin, dry mucous membranes, pupil dilation, urine retention) and anti-α effects (hypotension, sedation, cardiac depression)
Interactions	Sympathomimetics: May potentiate effects
	Central nervous system depressants: May potentiate effects
How Supplied	Tablet and capsule
Note	Ingestion of 1–2 g is potentially lethal and hard to treat
	Physostigmine (Antilirium), a cholinergic, may reverse some cholinergic symptoms
	Clinically related to phenothiazines
	Overdose effects may persist for days

Common Examples
Adapin
Anafranil
Asendin
Aventyl
Desyrel
Elavil
Etrafon
Limbitrol
Ludiomil

Norpramin
Pamelor
Pertofrane
Sinequan
Surmontil
Tofranil
Triadapin
Triptil
Vivactil

Antidiabetics: Insulins

Type(s)
Insulin (pancreatic hormone)

Actions
Facilitates glucose transmembrane transport and stimulates carbohydrate metabolism

Facilitates glucose storage (as glycogen), primarily in the liver, muscle, and kidney

Insulin type	Time (hour)		
	Onset	Peak	Duration
Short acting			
Regular (Toronto)	0.5–1	2.5–5	5–8
Similente	1–1.5	5–10	12–16
Intermediate acting			
NPH	1.5–2	4–12	24–48
Lente	2–2.5	7–15	22–48
Long acting			
PZI	4–7	10–30	36+
Ultralente	4–7	8–30	28–36+

Indications
Diabetes that cannot be controlled by diet alone:

Diabetics who cannot produce or excrete adequate amounts of insulin: usually type I (insulin-dependent diabetes mellitus), or juvenile diabetics

In place of oral hypoglycemic therapy in patients with complications

Adverse Effects
Other: Hypoglycemia, hypokalemia, and electrolyte depletion

Interactions
ETOH, β-blockers, monoamine oxidase inhibitors, anabolic steroids, salicylates: May potentiate hypoglycemic effects

Corticosteroids, thiazides, catecholamines: May diminish hypoglycemic effects

How Supplied
Multidose vial and penfill (subcutaneous or intramuscular injection); some are combination products

Note
Epinephrine may reverse hypoglycemic effects

May be on combination of different insulin preparations

Extracted from beef or pork pancreas or produced from genetic engineering

Insulin preparations differ primarily in onset, peak, and duration of action, which may vary slightly among manufacturers

Insulin is a protein and is destroyed in the gastrointestinal tract. It must be given parenterally. The abdomen, thigh, and arm are common sites.

| **Common Examples** | Humilin | Novolin |
| | Iletin | Velosulin |

Antidiabetics: Oral Hypoglycemics

Type(s)	Oral hypoglycemics (sulfonylureas)
Actions	Stimulates pancreatic beta cells to produce and secrete insulin
Indications	To control hyperglycemia in patients whose diabetes cannot be controlled by diet alone and when insulin therapy is inappropriate; usually type II (non-insulin-dependent diabetes mellitus or adult) diabetics
Adverse Effects	Severe and prolonged hypoglycemia (especially when accompanied by acute ETOH overdose); possible associated hypoglycemic seizure
Interactions	ETOH, anabolic steroids, monoamine oxidase inhibitors, oral anticoagulants, salicylates, sulfonamides, β-blockers: May potentiate hypoglycemic effects
	Corticosteroids, glucagon, thiazides, catecholamines: May diminish hypoglycemic effects
How Supplied	Tablet
Note	Provides an alternative to intravenous insulin
	Oral hypoglycemics differ primarily in onset, peak, and duration of action
	Hypoglycemia may persist despite intravenous dextrose or may recur (because oral hypoglycemics are longer lasting than dextrose)

Common Examples	Diabeta	Euglucon
	Diabinese	Mobenol
	Dimelor	Orinase

Antihypertensives

Type(s)	Various (vasodilators, sympatholytics, β-blockers, diuretics, and combination products)
Actions	Vasodilation (decreased blood pressure)
	ACE inhibitors (reduced vasoconstriction)
	Sympatholytics (reduced vessel tone)
	α-blockade (reduced SVR)
	Diuresis (decreased volume)

Indications	Hypertension, congestive heart failure
	Sodium retention, edema, ascites
Adverse Effects	*Cardiovascular system:* Orthostatic to profound hypotension, syncope, flushing, rebound hypertension, reflex tachycardia, arrhythmia, angina, and PVCs
	Central nervous system: Drowsiness, dizziness, confusion, sedation, and headache
	Other: Fluid and Na^+ retention, congestive heart failure, electrolyte imbalance, N/V/D, abdominal pain, and muscle cramps
Interactions	Monoamine oxidase inhibitors: May potentiate hypotensive effects
How Supplied	Tablet and capsule
Note	Some are combination products

Common Examples

Aldomet	Loniten
Capoten	Minipress
Catapres	Serparsil
Combipres	Viskazide

Antipsychotics

Type(s)	Primarily phenothiazines (major tranquilizers) (psychotropics)
Actions	Phenothiazines alter behavior in such a way as to enable the patient to cope with illness and function in daily activities without excessive sedation
	Some also have antiemetic or anticholinergic effects
Indications	Acute and chronic control of behavioral disorders resulting from mental illness:
	Schizophrenia, recurrent mania
	Psychotic disorders
	Anxiety disorders
	Prevention of N/V
Adverse Effects	*Cardiovascular system:* Hypotension, bradycardia, arrhythmia, and atrioventricular blocks
	Central nervous system: Respiratory depression, central nervous system depression, sedation, drowsiness, confusion, dizziness, weakness, tremor, seizure, and coma
	Other: Extrapyramidal effects (primarily muscle spasms) and anticholinergic effects (dry mouth, nasal congestion, blurred vision, salivation)
Interactions	Opiates, barbiturates, ETOH, and other central nervous system depressants: May potentiate effects
	"Epi": May be ineffective in reversing hypotension (may in fact potentiate the hypotension)

How Supplied	Tablet, solution, suspension, syrup, and suppository
Note	Diphenhydramine (Benadryl) or benztropine (Cogentin) may counteract some
	Tranquilizers induce calmness and sedation without excessively depressing level of consciousness

Common Examples		
Haldol	Peridol	Sparine
Haloperidol	Permitil	Stelazine
Mellaril	Quide	Trilafon
Nozinan	Serentil	

Beta-Blockers

Type(s)	Sympathetic blocker
Actions	Some selectively block β_1 (cardioselective) or β_2 (bronchoselective) receptors; some are nonselective
Indications	Mild to moderate hypertension
	Prevention of recurrent angina
	Prevention of recurring tachyarrhythmias
	Migraines
Adverse Effects	*Cardiovascular system:* May precipitate or aggravate chronic obstructive pulmonary disease, asthma, bronchospasm, increased airway resistance, hypotension, bradycardia, atrioventricular block, and congestive heart failure
	Central nervous system: Fatigue, headache, hallucinations, seizure, and coma
	Other: N/V, may induce hypoglycemia
Interactions	Sympathomimetics: Block β effects (patient may be unable to mount a tachycardic response to hypovolemia)
	Calcium blockers: Potentiate bradycardia and myocardial depression
	Cardiac glycosides: Potentiate bradycardia
	Epinephrine: Severe vasoconstriction
	Diuretics: May potentiate antihypertensive effects
How Supplied	Tablet
Note	Acute withdrawal may precipitate angina (due to increased sensitivity to catecholamines)
	Often used in combination therapy
	Selective β-blockers are usually dose dependent (tend to lose β selectivity in higher doses)

Common Examples	
Betaloc	Lopressor
Blocardren	Sotacor
Corgard	Tenormin
Inderal	Visken

Bronchodilators: Sympathomimetics

Type(s)	Sympathomimetics
Actions	Most are β selective (some are not)
	Bronchodilation (via β_2 stimulation)
	Some β effects
	Little or no α stimulation
Indications	Prevention or treatment of bronchospasm caused by reversible obstructive airway disease (chronic obstructive pulmonary disease, asthma, bronchitis, and emphysema)
Adverse Effects	*Cardiovascular system:* Excessive cardiac stimulation, tachycardia, palpitation, and hypertension; may precipitate angina, acute myocardial infarction, PVCs, and arrhythmia; and possible hypotension, sweating
	Central nervous system: Excessive central nervous system stimulation (anxiety to seizure), headache, dizziness, drowsiness, weakness, fatigue, and paresthesia
	Other: N/V, heartburn, bad taste, muscle cramps, and dry nose and throat; may cause severe paradoxical bronchospasm from repeated excessive use
Interactions	β-blocker: May block effects
	Monoamine oxidase inhibitors, tricyclic antidepressants: May potentiate effects
How Supplied	Aerosol, tablet, suppository, and nebulizer solution
Note	Aerosolized drugs may not reach the smaller airways, especially in the presence of bronchospasm and thick mucous plugs (the nebulizer solution will be much more effective)
	Aerosol sympathomimetics have the potential for patient tolerance and abuse
	These patients may also be on steroids and antibiotics
	Some are combination products
	Overdose effects may be reversed by a β-blocker such as propranolol (Inderal)
	Some are catecholamines, and some are not; they differ primarily in their onset and duration
	There is also a long-acting salbutamol called Serevent; it is not to be used for the compromised patient due to its longer onset of action
Common Examples	Alupent Bronkometer
	Berotec Bronkosol
	Brethaire Serevent
	Brethine Vaponefrin
	Bricanyl Ventolin
	Bronkaid

Bronchodilators: Theophyllines

Type(s)	Theophyllines
Actions	Bronchodilation and vasodilation
	Respiratory stimulation
	Diuresis
	(+) chronotropy, (+) inotropy
Indications	Prevention and treatment of bronchospasm caused by reversible obstructive airway disease (chronic obstructive pulmonary disease, asthma, bronchitis, emphysema) and related bronchospastic disorders
Adverse Effects	*Cardiovascular system:* Hypotension, angina, tachycardia, palpitation, arrhythmia, PVCs, and flushing
	Central nervous system: Headache, nervousness, irritability, anxiety, excitement, dizziness, mild delirium, insomnia, fever, tremor, seizure, coma, and increased respiratory rate
	Other: N/V/D, anorexia, abdominal cramps, hematemesis, diuresis, dehydration, and visual or auditory disturbances
Interactions	β-blockers: May oppose effects
	Barbiturates, phenytoin: May decrease theophylline blood levels
How Supplied	Tablet, aerosol, elixir, syrup, and suppository
Note	Children are very sensitive: Toxic-to-therapeutic ratio is small
	Some are combination products
Common Examples	Choledyl Somophyllin
	Phyllocontin Tedral
	Quibron Theo-Dur

Calcium Channel Blockers

Type(s)	Antiarrhythmic, antihypertensive, and antianginal
Actions	Blocks entry of calcium into the cell (especially cardiac and vascular smooth muscle):
	(−) chronotropy
	(−) inotropy
	(−) dromotropy
	Vasodilation (including coronary)
	Bronchodilation
	Inhibits coronary artery spasm
Indications	Nifedipine, verapamil, and diltiazem: Angina from coronary artery spasm and chronic stable angina (effort associated)
	Verapamil: PSVT, A-fib, A-flutter

Adverse Effects	**Diltiazem**
	Cardiovascular system: Conduction disturbances, arrhythmia, hypotension, bradycardia, congestive heart failure, flushing, and peripheral edema
	Central nervous system: Headache, fatigue, drowsiness, dizziness, nervousness, central nervous system depression, confusion, and insomnia
	Other: N/V/D/ and rash
	Verapamil and Nifedipine:
Interactions	Digoxin: May increase Digoxin blood levels
	β-blockers: May potentiate some effects
How Supplied	Tablet and capsule (oral and sublingual)
Note	Often used in combination therapy
	Verapamil's most potent activity is electrophysiological, and nifedipine's most potent activity is hemodynamic; diltiazem acts like a less potent combination of the two
Common Examples	Adalat Isoptin
	Cardizem

Cardiotonics: Cardiac Glycosides

Type(s)	Digitalis ("Dig") preparations
Actions	Promotes movement of calcium into the cell:
	(+) inotrope
	(−) chronotrope
	(−) dromotrope
	Improves atrial conduction
Indications	Congestive heart failure, after myocardial infarction
	A-fib, A-flutter
	SVTs
Adverse Effects	*Cardiovascular system:* May exacerbate congestive heart failure and almost any arrhythmia or conduction defect (usually conduction disturbances, PACs, PVCs, SVTs); hypotension
	Central nervous system: Fatigue, weakness, agitation, hallucinations, behavioral changes, headache, dizziness, vertigo, confusion, anxiety, paresthesia, and insomnia
	Other: N/V/D/, anorexia, malaise, visual disturbances, and hypokalemia
Interactions	Diuretics, Ca^{2+}, quinidine, Amiodarone, Ca^{2+} blockers, catecholamines: May precipitate digitalis toxicity
How Supplied	Tablet and capsule
Note	Toxicity is more frequent in patients with hypokalemia, hypocalcemia, or hypomagnesemia
	About 7 percent to 40 percent of patients on digitalis develop some symptoms of toxicity

Digitalized patients may develop more serious and resistant arrhythmias following cardioversion; use of very low energy levels and prophylactic lidocaine or phenytoin may prevent this

Digitalis glycosides vary in potency, onset, and duration of action; they are generally long acting

Common Examples	Cedilanid	Lanoxin
	Crystodigin	Novodigoxin
	Digitaline	

Diuretics

Type(s)	Various (primarily thiazides, Loop, and combination products with antihypertensives, β-blockers, and aldosterone antagonists)
Actions	Diuresis
	Promotes sodium (Na$^+$) excretion
	Vasodilation
Indications	Hypertension
	Chronic fluid overload (congestive heart failure, pulmonary, peripheral edema)
	Liver cirrhosis with ascites and edema
	Decreased renal function (impairment)
	Edema (drug induced or from renal origin)
Adverse Effects	*Cardiovascular system:* Hypovolemia, hypotension, tachycardia, and arrhythmia
	Central nervous system: Drowsiness, confusion, delirium, dizziness, weakness, seizure, and coma
	Other: Dehydration, electrolyte imbalance (most commonly K$^+$), hyperosmolality, dry mouth or thirst, cramps, N/V/D, and visual or auditory disturbances; may inhibit insulin release (hyperglycemia)
Interactions	Antihypertensives: Increased antihypertensive effects
How Supplied	Tablet, capsule, and suppository
Note	Also known as "water pills"
	These patients are often on potassium (K$^+$) supplements
	Electrocardiogram may show prominent P waves, diminished T waves, and presence of U waves
Common Examples	Aldactazide	Dyazide
	Aldactone	Lasix
	Duretic	Moduret

Sedatives and Hypnotics

Type(s)
Primarily barbiturates, benzodiazepines; also piperidines, carbamates

Actions
Sedatives induce central nervous system depression and sedation, and "calm the nerves"

Hypnotics induce and maintain sleep

Indications
Some are for daytime use, some are for nighttime use

Anxiety, tension, stress, apprehension, irritability, excitement, and insomnia

Chronic behavioral disorders

Psychotherapy

Seizure disorders

Adverse Effects
Cardiovascular system: Hypotension and pulmonary edema

Central nervous system: Central nervous system or respiratory depression, drowsiness, dizziness, weakness, confusion, delirium, headache, ataxia, slurred speech, hypnosis (paradoxical excitement in the elderly), possible paresthesia, seizure, coma, nightmares, and hangover

Other: Extrapyramidal reactions, anticholinergic effects, Parkinson-like reactions (especially in children), N/V/D, rash, and withdrawal syndrome

Interactions
ETOH, other central nervous system depressants: Excessive central nervous system and respiratory depression

Monoamine oxidase inhibitors: Inhibit barbiturate metabolism

How Supplied
Tablet, capsule, and suppository

Note
Some have potential for tolerance, abuse, and addiction from chronic use

Some are combination products

Duration of action varies with each drug; some may be extremely long acting

Common Examples

Amytal	Nembutal
Butisol	Nodular
Dalmane	Placidyl
Day-Barb	Plexonal
Doriden	Restoril
Halcion	Seconal
Mandrax	Tuinal
Mogadon	Tranxene

COMMON EXAMPLES OF HOME MEDICATIONS

Narcotic: Analgesics

Ancasal
Atasol
Codeine
Darvon
Demerol
Dilaudid
Empracet
Exdol

Morphine
Numorphan
Oxycocet
Oxycodan
Percocet
Percodan
Talwin
Tylenol with Codeine (Nos. 1, 2, 3, and 4)

Antianginals

Cardilate
Coronex
Isordil
Nitrobid
Nitrogard

Nitrol
Nitrolingual Spray
Nitrong
Nitrostablin
Nitrostat

Anxiolytic (Antianxiety)

Atarax
Ativan
Donnatal
Lectopam
Librium
Loftran
Mellaril

Multipax
Serax
Stelzine
Tranxene
Valium
Vivol
Xanax

Antiarrhythmics

Antiarrhythmics may be classified by their predominant electrophysiological effects (e.g., Vaughn-Williams-Singh Classification).

Class I	Class II	Class III
Biquin	*Primarily β-blockers*	Bretylate
Dilantin	Betaloc	Bretylol
Mexitil	Biocadren	Cordarone
Norpace	Corgard	
Procan	Inderal	
Pronestyl	Lopressor	
Prosedyl	Sotacor	
Quinate	Tenormin	
Quinidex	Visken	
Quinine		
Rhythmodan		
Tonocard		
Xylocaine		

Class IV
Ca²⁺ channel blockers

Adalat
Cardizem
Isoptin

Cardiac glycoside

Cedilanid
Crystodigin
Digitaline
Lanoxin
Novodigozin

Anticoagulants

Coumadin
Hepalean
Heparin

Minihep
Sintrom
Warfilone

Anticonvulsants

Celontin
Depakene
Dilantin
Epival
Mebaral
Mebroin
Mesantoin

Milontin
Mogadon
Mysoline
Rivotril
Tegretol
Zarontin

Antidepressants: Monamine Oxidase Inhibitors

Marplan
Nardil

Parnate

Antidepressants: Tricyclic Antidepressants

Adapin
Anafranil
Asendin
Aventyl
Desyrel
Elavil
Etrafon
Limbitrol
Ludiomil

Norpramin
Pamelor
Pertofrane
Sinequan
Surmontil
Tofranil
Triadapin
Triptil
Vivactil

Antidiabetics: Insulins

Humilin
Iletin

Novolin
Velosulin

Antidiabetics: Oral Hypoglycemics

Diabeta
Diabinese
Dimelor
Euglucon
Mobenol
Orinase

Antihypertensives

Aldomet
Capoten
Catapres
Combipres
Loniten
Minipress
Serparsil
Viskazide

Antipsychotics

Haldol
Haloperidol
Mellaril
Nozinan
Peridol
Permitil
Quide
Serentil
Sparine
Stelazine
Trilafon

Beta-Blockers

Betaloc
Blocardren
Corgard
Inderal
Lopressor
Sotacor
Tenormin
Visken

Bronchodilators: Sympathomimetics

Alupent
Berotec
Brethaire
Brethine
Bricanyl
Bronkaid
Bronkometer
Bronkosol
Vaponefrin
Ventolin

Bronchodilators: Theophyllines

Choledyl
Phyllocontin
Quibron
Somophyllin
Tedral
Theo-Dur

Calcium Channel Blockers

Adalat
Cardizem
Isoptin

Cardiotonics: Cardiac Glycosides

Cedilanid

Crystodigin

Lanoxin

Novodigoxin

Diuretics

Aldactazide

Aldactone

Duretic

Digitaline

Dyazide

Lasix

Moduret

Sedatives and Hypnotics

Amytal

Butisol

Dalmane

Day-Barb

Doriden

Halcion

Mandrax

Mogadon

Nembutal

Nodular

Placidyl

Plexonal

Restoril

Seconal

Tuinal

Tranxene

PEDIATRIC DRUG DOSAGES

PEDIATRIC EMERGENCY MEDICATION DOSAGES

Activated Charcoal

Dose	1 g/kg
Maximum Dose	60 g No Max.
Route	Oral, nasogastric
Remarks	If administered with ipecac, it will absorb the ipecac

Adenosine

Dose	0.1 mg/kg first dose
	0.2 mg/kg second dose
Maximum Dose	12 mg
Route	Intravenous, intraosseous
Remarks	Rapid intravenous bolus

Atropine

Dose	0.02 mg/kg
Route	Intravenous, intraosseous, endotracheal
Remarks	Minimum dose is 0.1 mg
	Maximum dose in child 0.5 mg; maximum total dose 1.0 mg
	Maximum dose in adolescent 1.0 mg; maximum total dose 2.0 mg

Bretylium

Remarks   Not recommended for pediatric patients

10 Percent Calcium Chloride

Dose   20 mg/kg repeated once if necessary
Maximum Dose   500 mg No Max.
Route   Intravenous, intraosseous
Remarks   Give slowly (<100 mg/min).

Dextrose

Dose   Neonates and infants up to 3 months old,
   $D_{10}W$ 2–6 mL/kg
   >3 months, $D_{25}W$ 2–4 mL/kg
Route   Intravenous, intraosseous
Remarks   If you do not have 25 percent, dilute $D_{50}W$ with sterile
   water 1:1.

Diazepam

Dose   0.5 mg/kg rectal
   0.1–0.3 mg/kg intravenous, intraosseous
Route   Intravenous, intraosseous, rectal
Remarks   Maximum dose is 5 mg for children under the age of 5
   years and 10 mg for children over the age of 5 years.

Diphenhydramine (Benadryl)

Dose   1 mg/kg repeated once
Route   Intravenous, intraosseous, intramuscular
Remarks   Monitor blood pressure; maximum single dose is 50 mg

Dobutamine

Dose   2–20 µg/kg/min
Route   Intravenous drip
Remarks   Titrate to desired effect

Dopamine

Dose   2–20 µg/kg/min
Route   Intravenous drip
Remarks   Titrate to desired effect

Epinephrine 1:1000 (Adrenalin)

Dose	0.01 mg/kg; 0.01 mL/kg
Route	Subcutaneous
Remarks	Do not exceed 0.5 mL

Epinephrine 1:10 000

Dose	0.01 mg/kg (0.1 mL/kg) intravenous 0.1 mg endotracheal
Route	Intravenous, endotracheal, intraosseous
Remarks	Dose may be repeated at 5-minute intervals High dose: 0.1 mg/kg

Fentanyl

Dose	1–3 µg/kg Repeat 0.5 µg/kg
Route	Intravenous, intraosseous
Remarks	Administer slow intravenous push

Furosemide (Lasix)

Dose	1 mg/kg
Route	Intravenous, intraosseous
Remarks	Administer slow intravenous push over 5–10 minutes

Glucagon

Dose	0.03 mg/kg
Route	Intravenous, intramuscular, subcutaneous
Remarks	Sufficient glycogen stores in liver are needed; increase in blood sugar maximum of 1 mg

Lidocaine (Xylocaine)

Dose	1 mg/kg
Route	Intravenous, endotracheal, intraosseous
Remarks	Slow intravenous push; may be repeated at 8–10 minutes but total dose should not exceed 3 mg/kg

Lorazepam (Ativan)

Dose	0.5 mg/kg 0.05 mg/kg
Route	Intravenous, intraosseous

Remarks   Administer slow intravenous push over 20–30 seconds
Maximum of 0.2 mg/kg
Dose may be repeated every 10–15 minutes.

Midazolam (Versed)

Dose   0.07–0.3 mg/kg (usually 0.1 mg/kg)
Oral: 0.3–0.5 mg/kg
Intramuscular: 0.2 mg/kg
Rectal: 0.4–0.5 mg/kg

Route   Intravenous, intraosseous
Remarks   Administer slow intravenous push over 20–30 seconds

Morphine

Dose   0.1 mg/kg
Route   Intravenous, endotracheal, intraosseous
Remarks   Monitor respirations and administer slow intravenous

Naloxone (Narcan)

Dose   <5 years: 0.1 mg/kg
>5 years: 2.0 mg

Route   Intravenous, endotracheal, intraosseous, intramuscular
Remarks   Slow intravenous push; if desired response is not
achieved, subsequent dose of 0.1 mg/kg may be given

Salbutamol (Ventolin)

Dose   <5 years: 1.25–2.5 mg
>5 years: 2.5–5.0 mg
Intravenous bolus 4 μg/kg over 2–5 minutes
Repeat once as needed
Infusion 0.2 μg/kg/min up to maximum 10 μg/kg/min

Route   Nebulizer mask
Remarks   Administer through a nebulizer mask using nonhumidified oxygen at approximately 8 L/min or until
mask starts to mist; administer drug with 2 mL of
normal saline if not premixed in nebules.

Sodium Bicarbonate

Dose   1 mEq/kg
Route   Intravenous
Remarks   Infuse slowly
Ensure adequate ventilations

PRECALCULATED PEDIATRIC DRUG DOSAGES

Drug Supplied and Dose		Atropine 0.1 mg/mL 0.02 mg/kg		Diazepam 5 mg/mL 0.2 mg/kg		Dextrose 25% or 50% 0.5 g/kg			Epinephrine 1:10 000 0.01 mg/kg	
Age	kg	mg	mL	mg	mL	g	%	mL	mg	mL
Birth	3	0.1	1.0	0.6	0.1	1.5	25	6	0.03	0.3
3 months	5	0.1	1.0	1.0	0.2	2.5	25	10	0.05	0.5
6 months	7	0.14	1.4	1.4	0.28	3.5	25	14	0.07	0.7
1 year	10	0.20	2.0	2.0	0.4	5	25	20	0.10	1.0
2 years	12	0.24	2.4	2.4	0.48	6	50	12	0.12	1.2
3 years	15	0.30	3.0	3.0	0.6	7.5	50	15	0.15	1.5
4 years	17	0.34	3.4	3.4	0.68	8.5	50	17	0.17	1.7
5 years	18	0.36	3.6	3.6	0.72	9	50	18	0.18	1.8
6 years	20	0.40	4.0	4.0	0.8	10	50	20	0.20	2.0
8 years	25	0.50	5.0	5.0	1.0	12.5	50	25	0.25	2.5
10 years	30	0.60	6.0	6.0	1.2	15	50	30	0.30	3.0
12 years	38	0.76	7.6	7.6	1.52	19	50	38	0.38	3.8
14 years	50	1.0	10.0	10	2	25	50	50	0.50	5.0

Drug Supplied Dose/kg		Lidocaine 20 mg/mL 1 mg/kg		Lorazepam 4 mg/mL 0.05 mg/kg		Naloxone 0.4 mg/mL 0.1 mg/kg		Bicarbonate 50 mEq/50 mL 1 mEq/kg	
Age	kg	mg	mL	mg	mL	mg	mL	mEq	mL
Birth	3	3	0.15	0.15	0.038	0.3	0.3	3.0	3.0
3 months	5	5	0.25	0.25	0.06	0.5	0.5	5.0	5.0
6 months	7	7	0.35	0.35	0.088	0.7	0.7	7.0	7.0
1 year	10	10	0.5	0.5	0.125	1.0	1.0	10.0	10.0
2 years	12	12	0.6	0.6	0.15	1.2	1.2	12.0	12.0
3 years	15	15	0.75	0.75	0.188	1.5	1.5	15.0	15.0
4 years	17	17	0.85	0.85	0.21	1.7	1.7	17.0	17.0
5 years	18	18	0.9	0.9	0.225	1.8	1.8	18.0	18.0
6 years	20	20	1.0	1	0.25	2.0	2.0	20.0	20.0
8 years	25	25	1.25	1.25	0.313	2.0	2.0	25.0	25.0
10 years	30	30	1.50	1.5	0.375	2.0	2.0	30.0	30.0
12 years	38	38	1.9	1.9	0.475	2.0	2.0	38.0	38.0
14 years	50	50	2.5	2.5	0.625	2.0	2.0	50.0	50.0

PEDIATRIC MEDICATION INFUSIONS

An infusion pump is highly recommended.

Aminophylline

How Supplied	Use 25 mg/mL solution
Dose	0.2 mL/kg in 100 D_5W, over 20–30 minutes
Maintenance	
Dose	0.5 mg/kg/hr
Remarks	To mix: Add 125 mg to 250 mL D_5W (or 50 mg in 100 mL D_5W)
Note	1 microdrop/kg/min of this solution = 0.5 mg/kg/hr

Dobutamine

How Supplied	Use 25 mg/mL solution
Dose	2–12 µg/kg/min
Remarks	To mix: Add 30 mg to 250 mL D_5W
Note	1 microdrop/kg/min of this solution = 2 µg/kg/min

Dopamine

How Supplied	Use 40 mg/mL solution
Dose	2–12 µg/kg/min
Remarks	To mix: Add 80 mg (2 mL) to 250 mL D_5W
Note	1 microdrop/kg/min of this solution = 5 µg/kg/hr

Epinephrine

How Supplied	Use 1:1000 solution, 1 mg/mL
Dose	0.1–1.0 µg/kg/min
Remarks	To mix: Add 1.5 mg (1.5 mL) to 250 mL D_5W
Note	1 microdrop/kg/min of this solution = 0.1 µg/kg/hr

Lidocaine

How Supplied	Use 2 percent solution, 20 mg/mL
Dose	20–50 µg/kg/min
Remarks	To mix: Add 300 mg (15 mL) to 250 mL D_5W
Note	1 microdrop/kg/min of this solution = 20 µg/kg/hr

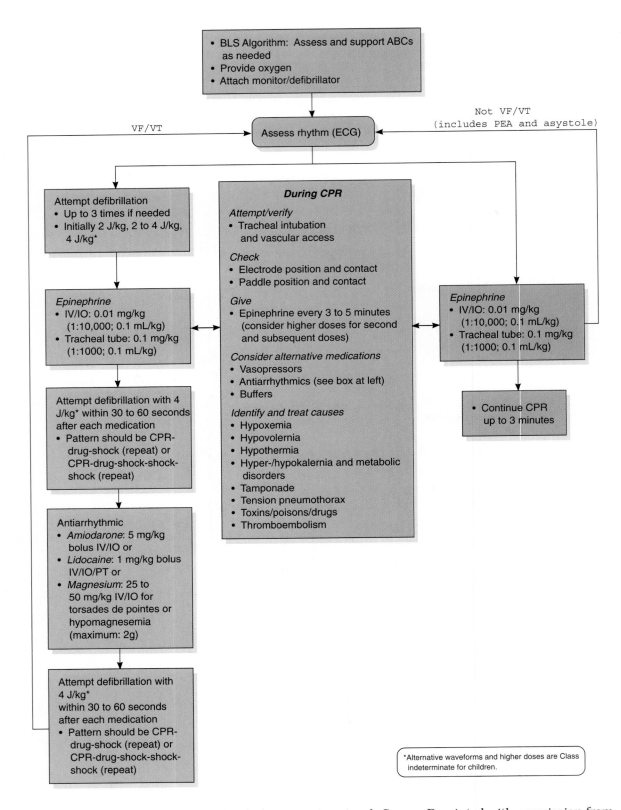

FIGURE E–1 Pediatric asystole and pulseless arrest protocol. *Source:* Reprinted with permission from *Journal of the American Medical Association* 268, no. 16 (October 28, 1992): 2171–2302. © 1992 by the American Medical Association.

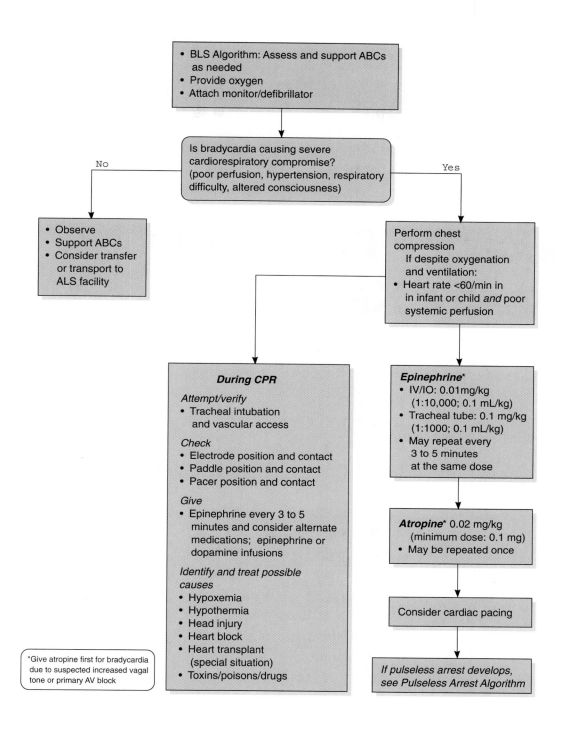

FIGURE E–2 Pediatric bradycardia protocol. *Source:* Reprinted with permission from *Journal of the American Medical Association* 268, no. 16 (October 28, 1992): 2171–2302. © 1992 by the American Medical Association.

PRACTICE PROBLEMS ANSWER KEY

SECTION 1

1.	1 g	=	1000 mg
2.	1 mg	=	1000 µg
3.	1 mg	=	0.001 g
4.	0.8 mg	=	800 µg
5.	1.5 L	=	1500 mL
6.	400 000 mg	=	400 g
7.	800 mg	=	0.8 g
8.	500 mL	=	0.5 L
9.	37 °C	=	98.6 °F
10.	104 °F	=	40 °C
11.	1/4 gr	=	16.25 mg
12.	2 Tbsp	=	30 mL
13.	180 lb	=	82 kg
14.	7 lb	=	3.2 kg
15.	25 kg	=	55 lb

SECTION 2

1. 10 mL
2. 4 mL
3. 5 mL
4. 100 mL
5. 2 mL
6. 0.33 mL
7. 1.5 mL
8. 2 mL
9. 8 mL
10. 50 mL

SECTION 3

1. 3.4 mL *This could be approximated to 3.5 mL. Check with your medical control.*
2. 6.8 mL
3. 0.59 mL *This could be approximated to 0.6 mL. Check with your medical control.*
4. 72 mL or 73 mL
5. 0.2 mL

SECTION 4

1. 800 mg/mL
2. 9 g
3. 5 mg/mL
4. 50 mg
5. 100 mg
6. 4 mg/mL
7. 1600 mg/mL
8. 3 mL
9. 4 mg/mL
10. 2 mg/mL

SECTION 5

1. 30 gtt/min
2. 60 gtt/min
3. 30 gtt/min
4. 30 gtt/min
5. 30 gtt/min
6. 5 gtt/min
7. 15 gtt/min
8. 23 gtt/min
9. 6 gtt/min
10. 60 gtt/min

SECTION 6

1. 30 gtt/min
2. 15 gtt/min
3. 30 gtt/min
4. 45 gtt/min
5. 45 gtt/min
6. 90 gtt/min
7. 15 gtt/min
8. 51–52 gtt/min
9. 10 mg/kg/min
10. 4 mg/kg/min

SECTION 7

1. 100 gtt/min
2. 50 gtt/min
3. 15 gtt/min
4. 100 gtt/min (first hour)
   25 gtt/min (over 8 hours)
5. 38 gtt/min

Drug Administration Skills

SUBCUTANEOUS DRUG ADMINISTRATION

Subcutaneous injection is a method of administering drugs directly into subcutaneous or fatty tissue, where they are absorbed into the general circulation (see Procedure G–1). Medication injected subcutaneously is typically absorbed more slowly than through the intravenous routes but faster than through the oral route. The subcutaneous injection of epinephrine may be lifesaving in severe cases of asthma or allergic reactions. Glucagon can also be administered subcutaneously for the treatment of insulin shock. The medication must be administered into the subcutaneous tissue and not into the more superficial dermis or deeper muscle, connective tissue, or blood vessels.

Epinephrine 1:1000 is the emergency drug most frequently given subcutaneously. The procedure is as follows:

1. Receive order.
2. Confirm the drug order, amount to be given, and route and write the information down.

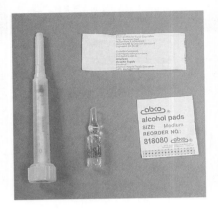

G–1a   Prepare the equipment.

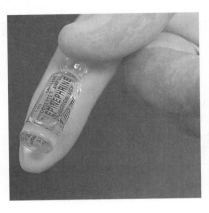

G–1b   Check the medication.

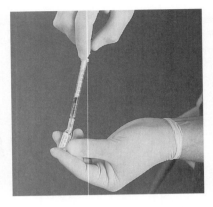

G–1c   Draw up the medication.

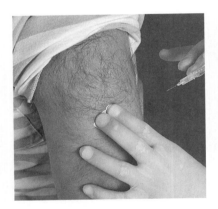

G–1d   Prep the site.

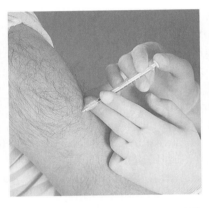

G–1e   Insert the needle at a 45° angle.

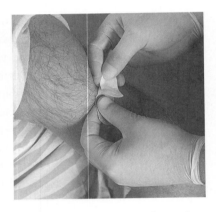

G–1f   Remove the needle and cover the puncture site.

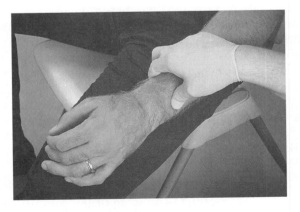

G–1g   Monitor the patient.

3. Prepare the necessary equipment and observe body substance isolation precautions (gloves):
   - 1 cc syringe
   - One needle (preferably 1 to $1\frac{1}{2}$ inches in length, 16 to 22 gauge) to withdraw medication
   - One needle (preferably $\frac{1}{2}$ to $\frac{5}{8}$ inch in length, 25 gauge) for drug administration
   - Alcohol or povidone-iodine preparation
   - 2 × 2 gauze pad
   - Medication
   - Sharps container
4. Explain to the patient what you are going to do and reconfirm that the patient is not allergic to the medication. Be sure to advise the patient of any complications that might result from the administration.
5. Examine the ampule of medication, including name and expiration date. Hold it up to the light and inspect for discoloration or particles in the solution. Do not administer if discolored or if particles are present.
6. "Shake down" the ampule. This will force the liquid to the lower portion of the ampule so that it can be broken without spillage of the drug.
7. Break the ampule using a 2 × 2 gauze pad to prevent injury.
8. Draw the medication into the syringe. Invert the syringe and expel any air present.
9. Choose a suitable site. The easiest and most accessible site is the subcutaneous tissue over the deltoid muscle in the arm.
10. Prepare the site by cleansing it with a povidone-iodine or alcohol preparation using a firm circular motion from the vein outward.
11. Pinch up the skin and insert the needle into the tissue at a 45-degree angle.
12. Inject the medication into the subcutaneous tissue slowly.
13. Remove the syringe. Do not recap the needle.
14. Apply pressure to the site with sterile gauze pad.
15. Dispose of the syringe and medication container.
16. Cover with an adhesive strip.
17. Confirm administration of the medication.
18. Closely monitor the patient for the desired therapeutic effect and possible side effects.
19. Document procedure and patient effects.

INTRAMUSCULAR INJECTION

Intramuscular (IM) injection is a method of administering drugs directly into muscle, where it is absorbed into the general circulation. Prehospital administration of IM drugs is relatively uncommon but is useful when other administration routes fail. Several prehospital drugs can be administered IM, the most common being diazepam, meperidine, morphine, and glucagon. Absorption by the IM route is slower than by the IV route; because it requires adequate perfusion, it may be ineffective in the hypotensive patient. IM

injections may be contraindicated in patients with coagulopathies (a defect in the clotting mechanism of the body) or those who take anticoagulants.
Several sites are used for intramuscular injections (see Figure G–1).

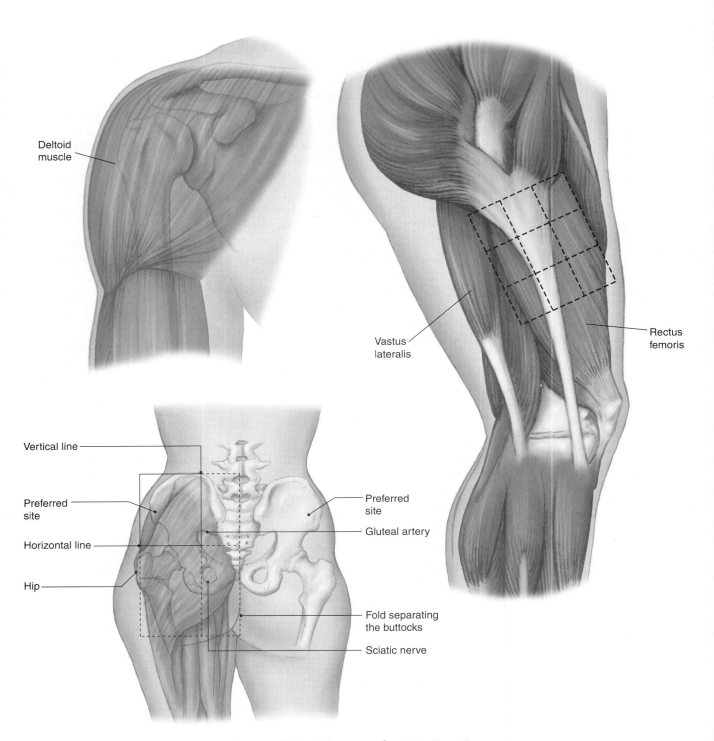

FIGURE G–1 Intramuscular injection sites.

The procedure for intramuscular medication administration is as follows (see Procedure G–2):

1. Receive order.
2. Confirm the drug order, amount to be given, and route and write the information down.
3. Prepare the necessary equipment and observe body substance isolation precautions (gloves):
   - Syringe of sufficient size to contain the medication
   - One needle (preferably 1 to 1½ inches in length, 16 to 22 gauge) to withdraw medication
   - One needle (preferably ¾ to 1 inch in length, 21 to 25 gauge) for drug administration
   - Alcohol or povidone-iodine preparation
   - 2 × 2 gauze pad
   - Medication
   - Sharps container
4. Explain to the patient what you are going to do and reconfirm that the patient is not allergic to the medication. Be sure to advise the patient of any complications that might result from the administration.
5. Examine the ampule of medication, including name and expiration date. Hold it up to the light and inspect for discoloration or particles in the solution. Do not administer if discolored or if particles are present.
6. "Shake down" the ampule. This will force the liquid to the lower portion of the ampule so that it can be broken without spillage of the drug.
7. Break the ampule using a 2 × 2 gauze pad to prevent injury.
8. Draw the medication into the syringe. Invert the syringe and expel any air present.
9. Choose a suitable site. The easiest and most accessible site is the deltoid muscle in the arm (see Figure G–3).
10. Prepare the site by cleansing it with a povidone-iodine or alcohol preparation using a firm circular motion from the vein outward.
11. Insert the needle into the tissue at a 90-degree angle (see Figure G–5).
12. Aspirate the syringe to ensure that you are not in a blood vessel. If you get any blood return, you should withdraw the needle and reattempt administration at another site.
13. Inject the medication slowly.
14. Remove the syringe. Do not recap the needle.
15. Apply pressure to the site.
16. Cover with an adhesive strip.
17. Confirm administration of the medication.
18. Closely monitor the patient for the desired therapeutic effect and possible undesired side effects.
19. Document procedure and patient effects.

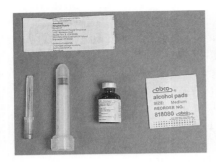

G–2a Prepare the equipment.

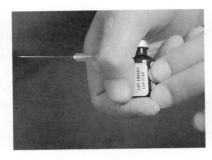

G–2b Check the medication.

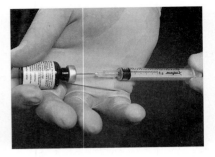

G–2c Draw up the medication.

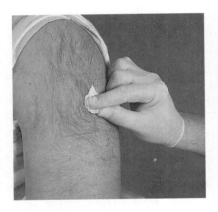

G–2d Prepare the site.

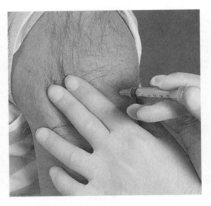

G–2e Insert the needle at a 90° angle.

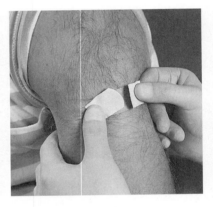

G–2f Remove the needle and cover the puncture site.

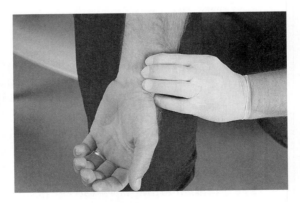

G–2g Monitor the patient.

(see Figure G–2 paramedic care)

1. Receive order.

2. Confirm the intravenous (IV) fluid, amount to be given, and route and write the information down.

3. Prepare the necessary equipment and observe body substance isolation precautions (gloves and goggles):
   - Appropriate IV fluid
   - Appropriate administration set
   - Appropriate indwelling catheter
   - Extension IV tubing if necessary

4. Remove the envelope from the IV fluid.

5. Inspect the fluid, making sure that it is not discolored and does not contain any particulate matter; check that it contains the correct amount of fluid. Do not administer if discolored, if particles are present, or if less than the indicated quantity of fluid is present.

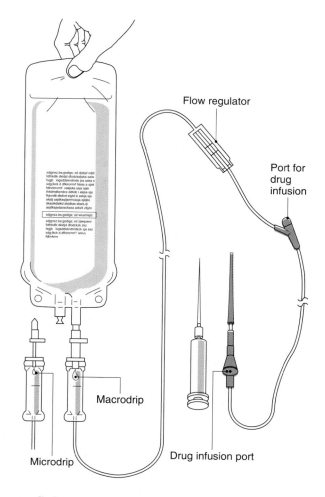

FIGURE G–2 Macrodrip and microdrip administration sets.

6. Open and inspect the IV tubing.

7. Attach the extension tubing.

8. Close the clamp on the tubing.

9. Remove the sterile cover from the IV fluid and the administration set.

10. Insert the administration set into the IV fluid.

11. Squeeze the drip chamber to fill it with fluid.

12. Bleed all of the air out of the IV tubing.

13. Hang the bag on an IV pole (or have a bystander hold it) at the appropriate height.

PROCEDURE FOR INTRAVENOUS CANNULATION

The procedure is as follows (see Procedure G–3):

1. Receive order.

2. Confirm the drug order, amount to be given, and route and write the information down.

3. Prepare the necessary equipment and observe body substance isolation precautions (gloves and goggles):

   - Appropriate IV fluid and administration set (previously set up)
   - Appropriate indwelling catheter (18 gauge for lifelines and 12 to 16 gauge for fluid administration)
   - Tourniquet
   - Povidone-iodine or alcohol preparation
   - Antibiotic ointment
   - 2 × 2 gauze pad
   - 1-inch tape
   - Short arm board
   - Sharps container

4. Explain to the patient what you are going to do. Be sure to advise the patient of any complications that might result from the procedure.

5. Place the tourniquet (or inflate blood pressure cuff to 20 mm Hg below systolic pressure) just above the elbow and place the arm in a dependent position.

6. Select a suitable vein and palpate it (see Chapter 5, Figures 5–6 and 5–7).

7. Select the most prominent vein on the hand, forearm, or antecubital space that is straight, on a flat surface, and not rolling. If possible, avoid veins over joints, using the antecubital veins as a last resort.

8. A vein may be distended for easier cannulation by gently tapping on it with the fingers.

9. Prepare the site by cleansing it with a povidone-iodine or alcohol preparation using a firm circular motion from the vein outward.

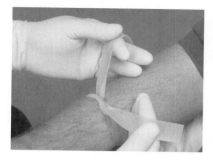

G–3a Place the constricting band.

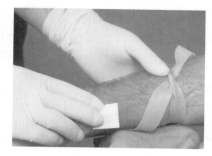

G–3b Cleanse the venipunture site.

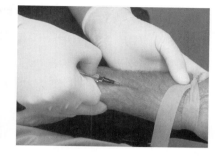

G–3c Insert the intravenous cannula into the vein.

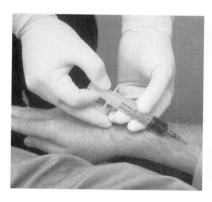

G–3d Withdraw any blood samples needed.

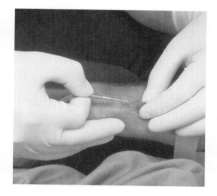

G–3e Connect the IV tubing.

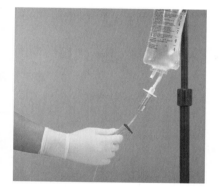

G–3f Turn on the IV and check the flow.

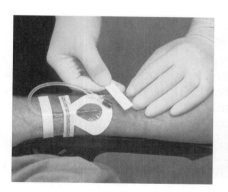

G–3g Secure the site.

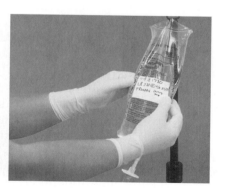

G–3h Label the intravenous solution bag.

10. Apply traction on the skin below the venipuncture site and stabilize the vein.

11. Tell the patient there will be a quick, painful stick.

12. With the bevel of the needle upward, puncture the skin using a 30- to 45-degree angle. Enter the vein directly from above or from the side.

13. When the vein is entered, you should feel a "pop" and see flashback into the catheter (see Chapter 5, Figures 5–8 through 5–10).

14. Carefully lower the catheter and advance the needle and catheter approximately 2 mm to stabilize the needle in the vein.

15. Slide the catheter off the needle into the vein and then remove the needle. Dispose of the needle in a puncture-proof (sharps) container.

16. Remove the tourniquet.

17. Connect the IV tubing and slowly open the valve.

18. Confirm that the fluid is flowing freely without any evidence of infiltration.

19. Apply povidone-iodine ointment or an antibiotic ointment over the puncture and cover with a sterile 2 × 2 gauze pad or adhesive bandage.

20. Securely tape the IV catheter to the skin using any acceptable technique.

21. Make a loop with the infusion tubing and tape the loop to the arm.

22. Adjust the flow rate.

23. If the vein is over a joint, immobilize with a short arm board to prevent dislodgment of the catheter.

24. Document the successful completion of the IV.

25. Monitor the patient for the desired effects and any undesired ones as well.

EXTERNAL JUGULAR VEIN CANNULATION

Intravenous Access in the External Jugular Vein

The external jugular vein is a large peripheral vein in the neck, between the angle of the jaw and the middle third of the clavicle. It connects into the central circulation of the subclavian vein. Since it lies so close to the central circulation, cannulation here offers many of the same benefits afforded central venous access. Fluids and medications rapidly reach the core of the body from this site.

Consider the external jugular vein only after you have exhausted other means of peripheral access or when a patient requires immediate fluid administration. This is an extremely painful site to access, so you typically will reserve its use for patients with a decreased or total loss of consciousness.

1. Receive order.

2. Confirm the drug order, amount to be given, and route and write the information down.

3. Prepare the necessary equipment and observe body substance isolation precautions (gloves and goggles):
   - Appropriate intravenous (IV) fluid and administration set (previously set up)
   - Appropriate indwelling catheter (18 gauge for lifelines and 12 to 16 gauge for fluid administration)
   - Povidone-iodine or alcohol preparation
   - Antibiotic ointment
   - 2 × 2 gauze pad
   - 1-inch tape
   - Sharps container

4. Explain to the patient what you are going to do (if the patient is conscious). Be sure to advise the patient of any complications that might result from the procedure.

5. Position the patient supine with feet elevated (when possible).

6. Turn the head in the direction away from the side to be cannulated.

7. Select a suitable vein and palpate it.

8. Prepare the site by cleansing it with a povidone-iodine or alcohol preparation.

9. Apply traction on the vein just below the clavicle.

10. Attach a 10 mL syringe to an IV catheter. Align the catheter and point the tip of the catheter toward the feet.

11. Tell the patient there will be a quick, painful stick.

12. With the bevel of the needle upward, puncture the skin using a 30-degree angle. The needle tip should enter midway between the angle of the jaw and the clavicle and should be aimed toward the shoulder on the same side as the vein. Apply suction to the syringe. As the vein is entered, note a flashback of blood.

13. Carefully lower the catheter and advance the needle and catheter approximately 2 mm to stabilize the needle in the vein.

14. Slide the catheter off the needle into the vein and then remove the needle. Dispose of the needle into a puncture-proof (sharps) container.

15. Connect the IV tubing and slowly open the valve.

16. Confirm that the fluid is flowing freely without any evidence of infiltration.

17. Apply povidone-iodine ointment or an antibiotic ointment over the puncture and cover with a sterile 2 × 2 gauze pad or adhesive bandage.

18. Securely tape the IV catheter to the skin using any acceptable technique.

19. Make a loop with the infusion tubing and tape the loop to the neck.

20. Adjust the flow rate.

21. Document the successful completion of the IV.

22. Monitor the patient for the desired effects and any undesired ones as well.

INTRAVENOUS BOLUS

Intravenous (IV) bolus, or IV push, is a method of administering drugs directly into the bloodstream (see Procedure G–4). This method provides a rapid route for medications. Because this is a rapid method of drug administration, it is the most commonly used route for life-threatening emergencies. These emergencies include the following:

- Ventricular dysrhythmias
- Supraventricular tachycardia
- Symptomatic bradycardia
- Hypoglycemia
- Metabolic acidosis
- Seizures
- Acute pulmonary edema
- Cardiopulmonary arrest
- Narcotic overdose
- Pain control

1. Receive order.
2. Confirm the drug order, amount to be given, and route and write the information down.
3. Prepare the necessary equipment and observe body substance isolation precautions (gloves):
   - Syringe of sufficient size to contain the medication (or prefilled syringe)
   - Needle (preferably 1 inch long, 18 gauge)
   - Alcohol or povidone-iodine preparation
   - 2 × 2 gauze pad
   - Medication
   - Sharps container
4. Explain to the patient what you are going to do and reconfirm that the patient is not allergic to the medication. Be sure to advise the patient of any complications that might result from the administration.
5. Examine the ampule of medication, including name and expiration date. Hold it up to the light and inspect for discoloration or particles in the solution. Do not administer if discolored or if particles are present.
6. "Shake down" the ampule. This will force the liquid to the lower portion of the ampule so that it can be broken without spillage of the drug.
7. Break the ampule using a 2 × 2 gauze pad to prevent injury.
8. Draw the medication into the syringe. Invert the syringe and expel any air.
9. Locate the medication port on the IV administration set and cleanse it with an alcohol swab.

Procedure G–4 Intravenous Bolus Administration

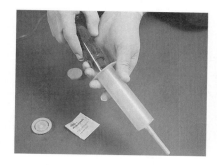

G–4a Prepare the equipment.

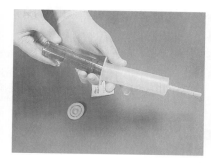

G–4b Prepare the medication.

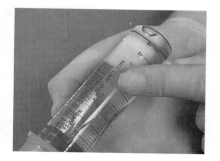

G–4c Check the label.

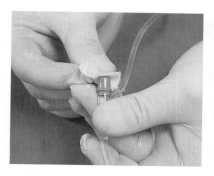

G–4d Select and clean an administration port.

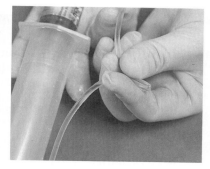

G–4e Pinch the line.

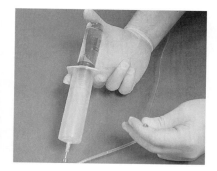

G–4f Administer the medication.

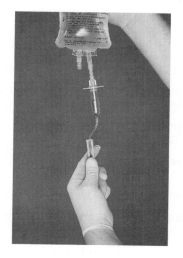

G–4g Adjust the IV flow rate.

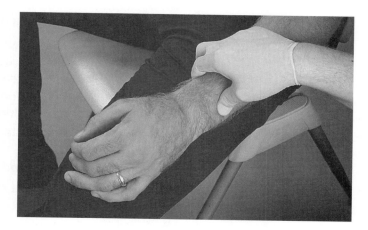

G–4h Monitor the patient.

10. Insert the needle into the medication port.

11. Pinch the IV line off above the medication port.

12. Administer the medication in a slow, deliberate fashion.

13. Remove the needle and wipe the medication port with an alcohol swab.

14. Release the pinched line.

15. Confirm administration of the medication.

16. Closely monitor the patient for the desired therapeutic effects as well as any undesired side effects.

INTRAVENOUS INFUSION ADMINISTRATION

Intravenous (IV) piggyback or IV drip infusion provides a route for continuous medication administration (see Procedure G–5). It offers the advantage of being easily titrated to increase or decrease the rate of flow or to discontinue the infusion based on the patient's response.

1. Receive order.

2. Confirm the drug order, amount to be given, and route and write the information down.

3. Prepare the necessary equipment and observe body substance isolation precautions (gloves):
   - Medication
   - Syringe to transfer the medication from the ampule to the diluent
   - Alcohol preparation or other antibacterial scrub
   - Two 18-gauge, 1-inch needles
   - Label for the bag

4. Explain to the patient what you are going to do and reconfirm that the patient is not allergic to the medication. Be sure to advise the patient of any complications that might result from the administration.

5. Examine the medication, including name and expiration date.

6. Assemble the equipment and attach the needle to the syringe if not preattached.

7. Calculate and draw up desired volume of drug into syringe.

8. Draw the medication into the syringe using aseptic technique. Invert and expel any air.

9. Cleanse the medication port on the IV bag into which the medication will be added.

10. Invert the bag and add the medication through the medication addition port.

11. Remove the needle and cleanse the medication addition port.

12. Invert the bag several times and place an administration set into it.

13. Bleed the air out of the administration set and attach a 1-inch, 18-gauge needle.

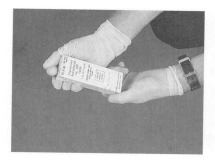

G–5a Select the drug.

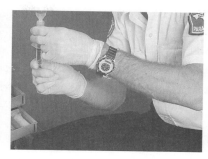

G–5b Draw up the drug.

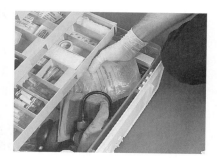

G–5c Select the IV fluid for dilution.

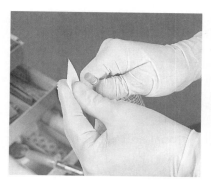

G–5d Clean the medication addition port.

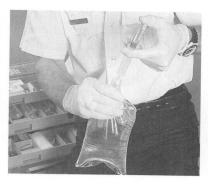

G–5e Inject the drug into the fluid.

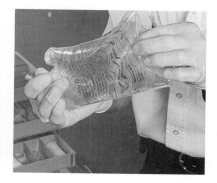

G–5f Mix the solution.

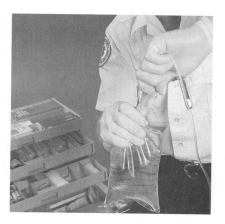

G–5g Insert an administration set and connect to main IV line with needle.

14. Cleanse the medication port on the administration set of the already established IV line and insert the needle.

15. Tape the needle securely.

16. Set the primary IV rate to TKVO.

17. Adjust the flow rate of the piggyback infusion to the desired dose.

18. Label the bag.

19. Confirm establishment of the infusion.

20. Closely monitor the patient for the desired therapeutic effects as well as any undesired side effects.

ENDOTRACHEAL TUBE ADMINISTRATION

Endotracheal bolus is a procedure that allows the delivery of a medication directly to the tracheobronchial tree and lung tissue via an endotracheal tube. The number of drugs administered via an endotracheal tube (ETT) is limited, and it is generally used during cardiac arrest when intravenous access is not available. The three medications most commonly administered via an ETT are atropine, epinephrine, and lidocaine. Although Narcan can be given via the ETT, other routes are available and may be preferable. There is some debate as to the exact amount of drug to be administered. However, the dose of drug should be at least equal to the IV dose and should be delivered in a volume of 5 to 10 mL.

The procedure is as follows:

1. Receive order.

2. Confirm the order, amount to be given, and route and write the information down.

3. Prepare the necessary equipment and observe body substance isolation precautions (gloves):
   - Prefilled syringe and needle or 18- or 19-gauge needle with syringe
   - Sterile saline or water for dilution

4. Examine the ampule of medication, including name and expiration date. Hold it up to the light and inspect for discoloration or particles in the solution. Do not administer if discolored or if particles are present.

5. Hyperventilate the patient in anticipation of administration.

6. Remove the bag-valve-mask unit and inject the medication down the tube.

7. Replace the bag-valve-mask unit and resume ventilation.

8. Monitor the patient for the desired therapeutic effect and any possible undesired side effects.

INTRAOSSEOUS INFUSION

Intraosseous (IO) infusion is a puncture into the medullary cavity of a bone that provides the paramedic with a rapid access route for fluids and medications. Generally IO infusion is indicated for the pediatric patient up to

6 years of age. The IO site is for temporary use only. Once the child's condition has stabilized, another form of intravenous therapy should be initiated. Prolonged use of IO infusion has led to infection more often than traditional intravenous (IV) lines. IOs are indicated in the following cases:

- Cardiac arrest
- Multisystem trauma associated with shock and/or severe hypovolemia; severe dehydration associated with vascular collapse and/or loss of consciousness
- Any child who is unresponsive and in need of immediate drug or fluid resuscitation (burns, status asthmaticus, status epilepticus, and sepsis)

The procedure is as follows:

1. Receive order.
2. Confirm the order, amount to be given, and route, and write the information down.
3. Prepare the necessary equipment and observe body substance isolation precautions (gloves):
   - Medication
   - Intravenous fluid and tubing
   - 10 mL syringe
   - Injectable saline
   - Intraosseous needle or 16- to 18-gauge spinal needle (see Figure G–3)
   - Povidone-iodine preparation
   - Antibiotic ointment
   - Several rolls of Kling
4. Examine the ampule of medication, including name and expiration date. Hold it up to the light and inspect for discoloration or particles in the solution. Do not administer if discolored or if particles are present.
5. Identify the landmark for insertion, preferably the anteromedial aspect of the proximal tibia, approximately 1 to 3 cm below the tibial tuberosity.
6. Prepare the area extensively with three povidone-iodine preparations in a circular fashion.
7. Replace your gloves with sterile gloves.

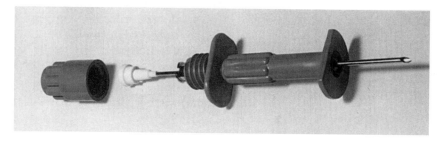

FIGURE G–3 Intraosseous needle or 16- to 18-gauge spinal needle.

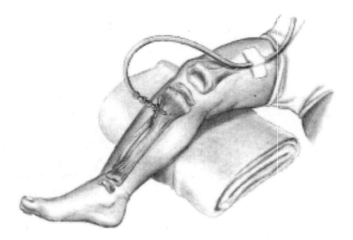

FIGURE G–4 Intraosseous infusion.

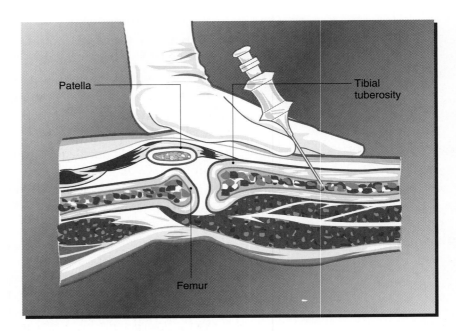

Patella

Tibial tuberosity

Femur

FIGURE G–5 Intraosseous infusion.

8. Take the sterile needle and insert it into the bone at a perpendicular angle or angled slightly inferior.

9. Using a twisting motion, introduce the needle using a 90-degree inferior puncture away from the joint and epiphyseal plate. There will be a decrease in resistance when the needle has been inserted. Stop insertion when a lack of resistance is felt (see Figures G–4 and G–5).

10. Remove the stylet, place a 10 mL syringe on the needle, and aspirate a small amount of marrow to verify the position of the needle.

11. Attach another 10 mL syringe filled with sterile saline. Inject 5 to 10 mL of saline to clear the lumen of the needle.

12. Attach the IV line and the desired fluid.

13. Place antibiotic ointment around the site and secure with tape.

14. Administer the medication.

15. Remove the syringe. Do not recap the needle. Dispose of the needle and syringe properly.

16. Following administration of a medication, 10 mL of saline should be administered to expedite absorption into the circulatory system.

17. Closely monitor the child for the desired effects as well as any side effects.

NEBULIZED INHALATION

Nebulized inhalation of drugs is a method of delivering medications via the tracheobronchial tree using a nebulizer. Nebulized inhalation mixes oxygen with a medication, which results in a vapor that the patient can inhale. Nebulized medication administration is used in the prehospital setting for asthma and chronic obstructive pulmonary disease (COPD). Commonly used medications include albuterol (Proventil), salbutamol (Ventolin), and metaproterenol (Alupent).

1. Receive order.

2. Confirm the order, amount to be given, and route and write the information down.

3. Prepare the necessary equipment and observe body substance isolation precautions (gloves, mask, and goggles):
   • Side-stream nebulizer
   • Oxygen tubing
   • Medication
   • Normal saline for dilution of the bronchodilator

4. Explain procedure to the patient.

5. Take the patient's vital signs and connect the patient to a cardiac monitor.

6. Assemble the nebulizer and place the bronchodilator and saline solution in the reservoir of the side-stream nebulizer.

7. Connect the device and administer oxygen at 6 to 12 L/min and start treatment.

8. Have the patient inhale normally through the mouthpiece or through the mask.

9. Have the patient take a deep breath every three to five inhalations.

10. Continue treatment until the solution is depleted.

11. Administer supplemental oxygen following treatment.

12. Reassess the patient's vital signs and monitor the electrocardiogram results.

BAG-VALVE NEBULIZED MEDICATION ADMINISTRATION

Nebulized medication administration may be required in patients with serious airway compromise due to a severe asthma attack. In these situations, the intubated patient may receive nebulized ventolin via the bag-valve device. Commonly used medications include albuterol (Proventil), salbutamol (Ventolin), and metaproterenol (Alupent).

1. Receive order.
2. Confirm the order, amount to be given, and route and write the information down.
3. Prepare the necessary equipment and observe body substance isolation precautions (gloves, mask, and goggles):
   - Side-stream nebulizer
   - Oxygen tubing
   - Bag-valve-mask device
   - Intubation equipment
   - Medication
   - Normal saline for dilution of the bronchodilator
4. Take the patient's vital signs and connect the patient to a cardiac monitor and O_2 saturation monitor.
5. Assemble the nebulizer and place the bronchodilator and saline solution in the reservoir of the side-stream nebulizer.
6. Connect the nebulizer to the bag-valve device and administer oxygen at 6 to 12 L/min and start treatment.
7. Ventilate the patient 12 to 20 times per minute.
8. Continue treatment until the solution is depleted.
9. Continue to assist ventilations following treatment.
10. Reassess the patient's vital signs, and monitor the electrocardiogram results.
11. Repeat treatment as necessary as per protocol.

SELF-ADMINISTERED NITROUS OXIDE

A 50:50 nitrous and oxygen mixture allows the patient to regulate his or her pain control by self-administering the gas. This mixture has a rapid effect on the central nervous system and depresses cortical function with no direct effects on the respiratory system. It has an extremely short half-life. Nitrous oxide is indicated in the following situations:

- Musculoskeletal trauma
- Thermal burns
- Childbirth

Nitrous oxide is contraindicated in the following situations:

- Altered mental status
- Alcohol intoxication

- Head injury
- Abdominal or chest trauma
- Shock
- Pneumothorax
- Pulmonary disease (chronic obstructive pulmonary disease or asthma)
- Inability to comprehend or respond to verbal commands
- Inability to self-administer
- Abdominal distention suggestive of bowel obstruction

    1. Receive order.

    2. Confirm the drug order, amount to be given, and route and write the information down.

    3. Prepare the necessary equipment and observe body substance isolation precautions (gloves):
- Medication tank(s)
- Face mask

    4. Invert the nitrous tank several times to create vaporization and mix the gases.

    5. Open the pressure valves on the oxygen and nitrous tanks

    6. Explain to the patient what you are going to do and reconfirm that the patient is not allergic to the medication. Be sure to advise the patient of any complications that might result from the administration.

    7. Instruct the patient on the use of the device.

    8. Place the patient in a sitting position (if possible) and instruct and assist the patient in creating a tight face mask seal.

    9. Coach the patient to inhale and exhale normally.

    10. If the patient feels uncomfortable for any reason during the procedure, the patient should remove the mask and breathe normally.

    11. No one should apply or hold the face mask to the patient except the patient.

    12. Monitor the patient for changes in level of consciousness and other vital signs.

EPINEPHRINE AUTOINJECTORS (EPI-PEN)

Patients who experience severe allergic reactions now carry epinephrine in autoinjectors. These injectors deliver an intramuscular dose of 0.3 mg of epinephrine for adults or 0.15 mg for children. These injectors are indicated for severe allergic reactions due to insect stings or bites, foods, drugs, or other allergens.

    1. Receive order.

    2. Confirm the order, amount to be given, and route and write the information down.

3. Prepare the necessary equipment and observe body substance isolation precautions (gloves):
   - Epinephrine autoinjector
   - Personal protective equipment
4. Explain to the patient what you are going to do and reconfirm that the patient is not allergic to the medication. Be sure to advise the patient of any complications that might result from the administration.
5. Assess need for epinephrine administration.
6. Examine the autoinjector for name, dose, and expiration date.
7. Remove safety cap from autoinjector.
8. Place autoinjector on outer thigh.
9. Press hard until you hear the injector function.
10. Hold autoinjector in place for several seconds.
11. Gently massage the injection area for 10 to 15 seconds.
12. Take the patient's vital signs, connect the patient to a cardiac monitor, and watch for a change in the patient's condition.

UMBILICAL VEIN CATHETERIZATION

Umbilical vein catheterization (UVC) is a method of gaining access by placing a special catheter or tubing into the umbilical vein of the neonatal umbilicus. This procedure allows the paramedic to administer fluids or medications when percutaneous cannulation into a small vein is impossible. Indications include a neonatal patient, less than 1 week of age, in need of intravenous (IV) access but without accessible peripheral veins.

The procedure is as follows:

1. Receive order.
2. Confirm the drug order, amount to be given and route and write the information down.
3. Prepare the necessary equipment and observe body substance isolation precautions (gloves and goggles):
   - Appropriate IV fluid and administration set (previously set up)
   - Appropriate indwelling catheter
   - Povidone-iodine or alcohol preparations
   - Antibiotic ointment
   - 2 × 2 gauze pad
   - 1-inch tape
   - Sharps container
4. Explain to the patient's parents what you are going to do. Be sure to advise the patient's parents of any complications that might result from the procedure.
5. Restrain the infant, if necessary.
6. Clean and drape the area. The umbilicus should be cleansed, using povidone-iodine solution.

7. Place a loose tie of umbilical tape around the base of the umbilicus.

8. Locate the two umbilical arteries and one umbilical vein. The vein has a thin wall and larger lumen compared with the thick walls and smaller lumen of the umbilical arteries. Trim the cord approximately 1 cm to provide a fresh opening.

9. Using a sterile hemostat, insert the tip of the hemostat into the lumen of the vein. Gently open the hemostat to dilate the vessel.

10. Introduce and advance a heparinized–saline flushed umbilical catheter approximately 2 to 4 inches. This will place the catheter into the inferior vena cava of the infant. You should note blood return after inserting the catheter. Do not force the catheter because severe hemorrhage or liver injury may occur.

11. Hook up the catheter to a three-way stopcock. Flush the catheter with 1 mL heparin solution.

12. Secure the catheter, using the piece of umbilical tape, by tying the tape around the umbilicus.

13. After securing the catheter, hook the IV tubing to the stopcock to allow for the administration of fluids and/or medications.

14. Monitor the umbilicus for bleeding. A dressing is usually not used in this situation, so that the umbilicus can be viewed.

A Guide to Herbal Supplements

Herb	Source: medicinal ingredients	Classification	Suggested uses
Alfalfa (*Medicago sativa*)	**Leaves and flowers:** Vitamins, minerals, proteins, enzymes	Diuretic, tonic	Helpful in stomach ailments including aiding peptic ulcers; Improves appetite; relieves urinary and bowel disorders; eliminates retained water
Aloe vera (*Aloe vera*)	**Leaves:** Polysaccharides, amino acids, vitamins, minerals, aloin	Emollient, purgative	Healing and soothing for the stomach; effective laxative; useful for bug bites, skin irritation, burns, minor cuts, and scratches; helps the body to eliminate waste material in adults with bronchial asthma
Bilberry (*Vaccinium myrtillus*)	**Fruit:** Anthocyanosides	Antiseptic, astringent	Improves nighttime vision, helps preserve eyesight, prevents eye damage, regulates bowel action, and stimulates appetite
Cascara sagrada (*Rhamnus purshiana*)	**Dried bark:** Hydroxianthracene derivative (HAD), free anthraquinone	Laxative, tonic	Acts on large intestine and stimulates peristalsis; useful in constipation, dyspepsia, and other digestive complaints; liver tonic *Caution: Contraindicated in lactating or pregnant women*

Herb	Source: medicinal ingredients	Classification	Suggested uses
Cat's claw (*Uncaria tomentosa*)	**Bark:** Proanthocyanidins, alkaloids, phytochemicals	Antiviral, antioxidant	Useful in stimulating the flow of gastric juices and pancreatic secretions; beneficial for irritable bowel syndrome, and Crohn's disease; anti-inflammatory, immune system booster
Cayenne (*Capsicum frutescens*)	**Fruit:** Capsaicin, carotenoids, capsicidins heat value 40,000 scovill units per gram	Stimulant, digestive	Used to stimulate appetite and aid digestion; increases production of gastric juices and relieves gas and bowel pains or cramps; irritating to hemorrhoids *Caution: Do not use in gastrointestinal problems*
Chamomile (*Maticaria chamomilla*)	**Flower:** Volatile oil, bisabolols, flavonoids	Anti-inflammatory, antispasmodic, anti-infective, mild sedative, calmative	Calms the nerves and upset stomach; reduces anxiety, soothes ulcers, and reduces mucous membrane inflammations; good antibacterial action; rare cases of allergic reaction in those with severe hypersensitivity to ragweed pollen
Coltsfoot (*Tussilago farfara*)	**Leaves:** Flavonoids, mucilage, tannin	Expectorant, anticatarrhal, antispasmodic, demulcent	Pulmonary coughs and colds; used for asthma, bronchitis, and emphysema
Cranberry (*Vaccinium macrocrarpon*)	**Twig and fruit:** Anthocyanidins	Antioxidant, bacteriostatic effect	Cleanses and stops infections in the urinary tract
Damiana (*Turnera aphrodisiaca*)	**Leaves and flowers:** Volatile oil, flavonoids, hydroquinine, glycoside	Tonic, nervine, aphrodisiac, antidepressant	Recommended as a laxative and as a general tonic; helps relieve anxiety and may enhance sexual performance *Caution: Damiana interferes with iron absorption*
Dandelion (*Taraxacum officinale*)	**Leaves and Roots:** Sesquiterpenes, triterpenes, phenolic acids, carotenoids	Used in kidney and liver disorders; a natural diuretic and digestive aid; reduces blood pressure, may help prevent iron deficiency, anemia, chronic rheumatism, gout, and stiff joints	Used in kidney and liver disorders; a natural diuretic and digestive aid; reduces blood pressure and may help prevent iron deficiency, anemia, chronic rheumatism, gout, and stiff joints

Herb	Source: medicinal ingredients	Classification	Suggested uses
Devil's claw (*Harpagophytum procumbens*)	**Root:** Harpogoside, beta-sitosterol	Anti-inflammatory, antirheumatic, analgesic, sedative	For arthritis and rheumatism; helpful to reduce swelling, relieve pain, and improve mobility in the joints *Caution: Contraindicated during pregnancy*
Dong quai (*Angelica sinensis*)	**Root:** Volatile aromatic oil, polysaccharides	Tonic immuno-stimulant, antispasmodic	Used to treat all symptoms of menopause as an alternative to estrogen therapy; regulates the hormonal system; overall tonic for female reproductive system; reduces high blood pressure and premenstrual syndrome *Caution: Contraindicated in pregnancy*
Echinacea (*Echinacea angustifolia* and *E. purpurea*)	**Root:** Echinacosides, polysaccharides, phytosterols	Antibiotic, antifungal immunostimulant	Stimulates and boosts immune function; has cortisone-like activity that helps wound healing; fights bacterial and viral infections *Caution: Contraindicated in pregnancy*
Evening primrose (*Oenothera biennis*)	**Plant:** Gamma-linolenic acid (GLA), mixed tocopherols	Antispasmodic	Used in treatment of multiple sclerosis and premenstrual syndrome; helps prevent heart disease and stroke and maintains healthy skin *Caution: Excess consumption can result in oily skin*
Eyebright (*Euphrasia officinalis*)	**Herb:** Iridoid glycosides, tannins, phenolic acids, volatile oil	Astringent, tonic	Strengthens the eye and assists in aiding the body to dissolve cataracts, heal lesions, and heal conjunctivitis
Fenugreek (*Trigonella foenum-graecum*)	**Seeds:** Flavonoids, saponin, vitamins	Demulcent, expectorant	Helpful in stomach and intestinal problems; good expectorant for coughs and colds
Feverfew (*Tanacetum parthenium*)	**Leaves:** Sesquiterpene lactones (parthenolide)	Anti-inflammatory, emmenagogue	Helps prevent migraine headaches and also useful against swelling and arthritis; stimulates digestion and improves liver function *Caution: Contraindicated in lactating or pregnant women*

Herb	Source: medicinal ingredients	Classification	Suggested uses
Ginger (*Zingiber officinale*)	**Root:** Volatile oil, phenylalkylketones	Diaphoretic, cholagogue, carminative, stimulant	Relieves indigestion and abdominal cramping; benefit in relieving motion sickness, dizziness, nausea, and colds; ginger lowers blood clotting
Ginkgo biloba (*Ginkgo biloba*)	**Leaves:** Flavoglycosides (quercetin, proanthocyanidins); also contains terpenes	Antiasthmatic, bronchodilator, platelet activating factor (PAF) inhibitor	Increases blood flow to the brain; decreases memory loss, Alzheimer's disease, cerebral vascular insufficiency, and blood clotting; has the ability to neutralize free radicals and also beneficial for asthma, stress, vertigo, and tinnitus *Caution: Potential drug interaction with warfarin and aspirin; take with food*
Ginseng (*Panax schin-seng*)	**Root:** Ginsenosides (triterpene saponins), glycosides	Tonic, stimulant, demulcent, stomachic	Stimulates both physical and mental activity; antifatigue (insomnia, nervousness, poor appetite); enhances immune system, inhibits exhaustion of adrenal gland; antistress *Caution: If you are pregnant or if you have high blood pressure, consult with your physician or health practitioner before using*
Goldenseal (*Hydrastis canadensis*)	**Root:** Alkaloids (hydrastine), fatty acids, volatile oil	Anti-inflammatory, tonic, mild laxative	Strengthens the immune system to help cold and flu symptoms; acts as an anti-inflammatory; helpful in constipation and in stomach disorders such as indigestion *Caution: Contraindicated during pregnancy*
Guggulipids (*Commiphora mukul*)	**Stem:** Essential oil, guggulsterone, oleoresin	Anticholesterenic	Lowers blood cholesterol by 14 to 27 percent and can lower triglycerides by 22 to 23 percent; helps reduce atherosclerotic plaques; improves the heart metabolism and increases liver metabolism of low-density lipoprotein cholesterol *Caution: Contraindicated during pregnancy*

Herb	Source: medicinal ingredients	Classification	Suggested uses
Hawthorn (*Crategus oxyacantha*)	**Berries:** Flavonoids, glycosides, saponins, catechins, tannins, procyanidins	Cardiac tonic, hypotensive, antisclerotic	Alleviates hypertension and high blood pressure and reduces the severity of angina attacks; sedative and antispasmodic effects
Horsetail (*Equisetum arvense*)	**Herb:** Silicic acid, minerals, silica, flavoglucosides, saponins, alkaloids	Astringent, diuretic	Genitourinary complaints, mild diuretic, broken nails, hair loss, skin; stimulates an increase in white blood cells; used for arteriosclerosis and inflamed or enlarged prostate
Licorice (*Glycyrrhiza glabra*)	**Root:** Glycyrrhizin, flavonoids	Demulcent, diuretic, expectorant, laxative	Gastric ulcers, adrenal insufficiency, and hypoglycemia; good for coughs and other bronchial complaints *Caution: Contraindicated for those with high blood pressure or if pregnant*
Milk thistle (*Siybum marianum*)	**Seeds and Leaves:** Flavonoids (silymarin)	Hepatoprotective, cholagogue	Promotes flow of bile; tonic for spleen, stomach, kidney, and gallbladder; beneficial for liver disease (jaundice, hepatitis, and cirrhosis)
Oats (*Avena sativa*)	**Stems and seeds:** Proteins, c-glycosyl flavones, avenacosides	Antidepressant, cardiac tonic, nervine	Lessens debility, depression, stress, and menopause symptoms; good for skin disease; tonic for impotence
Parsley (*Petroselinum sativum*)	**Leaves and seeds:** Volatile oil, coumarins, flavonoids	Carminative, diuretic, expectorant, antispasmodic	Relieves gas and is a natural diuretic; good for coughs, asthma, and suppressed or difficult menstruation
Peppermint (*Mentha piperita*)	**Leaves:** Essential oil, flavonoids, carotenes	Diaphoretic, carminative, antispasmodic	Aids in digestion, flatulence, colds, influenza, and migraines
Pumpkin (*Cucurbita pepo*)	**Seeds:** Linoleic acid, cucurbitacins, zinc	Diuretic, demulcent, taeniacide, anthelmintic	Effective in reducing the size and symptoms of an enlarged prostate. Helps to expel tapeworms
Pygeum (*Pygeum africanum*)	**Bark:** Phytosterols (sitosterols), terpenoids, ferulic esters	Anti-inflammatory, diuretic, antiedema	Prostatitis, benign prostatic hypertrophy (BPH), incontinence, painful urination, dysuria, cancer of the prostate, and urinary tract disorders

Herb	Source: medicinal ingredients	Classification	Suggested uses
Rosehips (*Rosa species*)	**Fruit:** Bioflavonoids, vitamins (C, B-complex)	Astringent, diuretic, tonic	Excellent source of vitamin C for nervous and stressful situations; helps prevent infections; blood purifier
Saw palmetto (*Serenoa serrulata*)	**Berries:** Saponins, phytosterols, fatty acids, volatile oil	Tonic, diuretic, sedative, endocrine agent	Benign prostatic hypotrophy, antiallergic and anti-inflammatory; urinary tract disorders, impotence, and infertility in women
Slippery elm (*Ulmus fulva*)	**Inner bark:** Mucilage: galactose, galacturonic acid	Demulcent, emollient, astringent, mucilage	Gastric or duodenal ulcers; inflammation of stomach, colitis, coughs, sore throat, and soothes skin disorders
St. John's wort (*Hypericum perforatum*)	**Herb:** Essential oil, glycosides (hypericin), flavonoids	Sedative, anti-inflammatory, astringent	Antidepressant; stress and irritability; immune support, anti-inflammatory, antiviral, AIDS *Caution: Avoid excessive exposure to sunlight since hypericin may render the skin photosensitive; note: Most resembles monoamine oxidase inhibitors*
Valerian (*Valeriana officinalis*)	**Root:** Valerinic acid, sequiterpenes, glycoside, essential oils	Sedative, hypnotic, nervine, hypotensive	Balancing agent for hyperexcitability and exhaustion; calms nervous disorders and acts as both sedative and tranquilizer; helps headaches, high blood pressure, and stomach and menstrual cramps *Caution: Contraindicated in pregnancy; high doses should be avoided over a long period of time*
White willow (*Salix alba*)	**Bark:** Salicin, tannins, flavonoid glycosides (quercetin)	Analgesic, anti-inflammatory, tonic	Soothes headaches and reduces fevers; helps stomach ailments and heartburn; mild analgesic for arthritic and rheumatic conditions
Wild yam (*Dioscorea villosa*)	**Root:** Diosgenins, saponins, glycosides	Anti-inflammatory, cholagogue, mild diaphoretic, spasmolytic	Menopause, menstrual cramps, ovarian pain; various types of rheumatism and intestinal colic

SPECIALTY PRODUCTS

Herb	Source: medicinal ingredients	Classification	Suggested uses
Bee pollen	**Bee pollen:** Vitamins, minerals, enzymes, amino acids	Supplement	Provides energy and essential nutrients; helpful in stomach ailments, hormonal system, allergies, hay fever, and exhaustion and builds resistance to diseases *Caution: Some people may be allergic to bee pollen; try small amounts of doses daily*
Coenzyme Q10	**CO Q10 Ubiquinone:** Japanese source	Supplement	Vital role in energy production at the cellular level and recommended in the treatment of cardiovascular disease; revitalizes the immune system
Flaxseed	**Seed:** Alpha-linolenic acid (ALA), omega-3 series of essential fatty acids	Purgative, demulcent, emollient	Helps lower cholesterol and blood triglyceride levels and helps prevent clot formation; digestive and urinary disorders
Glucosamine sulfate	**Crab shell:** Glucose, amino and sulfate group, mucopolysaccharides, glycoproteins	Supplement	Stimulates the synthesis of cartilage in the joints; relief from pain and inflammation around joints associated with osteoarthritis
Pycnogenol	**Pine bark extract:** Proanthocyanidins, natural soluble organic acids, glucose, bioflavonoid	Antioxidant	Strengthens blood vessels and useful for allergies; anti-inflammatory and antiaging; neutralizes existing free radicals in the blood

COMMON USES OF HERBAL EXTRACTS

Note: The following information should not be used for the diagnosis, treatment, or prevention of disease in humans. The information contained herein is in no way intended to be a guide to medical practice or a recommendation that herbs be used for medicinal purposes. This information is presented here for its educational value and as information for medical personnel.

Condition	Common herbs
Allergy	Nettles, echinacea, goldenseal, bee pollen
Antibacterial	Echinacea, garlic, angelica, barberry
Anticatarrhal	Elder, goldenseal, sandalwood, hyssop
Antidepressant	Lavender, St. John's wort, oats, damiana, rosemary, schizandra
Antifungal	Garlic, propolis, cinnamon, black walnut
Anti-inflammatory	Oak bark, thyme, peppermint, propolis, sage
Antiseptic	Peppermint, thyme, propolis, sage, oak bark, black walnut
Antispasmodic	Valerian, passion flower, peppermint, red clover, catnip, rosemary, motherwort, thyme
Antiviral	St. John's wort, echinacea, garlic, astragalus
Aphrodisiac	Schizandra, ginseng, damiana
Arthritis or rheumatism	Devil's claw, alfalfa, wild yam, white willow, black cohosh, sarsaparilla, glucosamine
Asthma	Mullein, coltsfoot, goldenseal, ginkgo biloba, horehound, licorice, elecampane, blessed thistle, wild cherry, blue cohosh
Astringent	Nettles, plantain, red raspberry, oak bark, goldenseal, rhubarb, sage, true unicorn, yellow dock, wild cherry bark, wood betony
Blood purifiers	Red clover, blessed thistle, burdock, sarsaparilla
Bronchial support	Schizandra, mullein, coltsfoot, fenugreek, horehound, hyssop, licorice, elecampane, thyme, myrrh, goldenseal
Cardiovascular	Hawthorn, fo-ti, oats, reishi, motherwort
Cholesterol	Hawthorn, reishi, linden, guggulipids
Circulatory	Ginkgo biloba, garlic, ginger, gotu kola, capsicum, prickly ash, hawthorn, bioflavonoids
Colds or flu	Echinacea, catnip, peppermint, boneset, elder, zinc lozenge
Cough	Wild cherry bark, licorice (daytime usage), slippery elm, coltsfoot, horehound
Diarrhea (*also see* Astringent)	Oak bark, plantain, thyme, chamomile
Digestive aids	Barberry, true unicorn, yellow dock, wild cherry bark, wood betony
Diuretics	Parsley, corn silk, couch grass, dandelion (also natural potassium source), buchu, uva ursi, rosehips, sandalwood
Earache	Mullein oil, garlic, sage (to swab in and around ear)
Eczema	Nettles, chickweed, goldenseal, red clover, burdock
Expectorant	Elecampane, fenugreek, plantain, thyme, horehound, hyssop, licorice, sage, mullein, garlic
Eyes	Eyebright, chamomile (eyewash)
Fever	Sage, thyme, echinacea, white willow, nettles, wild indigo, yarrow
Flatulence	Fennel, peppermint, ginger, sage
Hay fever	Nettles, echinacea (*see* Allergy)
Headache	White willow, peppermint, lavender, passion, flower, wood betony, linden, ginger, rosemary, valerian
High blood pressure	Garlic, hawthorne, yarrow
Immune support	Astragalus, reishi, nettles, shiitake, schizandra, echinacea, propolis, garlic, Pau D'Arco, cat's claw
Impotency	Oats, ginseng, damiana, sarsaparilla
Kidney or bladder	Couch grass, meadowsweet, uva ursi, cranberry
Laxative	Cascara sagrada, rhubarb
Liver	Yellow dock, milk thistle, boneset, fo-ti, blessed thistle, barberry, lipoic acid
Lymphatics	Echinacea, red clover
Male hormonals	Sarsaparilla, ginseng, damiana, oats
Menopause or premenstrual syndrome	Dong quai, evening primrose, licorice, black cohosh
Mental alertness	Ginkgo biloba, rosemary, gotu kola, periwinkle (helpful with senility)

Migraine headaches	Feverfew
Nausea	Peppermint, gingerroot, red raspberry
Nervine	Oats, passion flower, hops, chamomile, valerian, linden, reishi, rosemary, skullcap
Oral (mouthwash or antiseptics)	Myrrh gum, oak bark, goldenseal, chlorophyll
Pain (reduction)	Hops, white willow, valerian (also add immune herbal)
Prostate	Saw palmetto, pygeum, pumpkin seed
Psoriasis	Burdock, red clover, echinacea, chickweed, yellow dock, sarsaparilla
Respiratory	Horehound, mullein, myrrh, astragalus, goldenseal, elecampane
Shingles	Passion flower, echinacea, oats, (proper nutritional and stress support)
Sore throat	Sage, slippery elm, wild indigo, red raspberry, echinacea
Stomachic	Fennel, ginger, peppermint, chamomile
Thyroid	Bladderwrack
Tonic	Ginseng, reishi, schizandra, gotu kola, fo-ti, nettles, oat
Ulcers	Marshmallow, licorice, slippery elm (gastric peptic), meadowsweet, red clover.

GLOSSARY

Word	Definition
Alternative	Agents that gradually and favorably alter the condition of the body
Analgesic	Herbs that have the action of pain relief
Anthelmintic	Stimulating herbs that work against parasitic worms that may be present in the digestive system
Antibiotic	Substance that inhibits the growth of microorganisms
Anticatarrhal	Herbs that eliminate or counteract the formation of mucus
Antidepressant	An agent used in treating depression
Antifungal	Substance that is antagonistic to fungi
Anti-inflammatory	Substance that helps the body to combat inflammations
Antilithic	Herbs with the ability to remove or prevent the formation of stones or gravel in the urinary system
Antimicrobial	Herbs used to rid the body of microorganisms that have invaded it or act in the skin
Antineoplastic	Herbs that have the specific action of inhibiting and combating the development of tumors
Antioxidant	An agent that inhibits oxidation and thus prevents rancidity of oils or fats or the deterioration of other materials through oxidative processes
Antirheumatic	Herbs with a reputation for preventing, relieving, and curing rheumatic problems
Antiseptic	Substances that have a constricting or binding effect (herbs used to prevent or counteract the growth of disease germs)
Antispasmodic	Herbal remedies that rapidly reduce nervous tension that may be causing digestive spasms or colic
Antiviral	Substance that opposes a virus by weakening or abolishing its action
Aphrodisiac	Substance that arouses or increases sexual desire
Aromatic	Oils of aromatic herbs that penetrate into muscles, increasing circulation
Astringent	Substances that have a constricting or binding effect; aid in breaking down secretions
Bitter	Substance that promotes appetite and aids in digestion

Calmative	Any agent that allays excitement; often used as synonymous with sedative
Carminative	Herbs and spices taken to relieve gas and griping
Cathartic	Herbs that have a laxative effect
Cholagogue	Substance that promotes the flow and discharge of bile into the small intestine
Demulcent	Soothing substances taken internally to protect damaged tissue
Diaphoretic	Herbs used to induce sweating
Digestive	Substance that assists the process of digestion
Diuretic	Herbs that increase the flow of urine
Dysmenorrhea	Condition of menstruation accompanied by cramping pains that may be incapacitating in their intensity
Emmenagogue	Herbs that promote menstruation
Emollient	Substance that acts as a lubricant to the intestinal wall and softens the feces; emollients are applied to the skin to soften, soothe, or protect it
Expectorant	Herbs that assist in expelling mucus from the lungs and throat
Hepatic	Substance that strengthens, tones, and stimulates secretive functions of the liver
Laxative	Substance that has a moderate evacuating effect
Mucilage	Herbs that contain gelatinous constituents
Nervine	Herbs used to ease anxiety and stress and nourish the nerves
Purgative	Substances that promote bowel movement and increased intestinal peristalsis
Sedative	Herbs that quiet nervous excitement
Stimulant	Substance that quickens and enlivens the physiological function of the body
Tonic	Herbs that strengthen and enliven either specific organs or the whole body

Index